Personal Fitness and Wellness

ESS 1200

12th Edition

Werner W. K. Hoeger | Sharon A. Hoeger

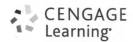

Australia • Brazil • Japan • Korea • Mexico • Singapore • Spain • United Kingdom • United States

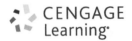

Personal Fitness and Wellness
ESS 1200

Executive Editors:
 Maureen Staudt
 Michael Stranz

Senior Project Development Manager:
 Linda deStefano

Marketing Specialist:
 Courtney Sheldon

Senior Production/Manufacturing Manager:
 Donna M. Brown

Production Editorial Manager:
 Kim Fry

Sr. Rights Acquisition Account Manager:
 Todd Osborne

Lifetime Personal Fitness and Wellness, Twelfth Edition
Werner W. K. Hoeger | Sharon A. Hoeger
© 2013, 2011 Cengage Learning. All rights reserved.

For product information and technology assistance, contact us at
Cengage Learning Customer & Sales Support, 1-800-354-9706

For permission to use material from this text or product,
submit all requests online at **cengage.com/permissions**
Further permissions questions can be emailed to
permissionrequest@cengage.com

This book contains select works from existing Cengage Learning resources and was produced by Cengage Learning Custom Solutions for collegiate use. As such, those adopting and/or contributing to this work are responsible for editorial content accuracy, continuity and completeness.

Compilation © 2012 Cengage Learning
ISBN-13: 978-1-285-11102-5

ISBN-10: 1-285-11102-8

Cengage Learning
5191 Natorp Boulevard
Mason, Ohio 45040
USA
Cengage Learning is a leading provider of customized learning solutions with office locations around the globe, including Singapore, the United Kingdom, Australia, Mexico, Brazil, and Japan. Locate your local office at:
international.cengage.com/region.

Cengage Learning products are represented in Canada by Nelson Education, Ltd.
For your lifelong learning solutions, visit **www.cengage.com/custom.**
Visit our corporate website at **www.cengage.com.**

Printed in the United States of America

Custom Contents

(* Note – this is a "custom" textbook that has been designed specifically for this course in a joint effort between you instructor and the publisher. Please note that some chapters have been removed intentionally.)

Physical Fitness and Wellness

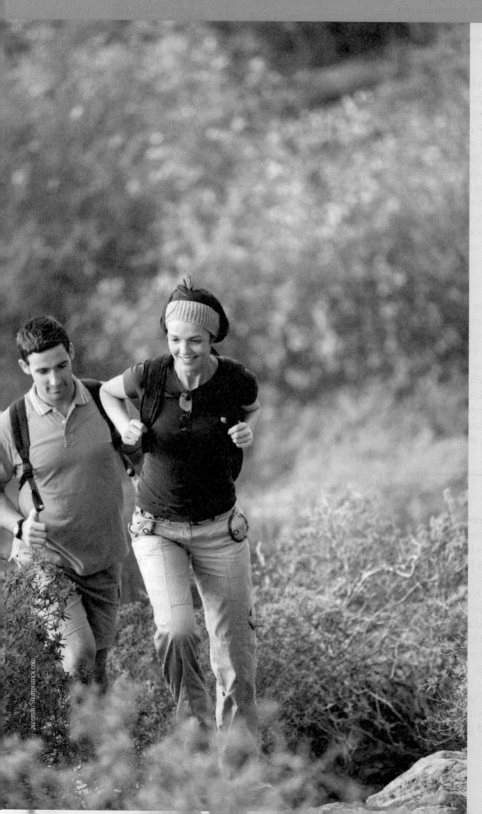

"The power of prevention is yours, it enables you to make lifestyle changes that will prevent disease and increase the quality and length of your life."

Objectives

▶ **Understand** the health and fitness consequences of physical inactivity.

▶ **Identify** the major health problems in the United States.

▶ **Learn** how to monitor daily physical activity.

▶ **Learn** the Federal Physical Activity Guidelines for Americans.

▶ **Define** wellness and list its dimensions.

▶ **Define** physical fitness and list health-related and skill-related components.

▶ **State** the differences among physical fitness, health promotion, and wellness.

▶ **Distinguish** between health fitness standards and physical fitness standards.

▶ **Understand** the benefits and significance of participating in a comprehensive wellness program.

▶ **List** key national health objectives for the year 2020.

▶ **Determine** if you can safely initiate an exercise program.

▶ **Learn** to assess resting heart rate and blood pressure.

CENGAGE brain

Visit **www.cengagebrain.com** to access course materials and companion resources for this text including: a daily exercise log, the Physical Activity Readiness Questionnaire (PAR-Q), the health history questionnaire, quiz questions designed to check your understanding of the chapter contents, and more! See the preface on page xv for more information.

Why should I take a fitness and wellness course?
Most people go to college to learn how to make a living, but a fitness and wellness course will teach you how to *live*— how to truly live life to its fullest potential. Some people seem to think that success is measured by how much money they make. Making a good living will not help you unless you live a wellness lifestyle that will allow you to enjoy what you earn. You may want to ask yourself: Of what value are a nice income, a beautiful home, and a solid retirement portfolio if at age 45 I suffer a massive heart attack that will seriously limit my physical capacity or end life itself?

Will the attainment of good physical fitness be sufficient to ensure good health? Regular participation in a sound physical fitness program will provide substantial health benefits and significantly decrease the risk of many chronic diseases. And although good fitness often motivates toward adoption of additional positive lifestyle behaviors, to maximize the benefits for a healthier, more productive, happier, and longer life we have to pay attention to all seven dimensions of wellness: physical, social, mental, emotional, occupational, environmental, and spiritual. These dimensions are interrelated, and one frequently affects the other. A wellness way of life requires a constant and deliberate effort to stay healthy and achieve the highest potential for well-being within all dimensions of wellness.

If a person is going to do only one thing to improve health, what would it be? This is a common question. It is a mistake to think, though, that you can modify just one factor and enjoy wellness. Wellness requires a constant and deliberate effort to change unhealthy behaviors and reinforce healthy behaviors. Although it is difficult to work on many lifestyle changes all at once, being involved in a regular physical activity program, proper nutrition, and avoidance of addictive behavior are lifestyle factors to work on first. Others should follow, depending on your current lifestyle behaviors.

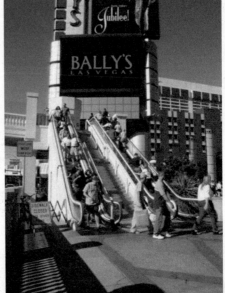

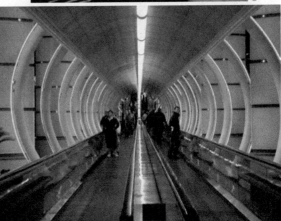

Modern-day conveniences lull people into a sedentary lifestyle.

Scientific findings have shown that physical inactivity and a negative lifestyle seriously threaten health and hasten the deterioration rate of the human body. Movement and physical activity are basic functions for which the human organism was created.

Advances in technology, however, have almost completely eliminated the necessity for physical exertion in daily life. Physical activity is no longer a natural part of our existence. We live in an automated society, where most of the activities that used to require strenuous exertion can be accomplished by machines with the simple pull of a handle or push of a button.

Most industrialized nations in the world are experiencing an epidemic of physical inactivity. In the United States, physical inactivity is the second greatest threat to

public health and has been termed "**Sedentary Death Syndrome**" or **SeDS** (the number-one threat is tobacco use—the largest cause of preventable deaths).

Widespread interest in **health** and preventive medicine in recent years, nonetheless, is motivating people to participate in organized fitness and wellness programs. The growing number of participants is attributed primarily to scientific evidence linking regular physical activity and positive lifestyle habits to better health, longevity, quality of life, and overall well-being.

At the beginning of the 20th century, **life expectancy** for a child born in the United States was only 47 years. The most common health problems in the Western world were infectious diseases, such as tuberculosis, diphtheria, influenza, kidney disease, polio, and other diseases of infancy. Progress in the medical field largely eliminated these diseases. Then, as more people started to enjoy the "good life" (**sedentary** living, alcohol, fatty

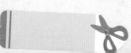

Ray's Experience

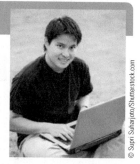

During our freshman year everyone at my school has to take a lifetime fitness and wellness class. When I first started the class, I thought it would be a piece of cake, with not that much work involved. I was taking hard math and writing classes, and I thought I would spend all my time studying for those courses and that the wellness class would just be something I barely had to think about, like high school PE. As the class got started, I found out that I had to do a lot more than I thought to get a good grade. I also became really interested in the subject! I started spending more time studying fitness and wellness and reading the textbook just because I wanted to know more. In my family, a lot of family members are really overweight and a couple of them have diabetes. As I began to learn more about those problems, I decided to be the one who breaks the trend and does not have the same health problems my relatives do. It has been six months since I finished the class and I am still continuing on with my healthy habits—eating well and exercising. I have lost 10 pounds and my last physical showed that my blood sugar, blood pressure, and cholesterol were all in the healthy range!

PERSONAL PROFILE

General Understanding of Fitness and Wellness

To the best of your ability, please answer the following questions. If you do not know the answer(s), this chapter will guide you through them.

   I. **Physical fitness implies making a constant and deliberate effort to stay healthy and achieve the highest potential for well-being.** _____ True   _____ False

   II. **The minimum requirement in the U.S. Federal Physical Activity Guidelines is that you accumulate _____ minutes of moderate-intensity aerobic activity or _____ minutes of vigorous-intensity aerobic activity on a weekly basis.**

   III. **Agility, balance, coordination, reaction time, power, and speed are the basic components of health-related fitness.** _____ True _____ False

   IV. **My current blood pressure is _____ /_____ mm Hg.**

   V. **Are you aware of potential risk factors in your life that may increase your chances of developing disease?** _____ Yes _____ No

---

foods, excessive sweets, tobacco, drugs), we saw a parallel increase in the incidence of **chronic diseases** such as cardiovascular disease, cancer, diabetes, and chronic respiratory diseases (Figure 1.1). According to the World Health Organization (WHO), chronic diseases account for 60 percent of all deaths worldwide.[1]

As the incidence of chronic diseases climbed, we recognized that prevention is the best medicine. Consequently, a fitness and wellness movement developed gradually in the 1980s. People began to realize that good health is mostly self-controlled and that the leading causes of premature death and illness could be prevented by adhering to positive lifestyle habits. We all desire to live a long life, and wellness programs seek to enhance the overall quality of life—for as long as we live.

There are three basic factors that determine our health and longevity: Genetics, the environment, and our behavior (Figure 1.2). Although we cannot change our genetic pool, we can exert control over the environment and our health behaviors so that we may reach our full physical potential based on our own genetic code. How we accomplish this goal will be thoroughly discussed through the chapters of this book.

Key Terms

Sedentary Death Syndrome (SeDS) Cause of deaths attributed to a lack of regular physical activity.

Health A state of complete well-being—not just the absence of disease or infirmity.

Life expectancy Number of years a person is expected to live based on the person's birth year.

Sedentary Description of a person who is relatively inactive and whose lifestyle is characterized by a lot of sitting.

Chronic diseases Illnesses that develop as a result of an unhealthy lifestyle and last a long time.

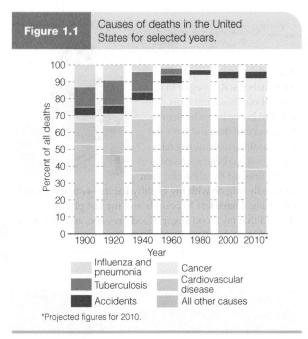

Figure 1.1 Causes of deaths in the United States for selected years.

Influenza and pneumonia
Cancer
Tuberculosis
Cardiovascular disease
Accidents
All other causes

*Projected figures for 2010.

SOURCE: National Center for Health Statistics, Division of Vital Statistics.

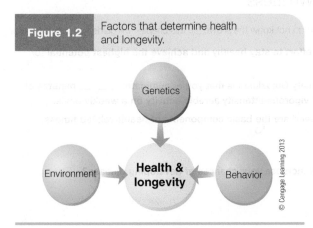

Figure 1.2 Factors that determine health and longevity.

© Cengage Learning 2013

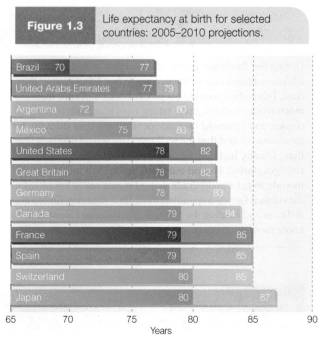

Figure 1.3 Life expectancy at birth for selected countries: 2005–2010 projections.

*Dark color is men; light color is women.

SOURCE: United Nations, Social Indicators: Indicators on Health, http://unstats.un. org/unsd/demographic/products/socind/health.htm. Downloaded March 31, 2011.

Life Expectancy

Based on the most recent data available, the average life expectancy in the United States is 78.3 years (75.7 years for men and 80.8 years for women). While in the past decade alone, life expectancy has increased by one year—the news is not all good. The data show that people now spend an extra 1.2 years with a serious illness and an extra two years of disability. Mortality has been postponed because medical treatments allow people to live longer with various chronic ailments (cardiovascular disease, cancer, diabetes).

Based on the WHO data, the United States ranks 38th in the world for life expectancy (see Figure 1.3). Between 2000 and 2010, U.S. male life expectancy slipped from 18th to 24th in the world and female life expectancy from 28th to 35th. Japan ranks first in the world with an overall life expectancy of 82.6 years.

Several factors may account for the current U.S. life expectancy ranking: the extremely poor health of some groups (such as Native Americans, rural African Americans, and the inner-city poor), the obesity epidemic, the low level of daily physical activity, the high incidence of tobacco use and coronary heart disease, and fairly high levels of violence (notably homicides).

Although life expectancy in the United States gradually increased by 30 years over the past century, scientists from the National Institute of Aging believe that in the coming decades the average lifespan may decrease by as much as five years. This decrease in life expectancy will be related primarily to the growing epidemic of obesity. According to estimates from the Centers for Disease Control and Prevention, 34 percent of the adult population in the United States is obese. If the current trend continues, the current generation of children may not outlive their parents. Additional information on the obesity epidemic and its detrimental health consequences is given in Chapter 5.

Leading Health Problems in the United States

The leading causes of death in the United States today are largely lifestyle related (Figure 1.4). The U.S. Surgeon General has stated that seven of ten Americans die of preventable chronic diseases.[2] Specifically, about 53 percent of all deaths in the United States are caused by cardiovascular disease and cancer.[3] Almost 80 percent of the latter deaths could be prevented through a healthy lifestyle program. The third and fourth leading causes of death, respectively, are chronic lower respiratory disease (CLRD) and accidents.

The most prevalent degenerative diseases in the United States are those of the cardiovascular system. About 30 percent of all deaths in this country are attributed to diseases of the heart and blood vessels. According to the American Heart Association (AHA), 81.1 million people in the United States are afflicted with diseases of the cardiovascular system, including 74.5 million with hypertension (high blood pressure) and 17.6 million with coronary heart disease (CHD). (Many of these people have more than one type of cardiovascular disease.) About 1.26 million people suffer from coronary heart disease each year, including 935,000 heart attacks and nearly 425,000 deaths from CHD and heart attacks. The estimated direct and indirect cost of cardiovascular disease in 2010 exceeded $503 billion.[4] A complete cardiovascular disease prevention program is outlined in Chapter 10.

The second leading cause of death in the United States is cancer. Even though cancer is not the number-one killer, it is the number-one health fear of the American people. Twenty-three percent of all deaths in the United States are attributable to cancer. More than 560,000 people died from this disease in 2010, and an estimated 1.5 million new cases were reported the same year.[5] The major contributor to the increase in the incidence of cancer during the past five decades is lung cancer, of which 87 percent is caused by tobacco use. Furthermore, smoking accounts for more than 30 percent of all deaths from cancer. Another 33 percent of deaths

Healthy Habits that Cut the Risk for Serious Disease

According to the Centers for Disease Control and Prevention, living four health habits can reduce your risk of chronic diseases such as heart disease, cancer, and diabetes by almost 80 percent:

- Get at least 30 minutes of daily moderate-intensity physical activity.
- Don't ever smoke.
- Eat a healthy diet (ample fruits and vegetables, whole grain products, and low meat consumption).
- Maintain a body mass index (BMI) less than 30.

are related to nutrition, physical inactivity, excessive body weight, and other faulty lifestyle habits.

The American Cancer Society maintains that the most influential factor in fighting cancer today is prevention through health education programs. Evidence indicates that as much as 80 percent of all human cancer can be prevented through positive lifestyle behaviors. A comprehensive cancer-prevention program is presented in Chapter 11.

CLRD, the third cause of death, is a general term that includes chronic obstructive pulmonary disease, emphysema, and chronic bronchitis (all diseases of the respiratory system). Although CLRD is related mostly to tobacco use (see Chapter 13 for discussion on how to stop smoking), lifetime nonsmokers also can develop CLRD.

Precautions to prevent CLRD include consuming a low-fat, low-sodium, nutrient-dense diet; staying physically active; not smoking and not breathing cigarette smoke; getting a pneumonia vaccine if over age 50 and a current or ex-smoker; and avoiding swimming pools for individuals sensitive to chlorine vapor.

Accidents are the fourth leading cause of death. Even though not all accidents are preventable, many are. Fatal accidents are often related to abusing drugs and not wearing seat belts. Furthermore, with the advent of cell phones, 1.6 million car accidents each year are caused by drivers using cell phones or reading/sending text messages.

Most people do not perceive accidents as a health problem. Even so, accidents affect the total well-being of millions of Americans each year. Accident prevention and personal safety are part of a health-enhancement program aimed at achieving a better quality of life. Proper nutrition, exercise, stress management, and abstinence from cigarette smoking are of little help if the person is involved in a disabling or fatal accident as a result of distraction, a single reckless decision, or not wearing seat belts properly.

Accidents do not just happen. We cause accidents, and we are victims of accidents. Although some factors in life, such as earthquakes, tornadoes, and airplane accidents, are completely beyond our control, more often

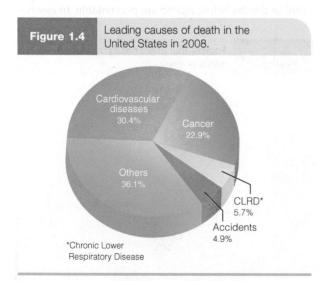

| **Figure 1.4** | Leading causes of death in the United States in 2008. |

Cardiovascular diseases 30.4%

Cancer 22.9%

Others 36.1%

CLRD* 5.7%

Accidents 4.9%

*Chronic Lower Respiratory Disease

SOURCE: U.S. Department of Health and Human Services, Centers for Disease Control and Prevention, National Center for Health Statistics, National Vital Statistics reports, *Deaths: Preliminary Data for 2008*, 59:2 (December 9, 2010).

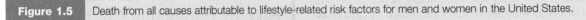

| Figure 1.5 | Death from all causes attributable to lifestyle-related risk factors for men and women in the United States. |

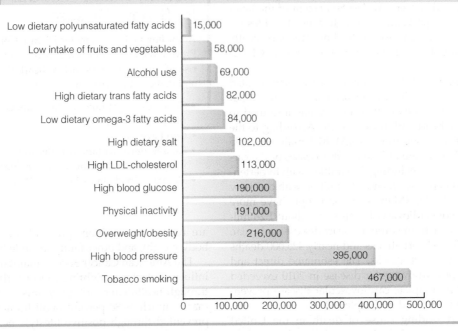

SOURCE: Danaei, G., et al. "The preventable causes of death in the United States: Comparative risk assessment of dietary, lifestyle, and metaboli risk factors," *PLoS Med* 6, 4 (2009): e1000058.doi:10.1371/journal.pmed.1000058.

than not, personal safety and accident prevention are a matter of common sense. Most accidents stem from poor judgment and confused mental states, which occur when people are upset, are not paying attention to the task at hand, or are abusing alcohol or other drugs.

Alcohol abuse is the number-one cause of all accidents. About half of accidental deaths and suicides in the United States are alcohol related. Further, alcohol intoxication is the leading cause of fatal automobile accidents. Other commonly abused drugs alter feelings and perceptions, generate mental confusion, and impair judgment and coordination, greatly enhancing the risk for accidental **morbidity** and mortality (Chapter 13).

The underlying causes of death attributable to leading **risk factors** in the United States (Figure 1.5) indicate that most factors are related to lifestyle choices we make. Of the approximately 2.4 million yearly deaths in the United States, the "big five" factors—tobacco smoking, high blood pressure, overweight and obesity, physical inactivity, and high blood glucose—are responsible for almost 1.5 million deaths each year.

Lifestyle as a Health Problem

As the incidence of chronic diseases rose, it became obvious that prevention was—and remains—the best medicine. According to the U.S. Surgeon General's of-

fice, more than half of the people who die in this country each year die because of what they do. Based on estimates, more than half of disease is lifestyle related, a fifth is attributed to the environment, and a tenth is influenced by the health care the individual receives. Only 16 percent is related to genetic factors (Figure 1.6). Thus, the individual controls as much as 84 percent of his or her vulnerability to disease—and thus quality of life. The same data indicate that 83 percent of deaths before age 65 are preventable. In essence,

| Figure 1.6 | Factors that affect health and well-being. |

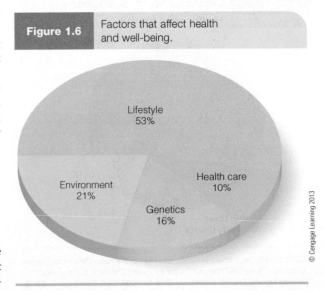

most people in the United States are threatened by the very lives they lead today.

Because of the unhealthy lifestyles that many young adults lead, their bodies may be middle-aged or older! Many physical education programs do not emphasize the skills necessary for young people to maintain a high level of fitness and health throughout life. The intent of this book is to provide those skills and help to prepare you for a lifetime of physical fitness and wellness. A healthy lifestyle is self-controlled, and you can learn how to be responsible for your own health and fitness. Healthy choices made today influence health for decades.

Physical Activity and Exercise Defined

Abundant scientific research over the past three decades has established a distinction between physical activity and exercise. **Physical activity** is bodily movement produced by skeletal muscles. It requires energy expenditure and produces progressive health benefits. Physical activity typically requires only a low to moderate intensity of effort. Examples of physical activity include walking to and from work, taking the stairs instead of elevators and escalators, gardening, doing household chores, dancing, and washing the car by hand. Physical inactivity, by contrast, implies a level of activity that is lower than that required to maintain good health.

Exercise is a type of physical activity that requires planned, structured, and repetitive bodily movement to improve or maintain one or more components of physical fitness. Examples of exercise are walking, running, cycling, aerobics, swimming, and strength training. Exercise is usually viewed as an activity that requires a vigorous-intensity effort.

Importance of Increased Physical Activity

The U.S. Surgeon General has stated that poor health as a result of lack of physical activity is a serious public health problem that must be met head-on at once. Regular **moderate physical activity** provides substantial benefits in health and well-being for the vast majority of people who are not physically active. For those who are already moderately active, even greater health benefits can be achieved by increasing the level of physical activity.

Among the benefits of regular physical activity and exercise are significantly reduced risks for developing or dying from heart disease, stroke, type 2 diabetes, colon and breast cancers, high blood pressure, and osteoporotic fractures.[6] Regular physical activity also is important for the health of muscles, bones, and joints, and it seems to reduce symptoms of depression and anxiety, improve mood, and enhance one's ability to

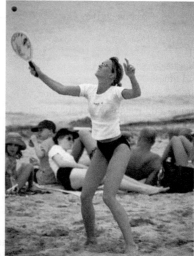

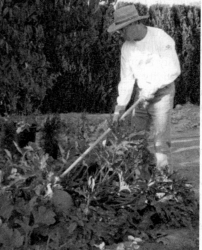

An active lifestyle increases health, quality of life, and longevity.

Key Terms

Morbidity A condition related to or caused by illness or disease.

Physical activity Bodily movement produced by skeletal muscles; requires expenditure of energy and produces progressive health benefits. Examples include walking, taking the stairs, dancing, gardening, house cleaning, snow shoveling, washing the car, and all forms of structured exercise.

Exercise A type of physical activity that requires planned, structured, and repetitive bodily movement with the intent of improving or maintaining one or more components of physical fitness.

Moderate physical activity Activity that uses 150 calories of energy per day, or 1,000 calories per week.

Table 1.1	Physical Activity Guidelines			
Benefits	Duration	Intensity	Frequency per Week	Weekly Time
Health	30 min	MI*	≥5 times	≥150 min
Health and fitness	≥20 min	VI*	≥3 times	≥75 min
Health, fitness, and weight gain prevention	60 min	MI/VI†	5–7 times	≥300 min
Health, fitness, and weight regain prevention	60–90 min	MI/VI†	5–7 times	≥450 min

*MI = moderate intensity, VI = vigorous intensity

†MI/VI = You may use MI or VI or a combination of the two

© Cengage Learning 2013

perform daily tasks throughout life. It also can help control health care costs and maintain a high quality of life into old age.

Moderate physical activity has been defined as any activity that requires an energy expenditure of 150 calories per day, or 1,000 calories per week. The general health recommendation is that people strive to accumulate at least 30 minutes of physical activity a minimum of 5 days per week (Table 1.1). Whereas 30 minutes of continuous activity is preferred, on days when time is limited, three activity sessions of at least 10 minutes each still provide substantial health benefits. Examples of moderate physical activity are brisk walking or cycling, playing basketball or volleyball, swimming, water aerobics, dancing fast, pushing a stroller, raking leaves, shoveling snow, washing or waxing a car, washing windows or floors, and even gardening. Light-intensity activities of daily living such as casual walking, self-care, shopping, or those lasting less than 10 minutes in duration cannot be included as part of the moderate physical activity recommendation.

Because of the ever-growing epidemic of obesity in the United States, the Institute of Medicine of the National Academy of Sciences increased the recommendation to 60 minutes of moderate-intensity physical activity every day.[7] This recommendation was based on evidence indicating that people who maintain healthy weight typically accumulate one hour of daily physical activity.

Subsequently, the Dietary Guidelines for Americans by the U.S. Department of Health and Human Services and the Department of Agriculture recommend that up to 60 minutes of moderate- to vigorous-intensity physical activity per day may be necessary to prevent weight gain, and between 60 and 90 minutes of moderate-intensity physical activity daily is recommended to sustain weight loss for previously overweight people.[8]

In sum, although health benefits are derived from 30 minutes of physical activity per day, people with a tendency to gain weight need to be physically active for an hour to an hour and a half daily to prevent weight gain. And 60 to 90 minutes of activity per day provides additional health benefits, including a lower risk for cardiovascular disease and diabetes.

National Initiatives to Promote Healthy and Active Lifestyles

Federal Guidelines for Physical Activity

Because of the importance of physical activity to our health, the U.S. Department of Health and Human Services has issued the Federal Physical Activity Guidelines for Americans. These guidelines complement the Dietary Guidelines for Americans (Chapter 3, pages 114–115) and further substantiate previous recommendations issued by the American College of Sports Medicine (ACSM) and the AHA in 2007,[9] and the U.S. Surgeon General in 1996.[10]

The federal guidelines provide science-based guidance on the importance of being physically active to promote health and reduce the risk for chronic diseases. The federal guidelines include the following recommendations[11]:

weekly recommendation

Adults between 18 and 64 years of age
- Adults should do 2 hours and 30 minutes a week of moderate-intensity aerobic (cardiorespiratory) physical activity, 1 hour and 15 minutes (75 minutes) a week of vigorous-intensity aerobic physical activity, or an equivalent combination of moderate- and vigorous-intensity aerobic physical activity (also see Chapter 6). When combining moderate- and vigorous-intensity activities, a person could participate in moderate-intensity activity twice a week for 30 minutes and high-intensity activity for 20 minutes on another two days. Aerobic activity should be performed in episodes of at least 10 minutes long each, preferably spread throughout the week.
- Additional health benefits are provided by increasing to 5 hours (300 minutes) a week of moderate-intensity aerobic physical activity, 2 hours and 30 minutes a week of vigorous-intensity physical activity, or an equivalent combination of both.
- Adults should also do muscle-strengthening activities that involve all major muscle groups, performed on two or more days per week.

Older adults (ages 65 and older)

- Older adults should follow the adult guidelines. If this is not possible due to limiting chronic conditions, older adults should be as physically active as their abilities allow. They should avoid inactivity. Older adults should do exercises that maintain or improve balance if they are at risk of falling.

Children 6 years of age and older and adolescents

- Children and adolescents should do 1 hour (60 minutes) or more of physical activity every day. Most of the 1 hour or more a day should be either moderate- or vigorous-intensity aerobic physical activity.
- As part of their daily physical activity, children and adolescents should do vigorous-intensity activity at least three days per week. They also should do muscle-strengthening and bone-strengthening activities at least three days per week.

Pregnant and postpartum women

- Healthy women who are not already doing vigorous-intensity physical activity should get at least 2 hours and 30 minutes (150 minutes) of moderate-intensity aerobic activity a week. Preferably, this activity should be spread throughout the week. Women who regularly engage in vigorous-intensity aerobic activity or high amounts of activity can continue their activity provided that their condition remains unchanged and they talk to their health care provider about their activity level throughout their pregnancy.

In a previous 2007 report, the ACSM and the AHA also released a joint statement on physical activity recommendations for healthy adults.[12] The ACSM/AHA report states that a greater amount of physical activity that exceeds the minimum recommendations provided above for adults between 18 and 64 years of age provides even greater benefits and is recommended for individuals who wish to further improve personal fitness, reduce the risk for chronic disease and disabilities, prevent premature mortality, or prevent unhealthy weight gain.

The ACSM/AHA report also states that only 49.1 percent of the adult population meets the recommendations. College graduates are more likely to adhere to the recommendations (about 53 percent of them), followed by individuals with some college education, then high school graduates; and the least likely to meet the recommendations are those with less than a high school diploma (37.8 percent).

In conjunction with the above report, the ACSM and the American Medical Association (AMA) have launched a nationwide "Exercise Is Medicine" program.[13] The goal of this initiative is to help improve the health and wellness of the nation through exercise prescriptions from physicians and health care providers. It calls on all physicians to assess and review every patient's physical activity program at every visit.

"Exercise is medicine and it's free." All physicians should be prescribing exercise to all patients and participate in exercise themselves. Exercise is considered to be the much-needed vaccine of our time to prevent chronic diseases. Physical activity and exercise are powerful tools for both the treatment and the prevention of chronic diseases and premature death. Additional information on this program can be obtained by consulting the following website: http://www.exerciseismedicine.org/.

Critical Thinking

Do you consciously incorporate physical activity into your daily lifestyle? Can you provide examples? Do you think you get sufficient daily physical activity to maintain good health?

National Health Objectives for the Year 2020

Every 10 years, the U.S. Department of Health and Human Services releases a list of objectives for preventing disease and promoting health. Since 1979, the Healthy People initiative has set and monitored national health objectives to meet a broad range of health needs, encourage collaborations across sectors, guide individuals toward making informed health decisions, and measure the impact of our prevention activity. Currently, Healthy People is leading the way to achieve increased quality and years of healthy life and to seek to eliminate health disparities among all groups of people. The objectives address three important points[14]:

1. *Personal responsibility for health behavior.* Individuals need to become ever more health conscious. Responsible and informed behaviors are the keys to good health.
2. *Health benefits for all people and all communities.* Lower socioeconomic conditions and poor health often are interrelated. Extending the benefits of good health to all people is crucial to the health of the nation.
3. *Health promotion and disease prevention.* A shift from treatment to preventive techniques will drastically cut health care costs and help all Americans achieve a better quality of life.

Developing these health objectives involves more than 10,000 people representing 300 national organizations, including the Institute of Medicine of the National Academy of Sciences, all state health departments, and the federal Office of Disease Prevention and Health

Figure 1.7   Selected Health Objectives for the Year 2020.

- Increase the proportion of persons with health insurance, a usual primary care provider, and coverage for clinical preventive services.
- Ensure that all people, including those with illnesses and chronic disability, participate daily in meaningful and freely chosen recreation, leisure, and physical activity, which directly influences well-being and quality of life.
- Reduce the proportion of adults who engage in no leisure-time physical activity.
- Increase the proportion of adolescents and adults who meet current Federal physical activity guidelines.
- Increase the proportion of adults who are at a healthy weight, and reduce the proportion of children, adolescents, and adults who are overweight or obese.
- Reduce coronary heart disease and stroke deaths.
- Reduce the mean total blood cholesterol levels among adults and the proportion of persons in the population with hypertension.
- Increase the proportion of adults aged 20 years and older who are aware of, and respond to, early warning symptoms and signs of a heart attack and stroke.
- Reduce the overall cancer death rate and provide counseling about cancer prevention.
- Reduce the diabetes death rate and the annual number of new cases of diagnosed diabetes in the population.

- Reduce infections caused by key pathogens commonly transmitted through food.
- Increase the proportion of sexually active persons who use condoms.
- Reduce the rate of HIV transmission among adults and adolescents, and reduce the number of deaths resulting from HIV infection.
- Increase the proportion of substance-abuse treatment facilities that offer HIV/AIDS education, counseling, and support.
- Increase school-based health promotion programs available to youth between the ages of 14 and 22 to decrease the rate of sexually transmitted diseases and teen pregnancy and to increase the proportion of adolescents who abstain from sexual intercourse or use condoms if sexually active.
- Reduce tobacco use by adults and adolescents, and reduce the initiation among children, adolescents, and young adults.
- Reduce average annual alcohol consumption, and increase the proportion of adolescents who disapprove of substance abuse.
- Increase the proportion, among persons who need alcohol and/or illicit drug treatment, of those who receive specialized treatment for abuse or dependence.
- Reduce drug-induced deaths.

© Cengage Learning 2013

Promotion. Figure 1.7 summarizes the key 2020 objectives. Living the fitness and wellness principles provided in this book will enhance the quality of your life and also will allow you to be an active participant in achieving the Healthy People 2020 Objectives.

National Physical Activity Plan

Newly established in 2010, the National Physical Activity Plan calls for policy, environmental, and cultural changes to help all Americans enjoy the health benefits of physical activity. It aims to increase physical activity among all segments of the population. The plan is a comprehensive private/public sector joint effort to create a culture that supports active lifestyles and enables everyone to meet physical activity guidelines throughout life.

The vision of the plan is that one day all Americans will be physically active, and they will live, work, and play in environments that facilitate regular physical activity. The plan complements the Federal Physical Activity Guidelines and the Healthy People 2020 objectives and comprises recommendations organized in eight sectors of societal influence: education; business and industry; health care; mass media; parks recreation, fitness, and sports; public health; volunteer and non-profit; and transportation, land use, and community design. Strategies to implement the plan include:

- Developing and implementing policies requiring school accountability for quality and quantity of physical education and physical activity.
- Encouraging early childhood education programs to have children as physically active as possible.
- Providing access to and opportunities for physical activity before and after school.
- Making physical activity a patient "vital sign" (tracking activity levels) that all health care providers assess and discuss with patients.
- Using routine performance measures by local, state, and federal agencies to set benchmarks for active travel (walking, biking, public transportation).
- Enhancing the existing parks and recreation infrastructure with effective policy and environmental changes to promote physical activity.
- Identifying and disseminating best practice models for physical activity in the workplace.
- Providing tax breaks for building owners or employers who provide amenities in workplaces and support active commuting, including showers in buildings, secure bicycle parking, free bicycles, or transit subsidies.
- Encouraging businesses to implement work policies that allow employees to get some physical activity before, during, or after work hours.

The implementation of the National Physical Activity Plan requires cooperation among school officials, city and county council members, state legislators, corporations, and Congress.

Figure 1.8	Prevalence of recommended physical activity in the United States.

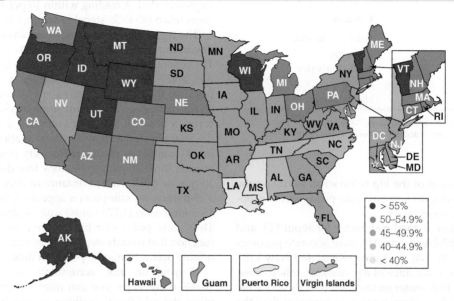

> 55%
50–54.9%
45–49.9%
40–44.9%
< 40%

Hawaii Guam Puerto Rico Virgin Islands

Note: Recommended physical activity is accumulation of 30 minutes per day of moderate-intensity activity a minimum of 5 days per week or 20 minutes per day of vigorous-intensity activity a minimum of 3 days per week.

SOURCE: Centers for Disease Control and Prevention.

Monitoring Daily Physical Activity

According to the Centers for Disease Control and Prevention, the majority of U.S. adults are not sufficiently physically active to promote good health. The most recent data indicate that only 49 percent of adults meet the minimal recommendation of 30 minutes of moderate physical activity at least 5 days per week, 24 percent report no leisure physical activity at all, and 14 percent are completely inactive (less than 10 minutes per week of moderate- or vigorous-intensity physical activity). The prevalence of physical activity by state in the United States is displayed in Figure 1.8.

Other than carefully monitoring actual time engaged in activity, an excellent tool to monitor daily physical activity is a **pedometer**. A pedometer is a small mechanical device that senses vertical body motion and is used to count footsteps. Wearing a pedometer throughout the day allows you to determine the total steps you take in a day. Some pedometers also record distance, calories burned, speeds, and actual time of activity each day. A pedometer is a great motivational tool to help increase, maintain, and monitor daily physical activity that involves lower-body motion (walking, jogging, running).

Before purchasing a pedometer, be sure to verify its accuracy. Many of the free and low-cost pedometers provided by corporations for promotion and advertisement purposes are inaccurate, so their use is discouraged. Pedometers also tend to lose accuracy at a very slow walking speed (slower than 30 minutes per mile) because the

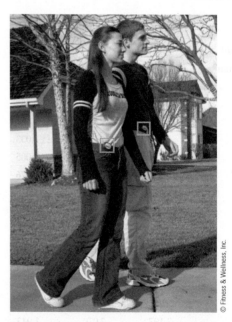

Pedometers are used to monitor daily physical activity; the recommendation is a minimum of 10,000 steps per day.

Key Terms

Pedometer An electronic device that senses body motion and counts footsteps. Some pedometers also record distance, calories burned, speeds, "aerobic steps," and time spent being physically active.

Table 1.2	Adult Activity Levels Based on Total Number of Steps Taken per Day
Steps per Day	**Category**
<5,000	Sedentary lifestyle
5,000–7,499	Low active
7,500–9,999	Somewhat active
10,000–12,499	**Active**
≥12,500	Highly active

SOURCE: C. Tudor-Locke and D. R. Basset, "How Many Steps/Day Are Enough? Preliminary Pedometer Indices for Public Health," *Sports Medicine* 34:1–8, 2004.

vertical movement of the hip is too small to trigger the spring-mounted lever arm inside the pedometer to properly record the steps taken.

You can obtain a good pedometer for about $25, and ratings are available online. The most accurate pedometer brands are Walk4Life, Yamax, Kenz, and New Lifestyles. To test the accuracy of a pedometer, follow these steps: Clip the pedometer on the waist directly above the kneecap, reset the pedometer to zero, carefully close the pedometer, walk exactly 50 steps at your normal pace, carefully open the pedometer, and look at the number of steps recorded. A reading within 10 percent of the actual steps taken (45 to 55 steps) is acceptable.

The typical male American takes about 6,000 steps per day, in comparison to women, who take about 5,300 steps. The general recommendation for adults is 10,000 steps per day, and Table 1.2 provides specific activity categories based on the number of daily steps taken.

All daily steps count, but some of your steps should come in bouts of at least 10 minutes, so as to meet the national physical activity recommendation of accumulating 30 minutes of moderate-intensity physical activity in at least three 10-minute sessions five days per week. A 10-minute brisk walk (a distance of about 1,200 yards at a 15-minute per mile pace) is approximately 1,300 steps. A 15-minute-mile (1,770 yards) walk is about 1,900 steps.[15] Thus, new pedometer brands have an "aerobic steps" function that records steps taken in excess of 60 steps per minute over a 10-minute period of time.

If you do not accumulate the recommended 10,000 daily steps, you can refer to Table 1.3 to determine the additional walking or jogging distance re-

Table 1.3	Estimated Number of Steps to Walk or Jog a Mile Based on Gender, Height, and Pace							
	Pace (min/mile)							
	Walking				Jogging			
Height	20	18	16	15	12	10	8	6
Women								
5'0"	2,371	2,244	2,117	2,054	1,997	1,710	1,423	1,136
5'2"	2,343	2,216	2,089	2,026	1,970	1,683	1,396	1,109
5'4"	2,315	2,188	2,061	1,998	1,943	1,656	1,369	1,082
5'6"	2,286	2,160	2,033	1,969	1,916	1,629	1,342	1,055
5'8"	2,258	2,131	2,005	1,941	1,889	1,602	1,315	1,028
5'10"	2,230	2,103	1,976	1,913	1,862	1,575	1,288	1,001
6'0"	2,202	2,075	1,948	1,885	1,835	1,548	1,261	974
6'2"	2,174	2,047	1,920	1,857	1,808	1,521	1,234	947
Men								
5'2"	2,310	2,183	2,056	1,993	1,970	1,683	1,396	1,109
5'4"	2,282	2,155	2,028	1,965	1,943	1,656	1,369	1,082
5'6"	2,253	2,127	2,000	1,937	1,916	1,629	1,342	1,055
5'8"	2,225	2,098	1,872	1,908	1,889	1,602	1,315	1,028
5'10"	2,197	2,070	1,943	1,880	1,862	1,575	1,288	1,001
6'0"	2,169	2,042	1,915	1,852	1,835	1,548	1,261	974
6'2"	2,141	2,014	1,887	1,824	1,808	1,521	1,234	947
6'4"	2,112	1,986	1,859	1,795	1,781	1,494	1,207	920

Prediction equations (pace in min/mile and height in inches):

Walking

Women: Steps/mile = $1{,}949 + [(63.4 \times \text{pace}) - (14.1 \times \text{height})]$

Men: Steps/mile = $1{,}916 + [(63.4 \times \text{pace}) - (14.1 \times \text{height})]$

Running

Women and men: Steps/mile = $1{,}084 + [(143.6 \times \text{pace}) - (13.5 \times \text{height})]$

SOURCE: Werner W. K. Hoeger et al., "One-Mile Step Count at Walking and Running Speeds." *ACSM's Health & Fitness Journal,* Vol 12(1):14–19, 2008.

quired to reach your goal. For example, if you are 5'8" tall, female, and you typically accumulate 5,200 steps per day, you would need an additional 4,800 daily steps to reach your 10,000-steps goal. You can do so by jogging 3 miles at a 10-minute-per-mile pace (1,602 steps x 3 miles = 4,806 steps) on some days, and you can walk 2.5 miles at a 15-minute-per-mile pace (1,941 steps x 2.5 miles = 4,853 steps) on other days. If you do not find a particular speed (pace) that you typically walk or jog at in Table 1.3, you can estimate the number of steps at that speed using the prediction equations at the bottom of this table.

The first practical application that you can undertake in this course is to determine your current level of daily activity. The log provided in Activity 1.1 will help you do this. Keep a 4-day log of all physical activities that you do daily. On this log, record the time of day, type and duration of the exercise/activity, and, if possible, steps taken while engaged in the activity. The results will indicate how active you are and serve as a basis to monitor changes in the next few months and years.

Wellness

Most people recognize that participating in fitness programs improves their quality of life. At the end of the 20th century, however, we came to realize that physical fitness alone was not always sufficient to lower the risk for disease and ensure better health. For example, individuals who run 3 miles (about 5 km) a day, lift weights regularly, participate in stretching exercises, and watch their body weight might be easily classified as having good or excellent fitness. Offsetting these good habits, however, might be risk factors including high blood pressure, smoking, excessive stress, drinking too much alcohol, and eating too many foods high in saturated fat. These factors place people at risk for cardiovascular disease and other chronic diseases of which they may not be aware. Thus, a new concept that is rapidly gaining popularity is **primordial prevention** or the prevention of the development of risk factors for disease.

Even though most people are aware of their unhealthy behaviors, they seem satisfied with life as long as they are free from symptoms of disease or illness. They do not contemplate change until they incur a major health problem. Nevertheless, present lifestyle habits dictate the health and well-being of tomorrow.

Good health should not be viewed simply as the absence of illness. The notion of good health has evolved considerably and continues to change as scientists learn more about lifestyle factors that bring on illness and affect wellness. Furthermore, once the idea took hold that fitness by itself would not always decrease the risk for disease and ensure better health, **health promotion** programs and the **wellness** concept followed.

Wellness implies a constant and deliberate effort to stay healthy and achieve the highest potential for well-being. Wellness requires implementing positive lifestyle habits to change behavior and thereby improve health and quality of life, prolong life, and achieve total well-being. Living a wellness way of life is a personal choice, but you may need additional support to achieve wellness goals. Thus, health promotion programs have been developed to educate people regarding healthy lifestyles and provide the necessary support to achieve wellness.

For example, you may be prepared to initiate an aerobic exercise program, but if you are not familiar with exercise prescription guidelines or places to exercise safely, or if you lack peer support or flexible scheduling to do so, you may have difficulty accomplishing your goal. Similarly, if you want to quit smoking but do not know how to do it and everyone else around you smokes, the chances for success are limited. To some extent, the environment limits your choices. Hence, the availability of a health promotion program would provide the much-needed support to get started and implement a wellness way of life.

The Seven Dimensions of Wellness

Wellness has seven dimensions: physical, emotional, mental, social, environmental, occupational, and spiritual (Figure 1.9). These dimensions are interrelated: One frequently affects the others. For example, a person who is emotionally "down" often has no desire to exercise, study, socialize with friends, or attend church, and he or she may be more susceptible to illness and disease.

The seven dimensions show how the concept of wellness clearly goes beyond the absence of disease. Wellness incorporates factors such as adequate fitness, proper nutrition, stress management, disease prevention, spirituality, not smoking or abusing drugs, personal safety, regular physical examinations, health education, and environmental support.

For a wellness way of life, individuals must be physically fit and manifest no signs of disease and they also must be free of risk factors for disease (such as hypertension, hyperlipidemia, cigarette smoking, negative stress, faulty nutrition, careless sex). The relationship between

---

Key Terms

Primordial prevention Prevention of the development of risk factors for disease.

Health promotion The science and art of enabling people to increase control over their lifestyle to move toward a state of wellness.

Wellness The constant and deliberate effort to stay healthy and achieve the highest potential for well-being. It encompasses seven dimensions—physical, emotional, mental, social, environmental, occupational, and spiritual—and integrates them all into a quality life.

Daily Physical Activity Log

Name: _____ Date: _____

Course: _____ Section: _____ Gender: _____ Age: _____

Date: [_____] Day of the Week: [_____]

Time of Day	Exercise/Activity	Duration	Number of Steps	Comments
[ ]	[ ]	[ ]	[ ]	[ ]
[ ]	[ ]	[ ]	[ ]	[ ]
[ ]	[ ]	[ ]	[ ]	[ ]
[ ]	[ ]	[ ]	[ ]	[ ]
[ ]	[ ]	[ ]	[ ]	[ ]
[ ]	[ ]	[ ]	[ ]	[ ]
[ ]	[ ]	[ ]	[ ]	[ ]
	Totals:	[ ]	[ ]	

Activity category based on steps per day (use Table 1.2, page 12): _____

Date: [_____] Day of the Week: [_____]

Time of Day	Exercise/Activity	Duration	Number of Steps	Comments
[ ]	[ ]	[ ]	[ ]	[ ]
[ ]	[ ]	[ ]	[ ]	[ ]
[ ]	[ ]	[ ]	[ ]	[ ]
[ ]	[ ]	[ ]	[ ]	[ ]
[ ]	[ ]	[ ]	[ ]	[ ]
[ ]	[ ]	[ ]	[ ]	[ ]
[ ]	[ ]	[ ]	[ ]	[ ]
	Totals:	[ ]	[ ]	

Activity category based on steps per day (use Table 1.2, page 12): _____

Daily Physical Activity Log (continued)

Date: _____   Day of the Week: _____

Time of Day	Exercise/Activity	Duration	Number of Steps	Comments
Totals:				

Activity category based on steps per day (use Table 1.2, page 12): _____

Date: _____   Day of the Week: _____

Time of Day	Exercise/Activity	Duration	Number of Steps	Comments
Totals:				

Activity category based on steps per day (use Table 1.2, page 12): _____

Briefly evaluate your current activity patterns, discuss your feelings about the results, and provide a goal for the weeks ahead.

_____

_____

_____

_____

_____

Figure 1.9 Dimensions of wellness.

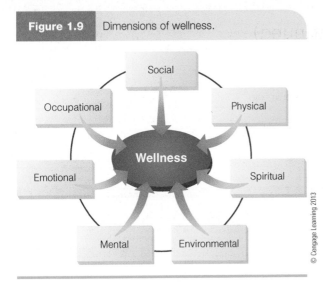

adequate fitness and wellness is illustrated in the continuum in Figure 1.10. Even though an individual tested in a fitness center may demonstrate adequate or even excellent fitness, indulging in unhealthy lifestyle behaviors will still increase the risk for chronic diseases and diminish the person's well-being.

Physical Wellness

Physical wellness is the dimension most commonly associated with being healthy. It entails confidence and optimism about one's ability to protect physical health and take care of health problems.

Physically well individuals are physically active, exercise regularly, eat a well-balanced diet, maintain recommended body weight, get sufficient sleep, practice safe sex, minimize exposure to environmental contaminants, avoid harmful drugs (including tobacco and excessive alcohol), and seek medical care and exams as needed. Physically well people also exhibit good cardiorespiratory endurance, adequate muscular strength and flexibility, proper body composition, and the ability to carry out ordinary and unusual demands of daily life safely and effectively.

Emotional Wellness

Emotional wellness involves the ability to understand your own feelings, accept your limitations, and achieve emotional stability. Furthermore, it implies the ability to express emotions appropriately, adjust to change, cope with stress in a healthy way, and enjoy life despite its occasional disappointments and frustrations.

Emotional wellness brings with it a certain stability, an ability to look both success and failure squarely in the face and keep moving along a predetermined course. When success is evident, the emotionally well person radiates the expected joy and confidence. When failure seems evident, the emotionally well person responds by making the best of circumstances and moving beyond the failure. Wellness enables you to move ahead with optimism and energy instead of spending time and talent worrying about failure. You learn from it, identify ways to avoid it in the future, and then go on with the business at hand.

Emotional wellness also involves happiness—an emotional anchor that gives meaning and joy to life. Happiness is a long-term state of mind that permeates the various facets of life and influences our outlook. Although there is no simple recipe for creating happiness, researchers agree that happy people are usually participants in some category of a supportive family unit where they feel loved. Healthy, happy people enjoy friends, work hard at something fulfilling, get plenty of exercise, and enjoy play and leisure time. They know how to laugh, and they laugh often. They give of themselves freely to others and seem to have found deep meaning in life.

An attitude of true happiness signals freedom from the tension and depression that many people endure. Emotionally well people are obviously subject to the same kinds of depression and unhappiness that occasionally plague us all, but the difference lies in the ability to bounce back. Well people take minor setbacks in stride and have the ability to enjoy life despite it all. They don't waste energy or time recounting the situation, wondering how they could have changed it, or dwelling on the past.

Mental Wellness

Mental wellness, also referred to as intellectual wellness, implies that you can apply the things you have learned, create opportunities to learn more, and engage your mind

Figure 1.10 Wellness continuum.

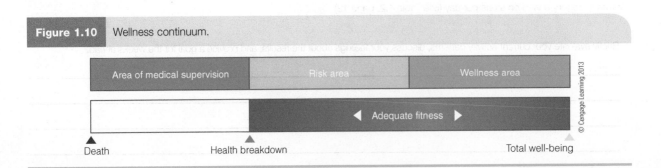

in lively interaction with the world around you. When you are mentally well, you are not intimidated by facts and figures with which you are unfamiliar, but you embrace the chance to learn something new. Your confidence and enthusiasm enable you to approach any learning situation with eagerness that leads to success.

Mental wellness brings with it vision and promise. More than anything else, mentally well people are open-minded and accepting of others. Instead of being threatened by people who are different from themselves, they show respect and curiosity without feeling they have to conform. They are faithful to their own ideas and philosophies and allow others the same privilege. Their self-confidence guarantees that they can take their place among others in the world without having to give up part of themselves and without requiring others to do the same.

Social Wellness

Social wellness, with its accompanying positive self-image, endows you with the ease and confidence to be outgoing, friendly, and affectionate toward others. Social wellness involves a concern for oneself and also an interest in humanity and the environment as a whole.

One of the hallmarks of social wellness is the ability to relate to others and to reach out to other people, both within one's family and outside it. Similar to emotional wellness, it involves being comfortable with your emotions and thus helps you understand and accept the emotions of others. Your own balance and sense of self allow you to extend respect and tolerance to others. Healthy people are honest and loyal. This dimension of wellness leads to the ability to maintain close relationships with other people.

Environmental Wellness

Environmental wellness refers to the effect that our surroundings have on our well-being. Our planet is a delicate **ecosystem**, and its health depends on the continuous recycling of its elements. Environmental wellness implies a lifestyle that maximizes harmony with the earth and takes action to protect the world around us.

Environmental threats include air pollution, chemicals, ultraviolet radiation in the sunlight, water and food contamination, secondhand smoke, noise, inadequate shelter, unsatisfactory work conditions, lack of personal safety, and unhealthy relationships. Health is affected negatively when we live in a polluted, toxic, unkind, and unsafe environment.

Unfortunately, a national survey of first-year college students showed that less than 20 percent were concerned about the health of the environment.[16] To enjoy environmental wellness, we are responsible for educating and protecting ourselves against environmental hazards and also protecting the environment so that we, our children, and future generations can enjoy a safe and clean environment.

Steps that you can take to live an environmentally conscious life include conserving energy (walk to your destination or ride on public transportation, do not drive unless absolutely necessary, turn off lights and computers when not in use); not littering and politely asking others not to do it either; recycling as much as possible (paper, glass, cans, plastics, cardboard); conserving paper and water (take shorter showers, don't let the water run while brushing your teeth); not polluting the air, water, or earth if you can avoid doing so; not smoking; planting trees and keeping plants and shrubs alive; evaluating purchases and conveniences based on their environmental impact; donating old clothes to Goodwill, veterans' groups, or other charities; and enjoying, appreciating, and spending time outdoors in natural settings.

Occupational Wellness

Occupational wellness is not tied to high salary, prestigious position, or extravagant working conditions. Any job can bring occupational wellness if it provides rewards that are important to the individual. To one person, salary might be the most important factor, whereas another might place much greater value on creativity. Those who are occupationally well have their own "ideal" job, which allows them to thrive.

People with occupational wellness face demands on the job, but they also have some say over demands placed on them. Any job has routine demands, but in occupational wellness, routine demands are mixed with new, unpredictable challenges that keep a job exciting. Occupationally well people are able to maximize their skills, and they have the opportunity to broaden their existing skills or gain new ones. Their occupation offers the opportunity for advancement and recognition for achievement. Occupational wellness encourages collaboration and interaction among coworkers, which fosters a sense of teamwork and support.

Key Terms

Physical wellness Good physical fitness and confidence in your personal ability to take care of health problems.

Emotional wellness The ability to understand your own feelings, accept your limitations, and achieve emotional stability.

Mental wellness A state in which your mind is engaged in lively interaction with the world around you.

Social wellness The ability to relate well to others, both within and outside the family unit.

Environmental wellness The capability to live in a clean and safe environment that is not detrimental to health.

Ecosystem A community of organisms interacting with each other in an environment.

Occupational wellness The ability to perform your job skillfully and effectively under conditions that provide personal and team satisfaction and adequately reward each individual.

Spiritual Wellness

Spiritual wellness provides a unifying power that integrates all dimensions of wellness. Basic characteristics of spiritual people include a sense of meaning and direction in life and a relationship to a higher being. Pursuing these avenues may lead to personal freedom, including prayer, faith, love, closeness to others, peace, joy, fulfillment, and altruism.

Several studies have reported positive relationships among spiritual well-being, emotional well-being, and satisfaction with life. Spiritual health is somehow intertwined with physical health. People who attend church and regularly participate in religious organizations enjoy better health, have a lower incidence of chronic diseases, are more socially integrated, handle stress more effectively, and appear to live longer.[17] Other studies have shown that spirituality strengthens the immune system, is good for mental health, prevents age-related memory loss, decreases the incidence of depression, leads to fewer episodes of chronic inflammation, and decreases the risk of death and suicide.

Prayer is a signpost of spirituality at the core of most spiritual experiences. It is communication with a higher power. At least 200 studies have been conducted on the effects of prayer on health. About two-thirds of these studies have linked prayer to positive health outcomes—as long as these prayers are offered with sincerity, humility, love, empathy, and compassion. Some studies have shown faster healing time and fewer complications in patients who didn't even know they were being prayed for, compared with patients who were not prayed for.[18]

Altruism, a key attribute of spiritual people, seems to enhance health and longevity. Studies indicate that people who regularly volunteer live longer. Research has found that health benefits of altruism are so powerful that doing good for others is good for oneself, especially for the immune system.

Researchers believe that there seems to be a strong connection among the mind, spirit, and body. As one improves, the others follow. The relationship between spirituality and wellness is meaningful in our quest for a better quality of life. As with the other dimensions, development of the spiritual dimension to its fullest potential contributes to wellness. Wellness requires a balance among all seven dimensions.

Critical Thinking

Now that you understand the seven dimensions of wellness, rank them in order of importance to you and explain your rationale in doing so.

Wellness, Fitness, and Longevity

During the second half of the 20th century, scientists began to realize the importance of good fitness and improved lifestyle in the fight against chronic diseases,

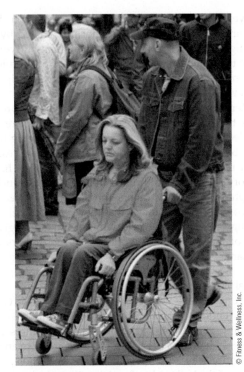

Altruism enhances health and well-being.

particularly those of the cardiovascular system. Because of more participation in wellness programs, cardiovascular mortality rates dropped. The decline began in about 1963, and between 1960 and 2000, the incidence of cardiovascular disease dropped by 26 percent. Additionally, heart attack and death rates from them have further declined by 24 percent between 1999 and 2008. This decrease is credited to higher levels of wellness and better treatment modalities in the United States.

Furthermore, several studies showed an inverse relationship between physical activity and premature mortality rates. The first major study in this area was conducted in the 1980s among 16,936 Harvard alumni, and the results linked physical activity habits and mortality rates.[19] As the amount of weekly physical activity increased, the risk for cardiovascular deaths decreased. The largest decrease in cardiovascular deaths was observed among alumni who used more than 2,000 calories per week through physical activity.

A landmark study subsequently conducted at the Aerobics Research Institute in Dallas upheld the findings of the Harvard alumni study.[20] Based on data from 13,344 people followed over an average of eight years, the study revealed a graded and consistent inverse relationship between physical activity levels and mortality, regardless of age and other risk factors. As illustrated in Figure 1.11, the higher the level of physical activity, the longer the lifespan.

The death rate during the eight-year study from all causes for the low-fit men was 3.4 times higher than that of the high-fit men. For the low-fit women, the death rate

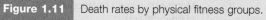

Figure 1.11 Death rates by physical fitness groups.

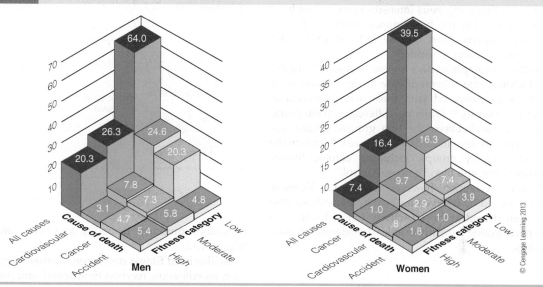

© Cengage Learning 2013

was 4.6 times higher than that of high-fit women. A most significant finding of this landmark study was the large drop in all-cause, cardiovascular, and cancer mortality when individuals went from low fitness to moderate fitness—a clear indication that moderate-intensity physical activity, achievable by most adults, does provide considerable health benefits and extends life. The data also revealed that the participants attained more protection by combining higher fitness levels with reduction in other risk factors such as hypertension, serum cholesterol, cigarette smoking, and excessive body fat.

Two additional studies reported in 2009 confirm that fitness improves wellness, quality of life, and longevity. The first study included 4,384 subjects and the results showed that the least-fit group had an almost twofold greater risk of all-cause and cardiovascular mortalities as compared with the moderately fit groups and a fourfold increased risk in comparison to the most-fit group.[21] The researchers concluded that the mortality rates between the least-fit and the other groups was most likely related to their **sedentary** lifestyle rather than differences in other health parameters.

The second study looked at four health-related factors among a group of more than 23,000 people.[22] These factors included lifetime nonsmoker, not considered obese (body mass index below 30), engaging in a minimum of 3.5 hours of weekly physical activity, and adherence to healthy nutrition principles (high consumption of whole-grain breads, fruits, and vegetables; and low consumption of red meat). Those who adhered to all four health habits were 78 percent less likely to develop chronic diseases (diabetes, heart disease, stroke, and cancer) during the almost eight-year study. Furthermore, the risk for developing a chronic disease progressively increased as the number of health factors decreased.

Currently, research on the benefits of physical activity and exercise on health and longevity is far too impressive to be ignored. A 2010 analysis of 33 studies involving more than 180,000 people quite clearly concluded that better aerobic fitness is associated with a substantial lower risk of all-cause mortality and cardiovascular disease.[23] In today's society, a person cannot afford not to participate in a lifetime physical fitness program.

While it is clear that moderate-intensity exercise does provide substantial health benefits, research data also show a dose-response relationship between physical activity and health. That is, greater health and fitness benefits occur at higher duration and/or intensity of physical activity. **Vigorous activity** and longer duration are preferable to the extent of one's capabilities because they are most clearly associated with better health and longer life.

Vigorous-intensity exercise seems to provide the best benefits.[24] As compared with prolonged moderate-intensity activity, vigorous-intensity exercise has been shown to provide the best improvements in aerobic capacity, coronary heart disease risk reduction, and overall cardiovascular health.[25]

Further, a comprehensive review of research studies found a lower rate of heart disease in vigorous-intensity exercisers as compared with those who exercised at moderate intensity.[26] While no differences were found in weight loss between the two groups, greater improvements are seen in cardiovascular risk factors in the vigorous-intensity groups, including aerobic fitness, blood pressure, and blood glucose control.

A word of caution, however, is in order. Vigorous exercise should be reserved for healthy individuals who have been cleared to do so (Activity 1.3) and who have been participating regularly in at least moderate-intensity activities.

Types of Physical Fitness

As the fitness concept grew at the end of the past century, it became clear that several specific components contribute to an individual's overall level of fitness. **Physical fitness** is classified into health-related and skill-related.

Health-related fitness relates to the ability to perform activities of daily living without undue fatigue and is conducive to a low risk of premature **hypokinetic diseases**. The health-related fitness components are cardiorespiratory (aerobic) endurance, muscular strength and

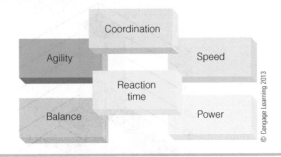

| **Figure 1.13** | Motor-skill-related components of physical fitness. |

endurance, muscular flexibility, and body composition (Figure 1.12).

Skill-related fitness components consist of agility, balance, coordination, reaction time, speed, and power (Figure 1.13). These components are related primarily to successful sports and motor skill performance. Participating in skill-related activities contributes to physical fitness, but in terms of general health promotion and wellness, the main emphasis of physical fitness programs should be on the health-related components.

Critical Thinking

What role do the four health-related components of physical fitness play in your life? Rank them in order of importance to you and explain the rationale you used.

| **Figure 1.12** | Health-related components of physical fitness. |

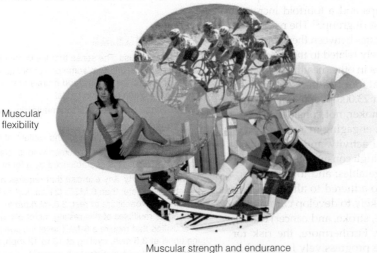

Cardiorespiratory endurance

Muscular flexibility

Body composition

Muscular strength and endurance

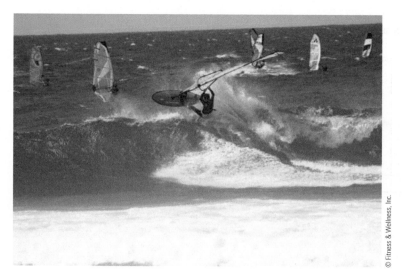

© Fitness & Wellness, Inc.

Good health-related fitness and skill-related fitness are required to participate in highly skilled activities.

Fitness Standards: Health versus Physical Fitness

A meaningful debate regarding age- and gender-related fitness standards has resulted in two standards: health fitness (also referred to as *criterion referenced*) and physical fitness. Following are definitions of both. The assessment of health-related fitness is presented in Chapters 4, 6, 7, and 8; where appropriate, physical fitness standards are included for comparison.

Health Fitness Standards

The **health fitness standards** proposed here are based on data linking minimum fitness values to disease prevention and health. Attaining the health fitness standard requires only moderate physical activity. For example, a two-mile walk in less than 30 minutes, five or six times a week, seems to be sufficient to achieve the health-fitness standard for cardiorespiratory endurance.

As illustrated in Figure 1.14, significant health benefits can be reaped with such a program, although fitness improvements, expressed in terms of maximum oxygen uptake, or VO_{2max} (explained next and in Chapter 6), are not as notable. Nevertheless, health improvements are quite striking. These benefits include reduction in blood lipids, lower blood pressure, weight loss, stress release, less risk for diabetes, and lower risk for disease and premature mortality.

More specifically, improvements in the **metabolic profile** (measured by insulin sensitivity, glucose tolerance, and improved cholesterol levels) can be notable despite little or no weight loss or improvement in aerobic capacity. Metabolic fitness can be attained through an active lifestyle and moderate-intensity physical activity.

An assessment of health-related fitness uses **cardiorespiratory endurance** measured in terms of the maximal amount of oxygen the body is able to utilize per minute of physical activity (VO_{2max})—essentially, a measure of how efficiently the heart, lungs, and muscles can operate during aerobic exercise (Chapter 6). VO_{2max} is commonly expressed in milliliters (mL) of oxygen (volume of oxygen) per kilogram (kg) of body weight per minute (mL/kg/min). Individual values can range from about 10 mL/kg/min in cardiac patients to more than 80 mL/kg/min in world-class runners, cyclists, and cross-country skiers.

Research data from the study presented in Figure 1.11 reported that achieving VO_{2max} values of 35 and 32.5 mL/kg/min for men and women, respectively, may be sufficient to lower the risk for all-cause mortality significantly. Although greater improvements in fitness yield an even lower risk for premature death, the largest drop is seen between the least fit and the moderately fit. Therefore, the 35 and 32.5 mL/kg/min values could be selected as the health fitness standards.

Physical Fitness Standards

Physical fitness standards are set higher than health fitness standards and require a more intense exercise program. Physically fit people of all ages have the

---

Key Terms

Physical fitness The ability to meet the ordinary as well as unusual demands of daily life safely and effectively without being overly fatigued and still have energy left for leisure and recreational activities.

Health-related fitness Fitness programs that are prescribed to improve the individual's overall health.

Hypokinetic diseases "Hypo" denotes "lack of"; therefore, illnesses related to lack of physical activity.

Skill-related fitness Fitness components important for success in skillful activities and athletic events; encompasses agility, balance, coordination, power, reaction time, and speed.

Health fitness standards The lowest fitness requirements for maintaining good health, decreasing the risk for chronic diseases, and lowering the incidence of muscular-skeletal injuries.

Metabolic profile A measurement of plasma insulin, glucose, lipid, and lipoprotein levels to assess risk for diabetes and cardiovascular disease.

Cardiorespiratory endurance The ability of the lungs, heart, and blood vessels to deliver adequate amounts of oxygen to the cells to meet the demands of prolonged physical activity.

Physical fitness standards A fitness level that allows a person to sustain moderate-to-vigorous physical activity without undue fatigue and the ability to closely maintain this level throughout life.

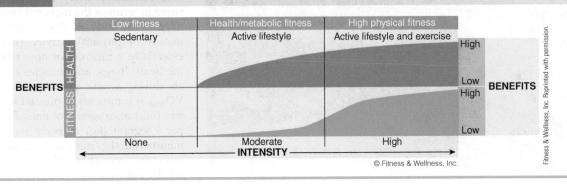

Figure 1.14 Health and fitness benefits based on the type of lifestyle and physical activity program.

© Fitness & Wellness, Inc.

Fitness & Wellness, Inc. Reprinted with permission.

Behavior Modification Planning

Financial Fitness Prescription

Although not one of the components of physical fitness, taking control of your personal finances is critical for your success and well-being. The sooner you start working on a lifetime personal financial plan, the more successful you will be in becoming financially secure and being able to retire early, in comfort, if you choose to do so. Most likely, you have not been taught basic principles to improve personal finance and enjoy "financial fitness." Thus, start today using the following strategies:

1. *Develop a personal financial plan.* Set short-term and long-term financial goals for yourself. If you do not have financial goals, you cannot develop a plan or work toward that end.

2. *Subscribe to a personal finance magazine or newsletter.* In the same way that you should regularly read reputable fitness/wellness journals or newsletters, you should regularly peruse a "financial fitness" magazine. If you don't enjoy reading financial materials, then find a periodical that is quick and to the point; there are many available. You don't have to force yourself to read the *Wall Street Journal* to become financially knowledgeable. Many periodicals have resources to help you develop a financial plan. Educate yourself and stay current on personal finances and investment matters.

3. *Set up a realistic budget and live on less than you make.* Pay your bills on time and keep track of *all* expenses. Then develop your budget so that you spend less than you earn. Your budget may require that you either cut back on expenses and services or figure out a way to increase your income. Balance your checkbook regularly and do not overdraft your checking account.

4. *Learn to differentiate between wants and needs.* It is fine to reward yourself for goals that you have achieved (see Chapter 2), but limit your spending to items that you truly need. Avoid simple impulse spending because "it's a bargain" or something you just want to have.

5. *Pay yourself first; save 10 percent of your income each month.* Before you take any money out of your paycheck, put 10 percent of your income into a retirement or investment account. If possible, ask for an automatic withdrawal at your bank from your paycheck to avoid the temptation to spend this money. This strategy may allow you to have a solid retirement fund or even provide for an early retirement. If you start putting away $100 a month at age 20, and earn a modest 6 percent interest rate, at age 65 you will have more than $275,000.

6. *Set up an emergency savings fund.* Whether you ultimately work for yourself or for someone else, there may be uncontrollable financial setbacks or even financial disasters in the future. So, as you are able, start an emergency fund equal to 3 to 6 months of normal monthly earnings. Additionally, start a second savings account for expensive purchases such as a car, a down payment on a home, or a vacation.

7. *Use credit, gas, and retail cards responsibly and sparingly.* As soon as you receive new cards, sign them promptly and store them securely. Due to the prevalence of identity theft (someone stealing your creditworthiness), cardholders should even consider a secure post office box, rather than a regular mailbox, for all high-risk mail. Shred your old credit cards, monthly statements, and any and all documents that contain personal information to avoid identity theft. Pay off all credit card debt monthly, and do not purchase on credit unless

freedom to enjoy most of life's daily and recreational activities to their fullest potentials. Current health fitness standards may not be enough to achieve these objectives.

Sound physical fitness gives the individual a degree of independence throughout life that many people in the United States no longer enjoy. Most adults should be able to carry out activities similar to those they conducted in their youth, though not with the same intensity. These standards do not require being a championship athlete, but activities such as changing a tire, chopping wood, climbing several flights of stairs, playing basketball, mountain biking, playing soccer with children or grandchildren, walking several miles around a lake, and hiking through a national park do require more than the current "average fitness" level of most Americans.

Which Program Is Best?

Your own personal objectives will determine the fitness program you decide to use. If the main objective of your fitness program is to lower the risk for disease, attaining the health fitness standards will provide substantial health benefits. If, however, you want to participate in vigorous fitness activities, achieving a high physical fitness standard is recommended. This book gives both health fitness and physical fitness standards for each fitness test so that you can personalize your approach.

Benefits of a Comprehensive Fitness Program

An inspiring story illustrating what fitness can do for a person's health and well-being is that of George Snell from Sandy, Utah. At age 45, Snell weighed approximately

---

you have the cash to pay it off when the monthly statement arrives. Develop a plan at this very moment to pay off your debt if you have such. Credit card balances, high interest rates, and frequent credit purchases lead to financial disaster. Credit card debt is the worst enemy to your personal finances!

8. *Understand the terms of your student loans.* Do not borrow more money than you absolutely need for actual educational expenses. Student loans are not for wants but needs (see item 4). Remember, loans must be repaid, with interest, once you leave college. Be informed regarding the repayment process and do not ever default on your loan. If you do, the entire balance (principal, interest, and collection fees) is due immediately and serious financial and credit consequences will follow.

9. *Eat out infrequently.* Besides saving money that you can then pay to yourself, you will eat healthier and consume fewer calories.

10. *Make the best of tax "motivated" savings and investing opportunities available to you.* For example, once employed, your company may match your voluntary 401(k) contributions (or other retirement plan), so contribute at least up to the match (you may use the 10 percent you "pay yourself first"—see item 5—or part of it). Also, under current tax law, maximize your Roth IRA contribution personally. Always pay attention to current tax rules that provide tax incentives for investing in retirement plans. If at all possible, *never* cash out a retirement account early. You may pay penalties in addition to tax, in most situations. As you are able, employ a tax professional or financial planner to avoid serious missteps in your tax planning.

11. *Stay involved in your financial accumulations.* You may seek professional advice, but you stay in control. Ultimately, no one will look after your interests as well as you. Avoid placing all your trust (and assets) in

one individual or institution. Spreading out your assets is one way to diversify your risk.

12. *Protect your assets.* As you start to accumulate assets, get proper insurance coverage (yes, even renter's insurance) in case of an accident or disaster. You have disciplined yourself and worked hard to obtain those assets, now make sure they are protected.

13. *Review your credit report.* The best way to ensure that your credit "identity" is not stolen and ruined is to regularly review your credit report, at least once a year, for accuracy.

14. *Contribute to charity and the needy.* Altruism (doing good for others) is good for heart health and emotional well-being. Remember the less fortunate and donate regularly to some of your favorite charitable organizations and volunteer time to worthy causes.

The Power of Investing Early

Jon and Jim are both 20 years old. Jon begins investing $100 a month starting on his 20th birthday. He stops investing on his 30th birthday (he has set aside a total of $12,000). Jim does not start investing until he's 30. He chooses to invest $100 a month as Jon had done, but he does so for the next 30 years (Jim invests a total of $36,000). Although Jon stopped investing at age 30, assuming an 8 percent annual rate of return in a tax-deferred account, by the time both Jon and Jim are 60, Jon will have accumulated $199,035, whereas Jim will have $150,029. At a 6 percent rate of return, they would both accumulate about $100,000, but Jim invested three times as much as Jon did.

Post these principles of financial fitness in a visible place at home where you can review them often. Start implementing these strategies as soon as you can and watch your financial fitness level increase over the years.

© David Johnson, CPA and Fitness & Wellness, Inc.

Table 1.4	Immediate (Acute) Benefits of Exercise

You can expect a number of benefits as a result of a single exercise session. Some of these benefits last as long as 72 hours following your workout. Exercise:

- increases heart rate, stroke volume, cardiac output, pulmonary ventilation, and oxygen uptake.
- begins to strengthen the heart, lungs, and muscles.
- enhances metabolic rate or energy production (burning calories for fuel) during exercise and recovery (for every 100 calories you burn during exercise, you can expect to burn another 15 during recovery).
- uses blood glucose and muscle glycogen.
- improves insulin sensitivity (decreasing the risk of type 2 diabetes).
- immediately enhances the body's ability to burn fat.
- lowers blood lipids.
- improves joint flexibility.
- reduces low grade (hidden) inflammation (see pages 351–352 in Chapter 10).
- increases endorphins (hormones), which are naturally occurring opioids that are responsible for exercise-induced euphoria.
- increases fat storage *in muscle,* which can then be burned for energy.

- improves endothelial function (endothelial cells line the entire vascular system, which provides a barrier between the vessel lumen and surrounding tissue–endothelial dysfunction contributes to several disease processes, including tissue inflammation and subsequent atherosclerosis).
- enhances mood and self-worth.
- provides a sense of achievement and satisfaction.
- decreases blood pressure the first few hours following exercise.
- decreases arthritic pain.
- leads to muscle relaxation.
- decreases stress.
- improves brain function.
- promotes better sleep (unless exercise is performed too close to bedtime).
- improves digestion.
- boosts energy levels.
- improves resistance to infections.

© Cengage Learning 2013

400 pounds, his blood pressure was 220/180, he was blind because of undiagnosed diabetes, and his blood glucose level was 487.

Snell had determined to do something about his physical and medical condition, so he started a walking/jogging program. After about eight months of conditioning, he had lost almost 200 pounds, his eyesight had returned, his glucose level was down to 67, and he was taken off medication. Just two months later—less than 10 months after beginning his personal exercise program—he completed his first marathon, a running course of 26.2 miles!

Health Benefits

Most people exercise because it improves their personal appearance and makes them feel good about themselves. Although many benefits accrue from participating in a regular fitness and wellness program, and active people generally live longer, *the greatest benefit of all is that physically fit individuals enjoy a better quality of life.* These people live life to its fullest, with far fewer health problems than inactive individuals.

The benefits derived by regularly participating in exercise are so extensive that it is difficult to compile an all-inclusive list. Many of these benefits are summarized in Table 1.5. As far back as 1982, the American Medical Association indicated that *"there is no drug in current or prospective use that holds as much promise for sustained health as a lifetime program of physical exercise."* Further-

more, researchers and sports medicine leaders have stated that *if the benefits of exercise could be packaged in a pill, it would be the most widely prescribed medication throughout the world today.*

While most of the chronic (long-term) benefits of exercise are well-established, what many people fail to realize is that there are *immediate benefits* derived by participating in just one single bout of exercise. Most of these benefits dissipate within 48 to 72 hours following exercise. The *immediate benefits,* summarized in Table 1.4, are so striking that it prompted Dr. William L. Haskell of Stanford University to state: *"Most of the health benefits of exercise are relatively short term, so people should think of exercise as a medication and take it on a daily basis."* Of course, as you regularly exercise a minimum of 30 minutes five times per week, you will realize the impressive long-term benefits listed in Table 1.5.

Exercise and Brain Function

If the previous benefits of exercise still have not convinced you to start a regular exercise program, you may want to consider the effects of exercise on brain function and academic performance. Physical activity is related to better cognitive health and effective functioning across the lifespan.

While much of the research is still in its infancy, even in 400 years BC, the Greek philosopher Plato stated: *"In*

Table 1.5	Long-term Benefits of Exercise

Regular participation in exercise:

- improves and strengthens the cardiorespiratory system.
- maintains better muscle tone, muscular strength, and endurance.
- improves muscular flexibility.
- enhances athletic performance.
- helps maintain recommended body weight.
- helps preserve lean body tissue.
- increases resting metabolic rate.
- improves the body's ability to use fat during physical activity.
- improves posture and physical appearance.
- improves functioning of the immune system.
- lowers the risk for chronic diseases and illnesses (including heart disease, stroke, and certain cancers).
- decreases the mortality rate from chronic diseases.
- thins the blood so it doesn't clot as readily, thereby decreasing the risk for coronary heart disease and stroke.
- helps the body manage cholesterol levels more effectively.
- prevents or delays the development of high blood pressure and lowers blood pressure in people with hypertension.
- helps prevent and control type 2 diabetes.

- helps achieve peak bone mass in young adults and maintain bone mass later in life, thereby decreasing the risk for osteoporosis.
- helps people sleep better.
- helps prevent chronic back pain.
- relieves tension and helps in coping with life stresses.
- raises levels of energy and job productivity.
- extends longevity and slows the aging process.
- improves and helps maintain cognitive function.
- promotes psychological well-being, including higher morale, self-image, and self-esteem.
- reduces feelings of depression and anxiety.
- encourages positive lifestyle changes (improving nutrition, quitting smoking, controlling alcohol and drug use).
- speeds recovery time following physical exertion.
- speeds recovery following injury or disease.
- regulates and improves overall body functions.
- improves physical stamina and counteracts chronic fatigue.
- reduces disability and helps to maintain independent living, especially in older adults.
- enhances quality of life: People feel better and live a healthier and happier life.

order for man to succeed in life, God provided him with two means, education and physical activity. Not separately, one for the soul and the other for the body, but for the two together. With these two means, man can attain perfection."

Data on more than 2.4 million students in the state of Texas have shown consistent and significant associations between physical fitness and various indicators of academic achievement; in particular, higher levels of fitness were associated with better academic grades. Cardiorespiratory fitness was shown to have a dose-response association with academic performance (better fitness, better grades), independent of other sociodemographic and fitness variables.[27]

Emerging research shows that exercise allows the brain to function at its best because it increases blood and oxygen flow to the brain and leads to biological processes that instigate brain cells to bind one to another. These connections are critical for learning to take place. Exercise provides the necessary stimulus for brain neurons to interconnect, creating the perfect environment in which the brain is ready, willing, and able to learn.[28] Second, muscular activity generates growth factors (e.g., vascular endothelial growth factor and insulin-like growth factor) that are used to create new nerve cells, to increase the strength of the synaptic transmission (transmission between neurons), and in the mechanisms involved in the highest thought processes.

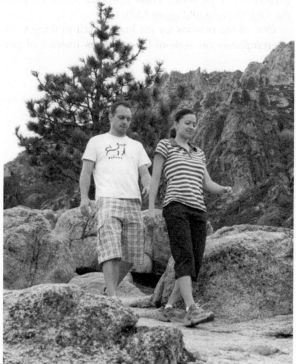

No current drug or medication provides as many health benefits as a regular physical activity program.

© Fitness & Wellness, Inc.

Exercise also increases the neurotransmitters dopamine, glutamate, norepinephrine, and serotonin, all of which are vital in the generation of thought and emotion. Low levels of serotonin have been linked to depression, and exercise has repeatedly been shown to be effective in treating depression. Furthermore, physical activity, and aerobic exercise in particular, protect against age-related loss of cognitive function (memory, thought process, and information processing).

Economic Benefits

Sedentary living can have a strong impact on a nation's economy. As the need for physical exertion in Western countries decreased steadily during the past century, health care expenditures increased dramatically. Health care costs in the United States rose from $12 billion in 1950 to $2.3 trillion in 2008 (Figure 1.15), or about 16 percent of the gross domestic product (GDP). This figure represents the highest of any country in the Organisation for Economic Co-operation and Development (OECD). The next closest country is France at 11.0 percent and Canada ranks sixth at 10.1 percent of the GDP (Figure 1.16). In 1980, health care costs in the United States represented 8.8 percent of the GDP, and if the current trend continues, they are projected to reach 19.3 percent by the year 2019.

In terms of yearly health care costs per person, the United States spends more per person than any other industrialized nation. Per capita U.S. health care costs exceed $7,000 per year. These costs are about 2.5 times the OECD average (Figure 1.17).

One of the reasons for the low overall ranking is the overemphasis on state-of-the-art cures instead of prevention programs. The United States is the best place in the world to treat people once they are sick, but the system does a poor job of keeping people healthy in the first place. Ninety-five percent of our health care dollars are spent on treatment strategies, and less than 5 percent is spent on prevention.

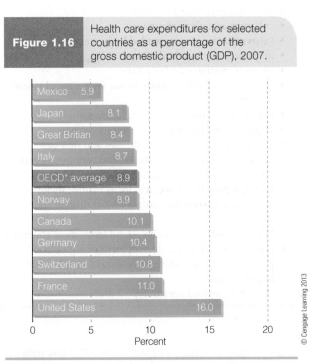

Figure 1.16 Health care expenditures for selected countries as a percentage of the gross domestic product (GDP), 2007.

*Organisation for Economic Co-operation and Development

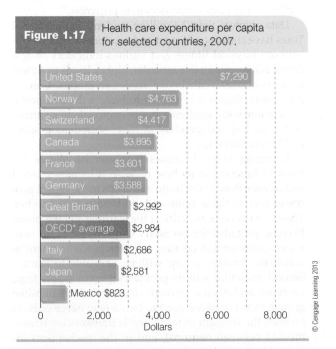

Figure 1.17 Health care expenditure per capita for selected countries, 2007.

*Organisation for Economic Co-operation and Development

Figure 1.15 U.S. health care cost increments since 1950.

Unhealthy behaviors also contribute to the staggering U.S. health care costs. Risk factors for disease such as obesity and smoking carry a heavy price tag. An estimated 1 percent of the people account for 30 percent of health care costs.[29] Half of the people use up about 97 percent of health care dollars. Without reducing the current burden of disease, real health care reform will most likely be impossible. True health care reform will require a nationwide call for action by everyone against chronic disease.

Scientific evidence links participation in fitness and wellness programs to better health, in addition to lower medical costs and higher job productivity. As a result of the staggering rise in medical costs, many organizations offer health-promotion programs, because keeping employees healthy costs less than treating them once they are sick.

The Wellness Challenge for Our Day

Because a better and healthier life is something that every person should strive for, our biggest health challenge today is to teach people how to take control of their personal health habits and adhere to a positive lifestyle. A wealth of information on the benefits of fitness and wellness programs indicates that improving the quality and possible length of our lives is a matter of personal choice.

Even though people in the United States believe a positive lifestyle has a great impact on health and longevity, most people do not reap the benefits because they simply do not know how to implement a safe and effective fitness and wellness program. Others are exercising incorrectly and, therefore, are not reaping the full

---

Behavior Modification Planning

Healthy Lifestyle Habits

Research indicates that adherence to the following 12 lifestyle habits will significantly improve health and extend life:

1. **Participate in a lifetime physical activity program.** Attempt to accumulate 60 minutes of moderate-intensity physical activity most days of the week. The 60 minutes should include 20 to 30 minutes of aerobic exercise (vigorous-intensity) at least three times per week, along with strengthening and stretching exercises two to three times per week.

2. **Do not smoke cigarettes.** Cigarette smoking is the largest preventable cause of illness and premature death in the United States. If we include all related deaths, smoking is responsible for more than 440,000 unnecessary deaths each year.

3. **Eat right.** Eat a good breakfast and two additional well-balanced meals every day. Avoid eating too many calories, processed foods, and foods with a lot of sugar, fat, and salt. Increase your daily consumption of fruits, vegetables, and whole-grain products.

4. **Avoid snacking.** Refrain from frequent high-sugar snacks between meals. Insulin is released to remove sugar from the blood, and frequent spikes in insulin may contribute to the development of heart disease.

5. **Maintain recommended body weight through adequate nutrition and exercise.** This is important in preventing chronic diseases and in developing a higher level of fitness.

6. **Sleep 7 to 8 hours every night.**

7. **Lower your stress levels.** Reduce your vulnerability to stress and practice stress management techniques as needed.

8. **Be wary of alcohol.** Drink alcohol moderately or not at all. Alcohol abuse leads to mental, emotional, physical, and social problems.

9. **Surround yourself with healthy friendships.** Unhealthy friendships contribute to destructive behaviors and low self-esteem. Associating with people who strive to maintain good fitness and health reinforces a positive outlook in life and encourages positive behaviors. Mortality rates are much higher among people who are socially isolated.

10. **Be informed about the environment.** Seek clean air, clean water, and a clean environment. Be aware of pollutants and occupational hazards: asbestos fibers, nickel dust, chromate, uranium dust, and so on. Take precautions when using pesticides and insecticides.

11. **Increase education.** Data indicate that people who are more educated live longer. As education increases, so do the number of connections between nerve cells. An increased number of connections helps the individual make better survival (i.e., healthy lifestyle) choices.

12. **Take personal safety measures.** Although not all accidents are preventable, many are. Taking simple precautionary measures—such as using seat belts and keeping electrical appliances away from water—lessens the risk for avoidable accidents.

Try It Look at the list above and indicate which habits are already a part of your lifestyle. What changes could you make to incorporate some additional healthy habits into your daily life?

benefits of their program. How, then, can we meet the health challenges of the 21st century? That is the focus of this book—to provide the necessary tools that will enable you to write, implement, and regularly update your personal lifetime fitness and wellness program.

> **Critical Thinking**
>
> What are your thoughts about lifestyle habits that enhance health and longevity? How important are they to you? What obstacles keep you from adhering to these habits or incorporating new habits into your life?

Wellness Education: Using This Book

Although everyone would like to enjoy good health and wellness, most people don't know how to reach this objective. Lifestyle is the most important factor affecting personal well-being. Granted, some people live long because of genetic factors, but quality of life during middle age and the "golden years" is more often related to wise choices initiated during youth and continued throughout life. In a few short years, lack of wellness can lead to a loss of vitality and gusto for life, as well as premature morbidity and mortality.

A Personalized Approach

Because fitness and wellness needs vary significantly from one individual to another, all exercise and wellness prescriptions must be personalized to obtain the best results. The Wellness Lifestyle Questionnaire in Activity 1.2 will provide an initial rating of your current efforts to stay healthy and well. Subsequent chapters of this book and their respective activities discuss the components of a wellness lifestyle and set forth the necessary guidelines that will allow you to develop a personal lifetime program to improve fitness and promote your own preventive health care and personal wellness.

The activities in this book have been prepared on tear-out sheets so that they can be turned in to class instructors. As you study this book and complete the worksheets, you will learn to:

- Implement motivational and behavior modification techniques to help you adhere to a lifetime fitness and wellness program
- Determine whether medical clearance is needed for your safe participation in exercise
- Conduct nutritional analyses and follow the recommendations for adequate nutrition
- Write sound diet and weight-control programs
- Assess the health-related components of fitness

- Write exercise prescriptions for cardiorespiratory endurance, muscular strength and endurance, and muscular flexibility
- Understand the relationship between fitness and aging
- Determine your levels of tension and stress, reduce your vulnerability to stress, and implement a stress management program if necessary
- Determine your potential risk for cardiovascular disease and implement a risk-reduction program
- Follow a cancer risk-reduction program
- Implement a smoking cessation program, if applicable
- Avoid chemical dependency and know where to find assistance if needed
- Learn the health consequences of sexually transmitted infections (STIs), including HIV/acquired immune deficiency syndrome (AIDS), and guidelines for preventing STIs
- Write goals and objectives to improve your fitness and wellness and learn how to chart a wellness program for the future
- Differentiate myths from facts about exercise and health-related concepts

Exercise Safety

Even though testing and participation in exercise are relatively safe for most apparently healthy individuals, the reaction of the cardiovascular system to higher levels of physical activity cannot be totally predicted. Consequently, a small but real risk exists for exercise-induced abnormalities in people with a history of cardiovascular problems, certain chronic conditions, and those who are at higher risk for disease. Among the exercise-induced abnormalities are abnormal blood pressure, irregular heart rhythm, fainting, and, in rare instances, a heart attack or cardiac arrest.

Before you engage in an exercise program or participate in any exercise testing, at a minimum you should fill out the Physical Activity Readiness Questionnaire (PAR-Q & YOU) found in Activity 1.3. Additional information can be obtained by filling out the Health History Questionnaire also given in Activity 1.3. Exercise testing and participation are not wise under some of the conditions listed in this activity and may require a medical evaluation, including a stress electrocardiogram (ECG) test for a few individuals. If you have any questions regarding your current health status, consult your doctor before initiating, continuing, or increasing your level of physical activity.

Now that you are about to embark in a wellness lifestyle program, sit down and subjectively determine where you are at on each of the seven dimensions of wellness. Use Activity 1.5 to help you with this exercise. Record the date at the top of the respective column. Next, write a goal for each wellness dimension to

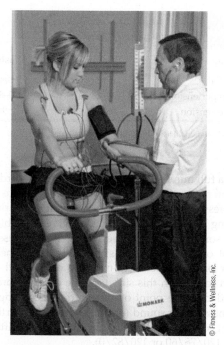

An exercise tolerance test with 12-lead electrocardiographic monitoring (stress ECG test) may be required of some individuals prior to initiating an exercise program.

Table 1.6	Resting Heart Rate Ratings
Heart Rate (bpm)	**Rating**
≤59	Excellent
60–69	Good
70–79	Average
80–89	Fair
≥90	Poor

accomplish prior to the end of this course. Also, list three specific objectives that will help you accomplish each goal.

As you continue to study the content of this book, use this same form to monitor your progress. About once a month reassess your status and make adjustments in your specific objectives so you may reach the desired goals. Modifying unhealthy behaviors and developing new positive habits take time. The plan of action that you are about to develop will help you achieve the desired outcomes.

Assessment of Resting Heart Rate and Blood Pressure

Heart rate can be obtained by counting your pulse either on the wrist over the radial artery or over the carotid artery in the neck (Chapter 6, page 195). In Activity 1.4 you will have an opportunity to determine your heart rate and blood pressure and calculate the extra heart rate life years an increase in exercise may produce.

You may count your pulse for 30 seconds and multiply by 2 or take it for a full minute. The heart rate usually is at its lowest point (resting heart rate) late in the evening after you have been sitting quietly for about half an hour watching a relaxing TV show or reading in bed, or

early in the morning just before you get out of bed. Your pulse should have a consistent (regular) rhythm. A pulse that misses beats or speeds up or slows down may be an indication of heart problems and should be followed up by a physician.

Unless you have a pathological condition, a lower resting heart rate indicates a stronger heart. To adapt to cardiorespiratory or aerobic exercise, blood volume increases, the heart enlarges, and the muscle gets stronger. A stronger heart can pump more blood with fewer strokes.

Resting heart rate categories are given in Table 1.6. Although resting heart rate decreases with training, the extent of **bradycardia** depends not only on the amount of training but also on genetic factors. Although most highly trained athletes have a resting heart rate around 40 beats per minute, occasionally one of these athletes has a resting heart rate in the 60s or 70s even during peak training months of the season. For most individuals, however, the resting heart rate decreases as the level of cardiorespiratory endurance increases.

Blood pressure is assessed using a **sphygmomanometer** and a stethoscope. Use a cuff of the appropriate size to get accurate readings. Size is determined by the width of the inflatable bladder, which should be about 80 percent of the circumference of the midpoint of the arm.

Blood pressure usually is measured while the person is in the sitting position, with the forearm and the manometer at the same level as the heart. The arm should be flexed slightly and placed on a flat surface. At first, the pressure is recorded from each arm, and after that from the arm with the highest reading.

The cuff should be applied approximately an inch above the antecubital space (natural crease of the elbow), with the center of the bladder directly over the medial (inner) surface of the arm. The stethoscope head should be applied firmly, but with little pressure, over the brachial artery in the antecubital space.

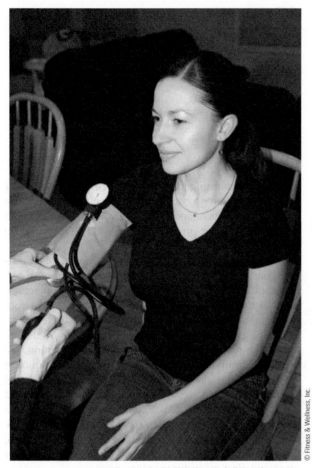

© Fitness & Wellness, Inc.

Assessment of resting blood pressure with an aneroid manometer.

To determine how high the cuff should be inflated, the person recording the blood pressure monitors the subject's radial pulse with one hand and, with the other hand, inflates the manometer's bladder to about 30 to 40 mm Hg above the point at which the feeling of the pulse in the wrist disappears. Next, the pressure is released, followed by a wait of about one minute, then the bladder is inflated to the predetermined level to take the blood pressure reading. The cuff should not be overinflated, as this may cause blood vessel spasm, resulting in higher blood pressure readings. The pressure should be released at a rate of 2 to 4 mm Hg per second.

As the pressure is released, **systolic blood pressure (SBP)** is recorded as the point where the sound of the pulse becomes audible. The **diastolic blood pressure (DBP)** is the point where the sound disappears. The recordings should be expressed as systolic over diastolic pressure—for example, 124/80.

If you take more than one reading, be sure the bladder is completely deflated between readings and allow at

Table 1.7	Resting Blood Pressure Guidelines (expressed in mm Hg)	
Rating	**Systolic**	**Diastolic**
Normal	≤120	≤80
Prehypertension	120–139	80–89
Hypertension	≥140	≥90

SOURCE: National Heart, Lung, and Blood Institute.

least a full minute before making the next recording. The person measuring the pressure also should note whether the pressure was recorded from the left or the right arm. Resting blood pressure ratings are given in Table 1.7.

In some cases, the pulse sounds become less intense (point of muffling sounds) but still can be heard at a lower pressure (50 or 40 mm Hg) or even all the way down to zero. In this situation, the diastolic pressure is recorded at the point of a clear, definite change in the loudness of the sound (also referred to as fourth phase) and at complete disappearance of the sound (fifth phase) (e.g., 120/78/60 or 120/82/0).

Mean Blood Pressure

During a normal resting contraction/relaxation cycle of the heart, the heart spends more time in the relaxation (diastolic) phase than in the contraction (systolic) phase. Accordingly, mean blood pressure (MBP) cannot be computed by taking an average of the SBP and DBP blood pressures. The equations used to determine MBP are shown in Activity 1.4.

When measuring blood pressure, be aware that a single reading may not be an accurate value because of the various factors (rest, stress, physical activity, food) that can affect blood pressure. Thus, if you are able, ask different people to take several readings at different times of the day to establish the real values. You can record the results of your resting heart rate and your SBP, DBP, and MBP assessments in Activity 1.4. You can also calculate the effects of aerobic activity on resting heart rate in this activity.

Key Terms

Systolic blood pressure (SBP) Pressure exerted by blood against walls of arteries during forceful contraction (systole) of the heart.

Diastolic blood pressure (DBP) Pressure exerted by the blood against the walls of the arteries during the relaxation phase (diastole) of the heart.

Assess Your Behavior

Log on to www.cengagebrain.com to access CengageNOW and the Behavior Change Planner where you can assess the behaviors that might benefit you most from healthy change.

1. Are you aware of your family health history and life-style factors that may negatively impact your health?

2. Do you accumulate at least 30 minutes of moderate-intensity physical activity five days per week?

3. Do you make a constant and deliberate effort to stay healthy and achieve the highest potential for well-being?

Assess Your Knowledge

Evaluate how well you understand the concepts presented in this chapter using the chapter-specific quizzing available in the online materials at www.cengagebrain.com.

1. Advances in modern technology
   a. help people achieve higher fitness levels.
   b. have led to a decrease in chronic diseases.
   c. have almost completely eliminated the necessity for physical exertion in daily life.
   d. help fight hypokinetic disease.
   e. make it easier to achieve good aerobic fitness.

2. Most activities of daily living in the United States help people
   a. get adequate physical activity on a regular basis.
   b. meet health-related fitness standards.
   c. achieve good levels of skill-related activities.
   d. Choices a, b, and c are correct.
   e. None of the choices is correct.

3. The leading cause of death in the United States is
   a. cancer.
   b. accidents.
   c. CLRD.
   d. diseases of the cardiovascular system.
   e. drug abuse.

4. Bodily movement produced by skeletal muscles is called
   a. physical activity.
   b. kinesiology.
   c. exercise.
   d. aerobic exercise.
   e. muscle strength.

5. Among the long-term benefits of regular physical activity and exercise are significantly reduced risks for developing or dying from
   a. heart disease.
   b. type 2 diabetes.
   c. colon and breast cancers.
   d. osteoporotic fractures.
   e. All are correct choices.

6. To be ranked in the "active" category, an adult has to take between
   a. 3,500 and 4,999 steps per day.
   b. 5,000 and 7,499 steps per day.
   c. 7,500 and 9,999 steps per day.
   d. 10,000 and 12,499 steps per day.
   e. 12,500 and 15,000 steps per day.

7. The constant and deliberate effort to stay healthy and achieve the highest potential for well-being is defined as
   a. health.
   b. physical fitness.
   c. wellness.
   d. health-related fitness.
   e. physiological fitness.

8. Research on the effects of fitness on mortality indicates that the largest drop in premature mortality is seen between
   a. the average and excellent fitness groups.
   b. the low and moderate fitness groups.
   c. the high and excellent fitness groups.
   d. the moderate and good fitness groups.
   e. The drop is similar among all fitness groups.

9. Metabolic fitness can be achieved through
   a. a moderate-intensity exercise program.
   b. a high-intensity speed-training program.
   c. an increased basal metabolic rate.
   d. anaerobic training.
   e. an increase in lean body mass.

10. What is the greatest benefit of being physically fit?
    a. absence of disease
    b. a higher quality of life
    c. improved sports performance
    d. better personal appearance
    e. maintenance of recommended body weight

Correct answers can be found at the back of the book.

Wellness Lifestyle Questionnaire

Name:_____ Date:_____

Course:_____ Section:_____ Gender:_____ Age:_____

The purpose of this questionnaire is to analyze current lifestyle habits and help determine changes necessary for future health and wellness. Check the appropriate answer to each question, and obtain a final score according to the guidelines provided at the end of the questionnaire.

	Always	Nearly always	Often	Seldom	Never
1. I participate in vigorous-intensity aerobic activity for 20 minutes on 3 or more days per week, and I accumulate at least 30 minutes of moderate-intensity physical activity on a minimum of 2 additional days per week.	5	4	3	2	1
2. I participate in strength-training exercises, using a minimum of eight different exercises, 2 or more days per week.	5	4	3	2	1
3. I perform flexibility exercises a minimum of 2 days per week.	5	4	3	2	1
4. I maintain recommended body weight (includes avoidance of excessive body fat, excessive thinness, or frequent fluctuations in body weight).	5	4	3	2	1
5. Every day, I eat three regular meals that include a wide variety of foods.	5	4	3	2	1
6. I limit the amount of saturated fat and trans fats in my diet on most days of the week.	5	4	3	2	1
7. I eat a minimum of five servings of fruits and vegetables and six servings from grain products daily.	5	4	3	2	1
8. I regularly avoid snacks, especially those that are high in calories and fat and low in nutrients and fiber.	5	4	3	2	1
9. I avoid cigarettes or tobacco in any other form.	5	4	3	2	1
10. I avoid alcoholic beverages. If I drink, I do so in moderation (one daily drink for women and two for men), and I do not combine alcohol with other drugs.	5	4	3	2	1
11. I avoid addictive drugs and needles that have been used by others.	5	4	3	2	1
12. I use prescription drugs and over-the-counter drugs sparingly (only when needed), and I follow all directions for their proper use.	5	4	3	2	1
13. I readily recognize and act on it when I am under excessive tension and stress (distress).	5	4	3	2	1
14. I am able to perform effective stress-management techniques.	5	4	3	2	1
15. I have close friends and relatives with whom I can discuss personal problems and approach for help when needed and with whom I can express my feelings freely.	5	4	3	2	1
16. I spend most of my daily leisure time in wholesome recreational activities.	5	4	3	2	1
17. I sleep 7 to 8 hours each night.	5	4	3	2	1
18. I floss my teeth every day and brush them at least twice daily.	5	4	3	2	1
19. I get "safe sun" exposure—that is, 10 to 20 minutes of unprotected exposure to the face, neck, and arms on most days of the week between the hours of 10:00 a.m. and 4:00 p.m. I avoid overexposure to the sun, and I use sunscreen and appropriate clothing when I am out in the sun for an extended time.	5	4	3	2	1
20. I avoid using products that have not been shown by science to be safe and effective. (This includes drugs and unproven nutrient and weight loss supplements.)	5	4	3	2	1
21. I stay current with the warning signs for heart attack, stroke, and cancer.	5	4	3	2	1
22. I practice monthly breast/testicle self-exams, get recommended screening tests (blood lipids, blood pressure, Pap tests), and seek a medical evaluation when I am not well or when disease symptoms arise.	5	4	3	2	1
23. I have a dental checkup at least once a year, and I get regular medical exams according to age recommendations.	5	4	3	2	1
24. I am not sexually active. / I practice safe sex.	5	4	3	2	1
25. I can deal effectively with disappointments and temporary feelings of sadness, loneliness, and depression. If I am unable to deal with these feelings, I seek professional help.	5	4	3	2	1
26. I can work out emotional problems without turning to alcohol, other drugs, or violent behavior.	5	4	3	2	1

Wellness Lifestyle Questionnaire (continued)

	Always	Nearly always	Often	Seldom	Never
27. I associate with people who have a positive attitude about life.	5	4	3	2	1
28. I respond to temporary setbacks by making the best of the circumstances and by moving ahead with optimism and energy. I do not spend time and talent worrying about failures.	5	4	3	2	1
29. I wear a seat belt whenever I am in a car, I ask others in my vehicle to do the same, and I make sure that children are in an infant seat or wear a shoulder harness.	5	4	3	2	1
30. I do not drive under the influence of alcohol or other drugs, and I make an effort to keep others from doing the same.	5	4	3	2	1
31. I avoid being alone in public places, especially after dark; I seek escorts when I visit or exercise in unfamiliar places.	5	4	3	2	1
32. I seek to make my living quarters accident-free, and I keep doors and windows locked, especially when I am home alone.	5	4	3	2	1
33. I try to minimize environmental pollutants, and I support community efforts to minimize pollution.	5	4	3	2	1
34. I use energy conservation strategies and encourage others to do the same.	5	4	3	2	1
35. I study and/or work in a clean environment (including avoidance of secondhand smoke).	5	4	3	2	1
36. I participate in recycling programs for paper, cardboard, glass, plastic, and aluminum.	5	4	3	2	1

How to Score

Enter the score you have marked for each question in the spaces provided below. Next, total the score for each specific wellness lifestyle category and obtain a rating for each category according to the criteria provided below.

	Health-related fitness		Nutrition		Avoiding chemical dependency		Stress management		Personal hygiene/ health		Disease prevention		Emotional well-being		Personal safety		Environmental health & protection
	1.		5.		9.		13.		17.		21.		25.		29.		33.
	2.		6.		10.		14.		18.		22.		26.		30.		34.
	3.		7.		11.		15.		19.		23.		27.		31.		35.
	4.		8.		12.		16.		20.		24.		28.		32.		36.
Total:																	
Rating:																	

Category Rating

Excellent (E) = ≥17 Your answers show that you are aware of the importance of this category to your health and wellness. You are putting your knowledge to work for you by practicing good habits. As long as you continue to do so, this category should not pose a health risk. You are also setting a good example for family and friends to follow. Because you got a very high score on this part of the test, you may want to consider other categories in which your score indicates room for improvement.

Good (G) = 13–16 Your health practices in this area are good, but you have room for improvement. Look again at the items you answered with a 4 or lower and identify changes that you can make to improve your lifestyle. Even small changes often can help you achieve better health.

Needs Improvement (NI) = ≤12 Your health risks are showing. You may be taking serious and unnecessary risks with your health. Perhaps you are not aware of the risks or what to do about them. Most likely you need additional information and help in deciding how to successfully make the changes you desire. You can easily get the information that you need to improve, if you wish. The next step is up to you.

　Please note that no final overall rating is provided for the entire questionnaire because it may not be indicative of your overall wellness. For example, an excellent rating in most categories will not offset the immediate health risks and life-threatening consequences of using addictive drugs or not wearing a seat belt.

PAR-Q and Health History Questionnaire

Name _____ Date _____ Grade _____

Instructor _____ Course _____ Section _____

Necessary Lab Equipment None.

Objective To determine the safety of exercise participation.

Physical Activity Readiness
Questionnaire - PAR-Q
(revised 2002)

PAR-Q & YOU

(A Questionnaire for People Aged 15 to 69)

Regular physical activity is fun and healthy, and increasingly more people are starting to become more active every day. Being more active is very safe for most people. However, some people should check with their doctor before they start becoming much more physically active. If you are planning to become much more physically active than you are now, start by answering the seven questions in the box below. If you are between the ages of 15 and 69, the PAR-Q will tell you if you should check with your doctor before you start. If you are over 69 years of age, and you are not used to being very active, check with your doctor.

Common sense is your best guide when you answer these questions. Please read the questions carefully and answer each one honestly: check YES or NO.

YES	NO	
☐	☐	**1.** Has your doctor ever said that you have a heart condition <u>and</u> that you should only do physical activity recommended by a doctor?
☐	☐	**2.** Do you feel pain in your chest when you do physical activity?
☐	☐	**3.** In the past month, have you had chest pain when you were not doing physical activity?
☐	☐	**4.** Do you lose your balance because of dizziness or do you ever lose consciousness?
☐	☐	**5.** Do you have a bone or joint problem (for example, back, knee or hip) that could be made worse by a change in your physical activity?
☐	☐	**6.** Is your doctor currently prescribing drugs (for example, water pills) for your blood pressure or heart condition?
☐	☐	**7.** Do you know of <u>any other reason</u> why you should not do physical activity?

If you answered

YES to one or more questions

Talk with your doctor by phone or in person BEFORE you start becoming much more physically active or BEFORE you have a fitness appraisal. Tell your doctor about the PAR-Q and which questions you answered YES.

• You may be able to do any activity you want—as long as you start slowly and build up gradually. Or, you may need to restrict your activities to those which are safe for you. Talk with your doctor about the kinds of activities you wish to participate in and follow his/her advice.

• Find out which community programs are safe and helpful for you.

NO to all questions

If you answered NO honestly to all PAR-Q questions, you can be reasonably sure that you can:

• start becoming much more physically active – begin slowly and build up gradually. This is the safest and easiest way to go.

• take part in a fitness appraisal – this is an excellent way to determine your basic fitness so that you can plan the best way for you to live actively. It is also highly recommended that you have your blood pressure evaluated. If your reading is over 144/94, talk with your doctor before you start becoming much more physically active.

DELAY BECOMING MUCH MORE ACTIVE:
• if you are not feeling well because of a temporary illness such as a cold or a fever—wait until you feel better; or
• if you are or may be pregnant—talk to your doctor before you start becoming more active.

PLEASE NOTE: If your health changes so that you then answer YES to any of the above questions, tell your fitness or health professional. Ask whether you should change your physical activity plan.

<u>Informed Use of the PAR-Q</u>: The Canadian Society for Exercise Physiology, Health Canada, and their agents assume no liability for persons who undertake physical activity, and if in doubt after completing this questionnaire, consult your doctor prior to physical activity.

No changes permitted. You are encouraged to photocopy the PAR-Q but only if you use the entire form.

NOTE: If the PAR-Q is being given to a person before he or she participates in a physical activity program or a fitness appraisal, this section may be used for legal or administrative purposes.

"I have read, understood and completed this questionnaire. Any questions I had were answered to my full satisfaction."

NAME _____

SIGNATURE _____ DATE _____

SIGNATURE OF PARENT _____ WITNESS _____
or GUARDIAN (for participants under the age of majority)

Note: This physical activity clearance is valid for a maximum of 12 months from the date it is completed and becomes invalid if your condition changes so that you would answer YES to any of the seven questions.

© Canadian Society for Exercise Physiology   Supported by: ▮✦ Health Santé
Canada Canada

continued on other side...

Source: Physical Activity Readiness Questionnaire (PAR-Q) © 2002. Used with permission from the Canadian Society for Exercise Physiology, www.csep.ca

Computing the Effects of Aerobic Activity on Resting Heart Rate

Using your actual resting heart rate (RHR), compute the total number of times your heart beats each day and each year:

A. Beats per day = [　　　] (RHR bpm) × 60 (min per hour) × 24 (hours per day) = [　　　] beats per day

B. Beats per year = [　　　] (heart rate in beats per day, use item A) × 365 = [　　　] beats per year

If your RHR dropped 20 bpm through an aerobic exercise program, determine the number of beats that your heart would save each year at that lower RHR:

C. Beats per day = [　　　] (RHR, use your current RHR) − 20 × 60 × 24 = [　　　] beats per day

D. Beats per year = [　　　] (heart rate in beats per day, use item C) × 365 = [　　　] beats per year

E. Number of beats saved per year (B − D) = [　　　] − [　　　] = [　　　] beats saved per year

Assuming that you will reach the average U.S. life expectancy of 80 years for women or 75 for men, determine the additional number of "heart rate life years" available to you if your rhr was 20 bpm lower:

F. Years of life ahead = [　　　] (use 80 for women and 75 for men) − [　　　] (current age) = [　　　] years

G. Number of beats saved = [　　　] (use item E) × [　　　] (use item F) = [　　　] beats saved

H. Number of heart rate life years based on the lower RHR = [　　　] (use item G) ÷ [　　　] (use item D) = [　　　] years

Dimensions of Wellness: Setting Your Goals

Name:_____ Date:_____

Course:_____ Section:_____ Gender:_____ Age:_____

Instructions

1. In the Wellness Dimension chart below, record the date at the top of the first column, then fill in that column using the following scale to indicate your wellness rating for each dimension:

    poor = 5, fair = 4, average = 3, good = 2, excellent = 1

2. Next, write a goal that you want to accomplish prior to the end of this course for each wellness dimension, and list three specific objectives that will help you accomplish each goal.

3. Once a month, review this form, fill in another column of self-evaluation, and adjust your objectives as necessary.

Here's an example:

Social goal: | To improve my social life at school |

Specific objectives

1. Find study buddies. Ask each instructor and counselor about study groups.

2. Attend Friday night discussion groups in Student Center.

3. Locate activities I enjoy—basketball, chess, dancing—and start a conversation.

Wellness Dimension	Date				
Physical					
Emotional					
Social					
Environmental					
Mental					
Spiritual					
Occupational					

Goals and Objectives

Physical goal: [   ]

Specific objectives

1. _____

2. _____

3. _____

Emotional goal: [   ]

Specific objectives

1. _____

2. _____

3. _____

Social goal: [   ]

Specific objectives

1. _____

2. _____

3. _____

Environmental goal: [   ]

Specific objectives

1. _____

2. _____

3. _____

Mental goal: [   ]

Specific objectives

1. _____

2. _____

3. _____

Spiritual goal: [   ]

Specific objectives

1. _____

2. _____

3. _____

Occupational goal: [   ]

Specific objectives

1. _____

2. _____

3. _____

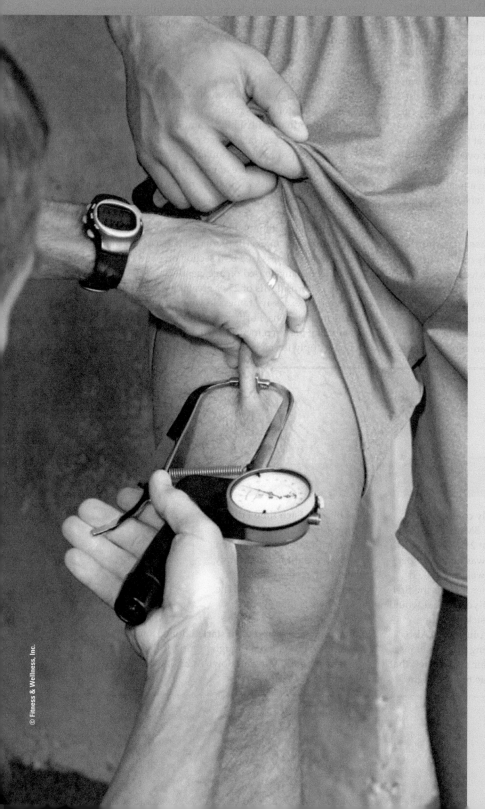

Body Composition

"You will rejoice in the way you feel if you follow a healthy diet, remain physically active, and maintain a lifetime exercise program."

Objectives

▶ **Define** body composition, and understand its relationship to assessment of recommended body weight.

▶ **Explain** the difference between essential fat and storage fat.

▶ **Describe** various techniques used to assess body composition.

▶ **Be able** to assess body composition using skinfold thickness and girth measurements.

▶ **Understand** the importance of body mass index (BMI) and waist circumference in the assessment of risk for disease.

▶ **Be able** to determine recommended weight according to recommended percent body fat values and BMI.

CENGAGE **brain**

Learn how to measure body composition. Assess your risks for potential disease. Visit **www.cengagebrain.com** to access course materials and companion resources for this text including quiz questions designed to check your understanding of the chapter contents. See the preface on page xv for more information.

© Fitness & Wellness, Inc.

What constitutes ideal body weight? There is no such thing as "ideal" body weight. Health/fitness professionals prefer to use the terms "recommended" or "healthy" body weight. Let's examine the question in more detail. For instance, 25 percent body fat is the recommended health fitness standard for a 40-year-old man. For the average "apparently healthy" individual, this body fat percentage does not constitute a threat to good health. Due to genetic and lifestyle conditions, however, if a person this same age at 25 percent body fat is prediabetic, prehypertensive, and with abnormal blood lipids (cholesterol and triglycerides—see Chapter 10), weight (fat) loss and a lower percent body fat may be recommended. Thus, what will work as recommended weight for most individuals may not be the best standard for individuals with disease risk factors. The current recommended or healthy weight standards (based on percent body fat or BMI) are established at the point where there appears to be a lower incidence for overweight-related conditions for most people. Individual differences have to be taken into consideration when making a final recommendation, especially in people with risk factors or a personal and family history of chronic conditions.

How accurate are body composition assessments? Most of the techniques to determine body composition require proper training on the part of the technician administering the test (skinfolds, hydrostatic weighing, DEXA, Bod Pod) and, in the case of hydrostatic weighing, proper performance on the part of the person being tested. As detailed in this chapter, body composition assessment is not a precise science. Some of the procedures are more accurate than others. Before undergoing body composition testing, make sure that you understand the accuracy of the technique (see standard error of estimates [SEEs] included under the description of each technique); and even more important, inquire about the training and experience of the person administering the test. We often encounter individuals who have been tested elsewhere by any number of assessments, particularly skinfolds, who come to our laboratory in disbelief (and rightfully so) because of the results that were given to them. To obtain the best possible results, look for trained and experienced technicians.

Is there a future trend in body composition assessment? Results of research data indicate that the area of the body where people store fat is more critical than how much is stored. Individuals with a higher amount of intra-abdominal or abdominal visceral fat (located around internal organs), as opposed to primarily abdominal fat stored beneath the skin (subcutaneous fat), are at greater risk for disease. Thus, to increase disease risk evaluation, future body composition tests will be designed to get a clearer view of where the abdominal fat lies.

Additionally, although not a body composition assessment, body mass index (BMI) guidelines to detect thinness and excessive fatness (see BMI section on page 127) will most likely change based on age, gender, and physical activity patterns. BMIs of 25 or greater are not accurate predictors of excessive fatness in younger people and in athletic populations. Furthermore, because of differences in essential fat between men and women, the same standard may not apply for men and women alike.

Real Life Story — Shondra's Experience

I was surprised at my results of the body composition assessments that we did in our lab. The BMI calculation told me I was at a healthy weight (about 24). But when we did the skinfold test, I found out that I was almost 29 percent body fat, which is considered overweight. I talked about it with my instructor, and I told her that for the first two years after starting college I had yo-yo dieted. I would eat a lot less, lose weight, and then get sick of dieting, eat what I wanted, and gain it all back, plus more. Also, I hated to exercise, so I didn't do anything other than just walking from class to class. My instructor said she felt that my higher percent body fat might be due to my weight loss history. Each time I dieted, I probably lost lean body mass along with fat, and then when I gained weight back, I mainly gained fat, so over time my percent body fat went up. The good news is that over the course of the year, I became much more active and even started doing some basic strength training. Even though I didn't lose any weight, my percent body fat went down to 23%, which is a lot healthier.

© Stephen Coburn/Shutterstock.com

Personal Body Composition Profile

Please answer the following questions to the best of your ability. If you cannot answer all of them at this time, you will be able to do so as you work through the chapter contents.

I. Do you understand the concept of body composition and its relationship to recommended body weight, proper weight management, and good health? _____ Yes _____ No

II. Current values

Body weight: _____ lb

Percent body fat is: _____%   Classification: _____

Lean body mass: _____ lb

Body Mass Index (BMI): Disease risk: _____   Classification: _____

Waist Circumference (WC): Disease risk: _____   Classification: _____

III. Goals for the end of the term:

Body weight: _____ lb

Percent body fat: _____%

BMI: _____ WC: _____

IV. Can you relate to Shondra's experience and what can you do in your life to avoid the same pitfalls?

To understand the concept of **body composition**, we must recognize that the human body consists of fat and non-fat components. The fat component is called fat mass or **percent body fat**. The non-fat component is termed **lean body mass**.

To determine **recommended body weight**, we need to find out what percent of total body weight is fat and what amount is lean tissue—in other words, assess body composition. Body composition should be assessed by a well-trained technician who understands the procedure being used.

Once the fat percentage is known, recommended body weight can be calculated from recommended body fat. Recommended body weight, also called "healthy weight," implies the absence of any medical condition that would improve with weight loss and a fat distribution pattern that is not associated with higher risk for illness.

Formerly, people relied on simple height/weight charts to determine their recommended body weight, but these tables can be highly inaccurate and fail to identify critical fat values associated with higher risk for disease. Standard height/weight tables, first published in 1912, were based on average weights (including shoes and clothing) for men and women who obtained life insurance policies between 1888 and 1905—a notably unrepresentative population. The recommended body weight on these tables was obtained according to gender, height, and frame size. Because no scientific guidelines were given to determine frame size, most people chose their frame size based on the column in which the weight came closest to their own!

The best way to determine whether people are truly **overweight** or falsely at recommended body weight is through assessment of body composition. **Obesity** is an excess of body fat. If body weight is the only criterion, an individual might easily appear to be overweight according to height/weight charts, yet not have too much body fat. Typical examples are football players, body builders, weight lifters, and other athletes with large muscle size. Some athletes who appear to be 20 or 30 pounds overweight really have little body fat.

The inaccuracy of height/weight charts was illustrated clearly when a young man who weighed about 225 pounds applied to join a city police force but was turned down without having been granted an inter-

Key Terms

Body composition The fat and non-fat components of the human body; important in assessing recommended body weight.

Percent body fat Proportional amount of fat in the body based on the person's total weight; includes both essential fat and storage fat; also termed fat mass.

Lean body mass Body weight without body fat.

Recommended body weight Body weight at which there seems to be no harm to human health; healthy weight.

Overweight An excess amount of weight against a given standard, such as height or recommended percent body fat.

Obesity An excessive accumulation of body fat, usually at least 30 percent above recommended body weight.

view. The reason? He was "too fat," according to the height/weight charts. When this young man's body composition was assessed at a preventive medicine clinic, it was determined that only 5 percent of his total body weight was in the form of fat—considerably less than the recommended standard. In the words of the director of the clinic, "The only way this fellow could come down to the chart's target weight would have been through surgical removal of a large amount of his muscle tissue."

At the other end of the spectrum, some people who weigh very little (and may be viewed as skinny or under-weight) actually can be classified as overweight because of their high body fat content. People who weigh as little as 120 pounds but are more than 30 percent fat (about one-third of their total body weight) are not rare. These cases are found more readily in the sedentary population and among people who are always dieting. Physical inactivity and a constant negative caloric balance both lead to a loss in lean body mass (see Chapter 5). These examples illustrate that body weight alone clearly does not tell the whole story.

Essential and Storage Fat

Total fat in the human body is classified into two types: **essential fat** and **storage fat**. Essential fat is needed for normal physiological function. Without it, human health and physical performance deteriorate. This type of fat is found within tissues such as muscles, nerve cells, bone marrow, intestines, heart, liver, and lungs. Essential fat constitutes about 3 percent of the total weight in men and 12 percent in women (see Figure 4.1). The percentage is higher in women because it includes sex-specific fat, such as that found in the breast tissue, the uterus, and other sex-related fat deposits.

Storage fat is the fat stored in adipose tissue, mostly just beneath the skin (subcutaneous fat) and around major organs in the body. This fat serves three basic functions:

1. As an insulator to retain body heat
2. As energy substrate for metabolism
3. As padding against physical trauma to the body

The amount of storage fat does not differ between men and women, except that men tend to store fat around the waist and women around the hips and thighs.

Techniques to Assess Body Composition

Body composition can be estimated through the several procedures described in the following pages. Each procedure includes a standard error of estimate (SEE), a measure of the accuracy of the prediction made through the regression equation for that specific technique. For example, if the SEE for a given technique is ±3.0 and the individual tests at a fat percentage of 18.0, the actual fat percentage may range from 15 to 21 percent.

Dual Energy X-ray Absorptiometry

Dual energy x-ray absorptiometry (DXA) is a method to assess body composition that is used most frequently in research and by medical facilities. A radiographic technique, DXA uses very low-dose beams of x-ray energy (hundreds of times lower than a typical body x-ray) to measure total body fat mass, fat distribution pattern (see "Waist Circumference" on page 129), and bone density. Bone density is measured to assess the risk for osteoporosis. The procedure itself is simple and

Figure 4.1	Typical body composition of an adult man and woman.

Male   **Female**

43% — 36%

3% — 12%

14% — 15%

15% — 12%

25% — 25%

■ Muscle   ■ Storage fat   ■ Other tissues
■ Essential fat   ■ Bone

© Cengage Learning 2013

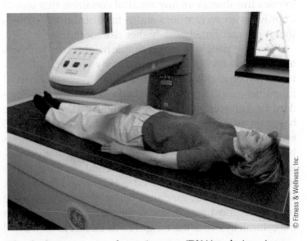

The dual-energy x-ray absorptiometry (DXA) technique is used to assess body composition and bone density.

© Fitness & Wellness, Inc.

takes less than 15 minutes to administer. Many exercise scientists consider DXA to be the standard technique to assess body composition. The SEE for this technique is ±1.8 percent.

Due to costs, DXA is not readily available to most fitness participants. Thus, other methods to estimate body composition are used. The most common of these follow:

1. Hydrostatic or underwater weighing
2. Air displacement
3. Skinfold thickness
4. Girth measurements
5. Bioelectrical impedance

Because these procedures yield estimates of body fat, each technique may yield slightly different values. Therefore, when assessing changes in body composition, be sure to use the same technique for pre- and post-test comparisons.

The most accurate techniques presently available in fitness laboratories is still hydrostatic weighing. Other techniques to assess body composition are available, but the equipment is costly and not easily accessible to the general population. In addition to percentages of lean tissue and body fat, some of these methods also provide information on total body water and bone mass. These techniques include air displacement, magnetic resonance imaging (MRI), computed tomography (CT), and total body electrical conductivity (TOBEC). In terms of predicting percent body fat, these techniques are not more accurate than hydrostatic weighing.

Hydrostatic Weighing

For decades, **hydrostatic weighing** has been the most common technique used in determining body composition in exercise physiology laboratories. In essence, a person's "regular" weight is compared with a weight taken underwater. Because fat is more buoyant than lean tissue, comparing the two weights can determine a person's percent of fat. Almost all other indirect techniques to assess body composition have been validated against hydrostatic weighing. The procedure requires a considerable amount of time, skill, space, and equipment and must be administered by a well-trained technician. The SEE for hydrostatic weighing is ±2.5 percent.

This technique has several drawbacks. First, because each individual assessment can take as long as 30 minutes, hydrostatic weighing is not feasible when testing a lot of people. Furthermore, the person's residual lung volume (amount of air left in the lungs following complete forceful exhalation) should be measured before testing. If residual volume cannot be measured, as is the case in some laboratories and health/fitness centers, it is estimated using the predicting equations, which may decrease the accuracy of hydrostatic weighing. Also, the requirement of being completely underwater makes hy-

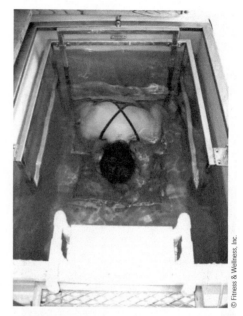

Hydrostatic or underwater weighing technique.

drostatic weighing difficult to administer to **aquaphobic** people. For accurate results, the individual must be able to perform the test properly.

For each underwater weighing trial, the person has to (a) force out all of the air in the lungs, (b) lean forward and completely submerge underwater for about 5 to 10 seconds (long enough to get the underwater weight), and (c) remain as calm as possible (chair movement makes reading the scale difficult). This procedure is repeated 8 to 10 times.

Forcing all of the air out of the lungs is not easy for everyone but is important to obtain an accurate reading. Leaving additional air (beyond residual volume) in the lungs makes a person more buoyant. Because fat is less dense than water, overweight individuals weigh less in water. Additional air in the lungs makes a person lighter in water, yielding a false, higher body fat percentage.

Key Terms

Essential fat Minimal amount of body fat needed for normal physiological functions; constitutes about 3 percent of total weight in men and 12 percent in women.

Storage fat Body fat in excess of essential fat; stored in adipose tissue.

Dual energy x-ray absorptiometry (DXA) Method to assess body composition that uses very low-dose beams of x-ray energy to measure total body fat mass, fat distribution pattern, and bone density.

Hydrostatic weighing Underwater technique to assess body composition; considered the most accurate of the body composition assessment techniques.

Aquaphobic Having a fear of water.

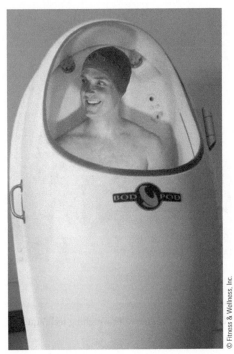

The Bod Pod, used for assessment of body composition.

Air Displacement

Air displacement (also known as air displacement plethysmography) is a newer technique that holds considerable promise. With this method, an individual sits inside a small chamber, commercially known as the **Bod Pod**. Computerized pressure sensors determine the amount of air displaced by the person inside the chamber. Body volume is calculated by subtracting the air volume with the person inside the chamber from the volume of the empty chamber. The amount of air in the person's lungs also is taken into consideration when determining the actual body volume. Body density and percent body fat then are calculated from the obtained body volume.

Initial research showed that this technique compares favorably with hydrostatic weighing, and it is less cumbersome to administer. The procedure takes only about 15 minutes. The published SEE for air displacement as compared with hydrostatic weighing is approximately ±2.2 percent; however, the SEE may actually be higher. Recent research has determined that percent body fat is about 5 percentage points higher with air displacement as compared to hydrostatic weighing.[1] The researchers concluded that further technical work is required to make air displacement an acceptable technique to determine body composition. Other investigators have also found this method to overestimate percent body fat.[2,3] Furthermore, research is required to determine its accuracy among different age groups, ethnic backgrounds, and athletic populations. At present, the Bod Pod is not readily available in most fitness centers and exercise laboratories.

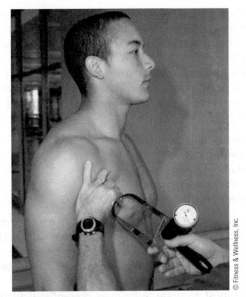

Skinfold thickness technique.

Skinfold Thickness

Because of the cost, time, and complexity of hydrostatic weighing and the expense of Bod Pod equipment, most health and fitness programs use **anthropometric measurement** techniques. These techniques, primarily skinfold thickness and girth measurements, allow quick, simple, and inexpensive estimates of body composition.

Assessing body composition using **skinfold thickness** is based on the principle that the amount of **subcutaneous fat** is proportional to total body fat. Valid and reliable measurements of this tissue give a good indication of percent body fat. The SEE for skinfold analysis is ±3.5 percent.

The skinfold test is done with the aid of pressure calipers. Several techniques requiring measurement of three to seven sites have been developed. The following three-site procedure is the most commonly used technique. The sites measured are as follows (also see Figure 4.2):

Women: triceps, suprailium, and thigh skinfolds
Men: chest, abdomen, and thigh

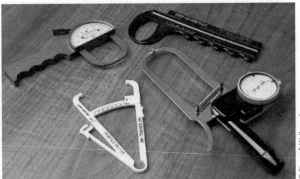

Various types of calipers used to assess skinfold thickness.

Figure 4.2	Procedure and anatomical landmarks for skinfold measurements.

Skinfold Measurement

1. Select the proper anatomical sites. For men, use chest, abdomen, and thigh skinfolds. For women, use triceps, suprailium, and thigh skinfolds. Take all measurements on the right side of the body with the person standing.

2. Measure each site by grasping a double thickness of skin firmly with the thumb and forefinger, pulling the fold slightly away from the muscular tissue. Hold the caliper perpendicular to the fold and take the measurement 1/2″ below the finger hold. Measure each site three times and read the values to the nearest .1 to .5 mm. Record the average of the two closest readings as the final value for that site. Take the readings without delay to avoid excessive compression of the skinfold. Release and refold the skinfold between readings.

3. When doing pre- and post-assessments, conduct the measurement at the same time of day. The best time is early in the morning to avoid water hydration changes resulting from activity or exercise.

4. Obtain percent fat by adding the skinfold measurements from all three sites and looking up the respective values in Tables 4.1, 4.2, or 4.3.

For example, if the skinfold measurements for an 18-year-old female are (a) triceps = 16, (b) suprailium = 4, and (c) thigh = 30 (total = 50), the percent body fat is 20.6%.

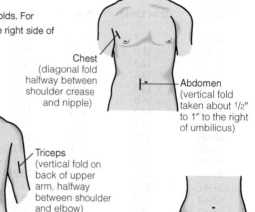

Chest
(diagonal fold halfway between shoulder crease and nipple)

Abdomen
(vertical fold taken about 1/2″ to 1″ to the right of umbilicus)

Triceps
(vertical fold on back of upper arm, halfway between shoulder and elbow)

Suprailium
(diagonal fold above crest of ilium, on the side of the hip)

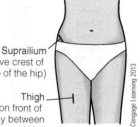

Thigh
(vertical fold on front of thigh, midway between knee and hip)

© Cengage Learning 2013

All measurements should be taken on the right side of the body.

With the skinfold technique, training is necessary to obtain accurate measurements. In addition, different technicians may produce slightly different measurements of the same person. Therefore, the same technician should take pre- and post-test measurements.

Measurements should be done at the same time of the day—preferably in the morning—because changes in water hydration from activity and exercise can affect skinfold girth. The procedure is given in Figure 4.2. If skinfold calipers are available, you may assess your percent body fat with the help of your instructor or an experienced technician (also see Activity 4.1). Then locate the percent fat estimates in Table 4.1, 4.2, or 4.3, as appropriate.

Girth Measurements

Another method that is frequently used to estimate body fat is to measure circumferences, or **girth measurements**, at various body sites. This technique requires only a stan-

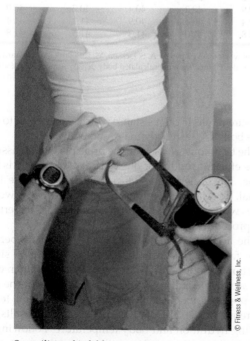

Suprailium skinfold assessment.

© Fitness & Wellness, Inc.

| Table 4.1 | | Skinfold Thickness Technique: Percent Fat Estimates for Women Calculated from Triceps, Suprailium, and Thigh | | | | | | | |

Sum of 3 Skinfolds	Age at Last Birthday								
	22 or Under	23 to 27	28 to 32	33 to 37	38 to 42	43 to 47	48 to 52	53 to 57	58 and Over
23–25	9.7	9.9	10.2	10.4	10.7	10.9	11.2	11.4	11.7
26–28	11.0	11.2	11.5	11.7	12.0	12.3	12.5	12.7	13.0
29–31	12.3	12.5	12.8	13.0	13.3	13.5	13.8	14.0	14.3
32–34	13.6	13.8	14.0	14.3	14.5	14.8	15.0	15.3	15.5
35–37	14.8	15.0	15.3	15.5	15.8	16.0	16.3	16.5	16.8
38–40	16.0	16.3	16.5	16.7	17.0	17.2	17.5	17.7	18.0
41–43	17.2	17.4	17.7	17.9	18.2	18.4	18.7	18.9	19.2
44–46	18.3	18.6	18.8	19.1	19.3	19.6	19.8	20.1	20.3
47–49	19.5	19.7	20.0	20.2	20.5	20.7	21.0	21.2	21.5
50–52	20.6	20.8	21.1	21.3	21.6	21.8	22.1	22.3	22.6
53–55	21.7	21.9	22.1	22.4	22.6	22.9	23.1	23.4	23.6
56–58	22.7	23.0	23.2	23.4	23.7	23.9	24.2	24.4	24.7
59–61	23.7	24.0	24.2	24.5	24.7	25.0	25.2	25.5	25.7
62–64	24.7	25.0	25.2	25.5	25.7	26.0	26.2	26.4	26.7
65–67	25.7	25.9	26.2	26.4	26.7	26.9	27.2	27.4	27.7
68–70	26.6	26.9	27.1	27.4	27.6	27.9	28.1	28.4	28.6
71–73	27.5	27.8	28.0	28.3	28.5	28.8	29.0	29.3	29.5
74–76	28.4	28.7	28.9	29.2	29.4	29.7	29.9	30.2	30.4
77–79	29.3	29.5	29.8	30.0	30.3	30.5	30.8	31.0	31.3
80–82	30.1	30.4	30.6	30.9	31.1	31.4	31.6	31.9	32.1
83–85	30.9	31.2	31.4	31.7	31.9	32.2	32.4	32.7	32.9
86–88	31.7	32.0	32.2	32.5	32.7	32.9	33.2	33.4	33.7
89–91	32.5	32.7	33.0	33.2	33.5	33.7	33.9	34.2	34.4
92–94	33.2	33.4	33.7	33.9	34.2	34.4	34.7	34.9	35.2
95–97	33.9	34.1	34.4	34.6	34.9	35.1	35.4	35.6	35.9
98–100	34.6	34.8	35.1	35.3	35.5	35.8	36.0	36.3	36.5
101–103	35.2	35.4	35.7	35.9	36.2	36.4	36.7	36.9	37.2
104–106	35.8	36.1	36.3	36.6	36.8	37.1	37.3	37.5	37.8
107–109	36.4	36.7	36.9	37.1	37.4	37.6	37.9	38.1	38.4
110–112	37.0	37.2	37.5	37.7	38.0	38.2	38.5	38.7	38.9
113–115	37.5	37.8	38.0	38.2	38.5	38.7	39.0	39.2	39.5
116–118	38.0	38.3	38.5	38.8	39.0	39.3	39.5	39.7	40.0
119–121	38.5	38.7	39.0	39.2	39.5	39.7	40.0	40.2	40.5
122–124	39.0	39.2	39.4	39.7	39.9	40.2	40.4	40.7	40.9
125–127	39.4	39.6	39.9	40.1	40.4	40.6	40.9	41.1	41.4
128–130	39.8	40.0	40.3	40.5	40.8	41.0	41.3	41.5	41.8

Body density is calculated based on the generalized equation for predicting body density of women developed by A. S. Jackson, M. L. Pollock, and A. Ward and published in *Medicine and Science in Sports and Exercise* 12 (1980): 175–182. Percent body fat is determined from the calculated body density using the Siri formula.

dard measuring tape. The limitation is that it may not be valid for athletic individuals (men or women) who participate actively in strenuous physical activity or for people who can be classified visually as thin or obese. The SEE for girth measurements is approximately ±4 percent.

The required procedure for girth measurements is given in Figure 4.3; conversion factors are in Tables 4.4 and 4.5. Measurements for women are the upper arm, hip, and wrist; for men, the waist and wrist.

Bioelectrical Impedance

The **bioelectrical impedance** technique is much simpler to administer, but its accuracy is questionable. In this technique, sensors are applied to the skin and a weak (totally painless) electrical current is run through the body to measure its electrical resistance which is then used to estimate body fat, lean body mass, and body water.

The technique is based on the principle that fat tissue is a less efficient conductor of electrical current than is lean tissue. The easier the conductance, the leaner the individual. Specialized equipment or simple body weight scales with sensors on the surface can be used to perform this procedure.

The accuracy of equations used to estimate percent body fat with this technique is questionable. A single equation cannot be used for everyone, but rather valid and accurate equations to estimate body fat for the specific population (age, gender, and ethnicity) being tested are required. Several factors can affect the results, including hydration and body temperature. Following all manufacturers' instructions will ensure the most accu-

| Table 4.2 | Skinfold Thickness Technique: Percent Fat Estimates for Men Under 40 Calculated from Chest, Abdomen, and Thigh |

Sum of 3 Skinfolds	Age at Last Birthday							
	19 or Under	20 to 22	23 to 25	26 to 28	29 to 31	32 to 34	35 to 37	38 to 40
8–10	.9	1.3	1.6	2.0	2.3	2.7	3.0	3.3
11–13	1.9	2.3	2.6	3.0	3.3	3.7	4.0	4.3
14–16	2.9	3.3	3.6	3.9	4.3	4.6	5.0	5.3
17–19	3.9	4.2	4.6	4.9	5.3	5.6	6.0	6.3
20–22	4.8	5.2	5.5	5.9	6.2	6.6	6.9	7.3
23–25	5.8	6.2	6.5	6.8	7.2	7.5	7.9	8.2
26–28	6.8	7.1	7.5	7.8	8.1	8.5	8.8	9.2
29–31	7.7	8.0	8.4	8.7	9.1	9.4	9.8	10.1
32–34	8.6	9.0	9.3	9.7	10.0	10.4	10.7	11.1
35–37	9.5	9.9	10.2	10.6	10.9	11.3	11.6	12.0
38–40	10.5	10.8	11.2	11.5	11.8	12.2	12.5	12.9
41–43	11.4	11.7	12.1	12.4	12.7	13.1	13.4	13.8
44–46	12.2	12.6	12.9	13.3	13.6	14.0	14.3	14.7
47–49	13.1	13.5	13.8	14.2	14.5	14.9	15.2	15.5
50–52	14.0	14.3	14.7	15.0	15.4	15.7	16.1	16.4
53–55	14.8	15.2	15.5	15.9	16.2	16.6	16.9	17.3
56–58	15.7	16.0	16.4	16.7	17.1	17.4	17.8	18.1
59–61	16.5	16.9	17.2	17.6	17.9	18.3	18.6	19.0
62–64	17.4	17.7	18.1	18.4	18.8	19.1	19.4	19.8
65–67	18.2	18.5	18.9	19.2	19.6	19.9	20.3	20.6
68–70	19.0	19.3	19.7	20.0	20.4	20.7	21.1	21.4
71–73	19.8	20.1	20.5	20.8	21.2	21.5	21.9	22.2
74–76	20.6	20.9	21.3	21.6	22.0	22.2	22.7	23.0
77–79	21.4	21.7	22.1	22.4	22.8	23.1	23.4	23.8
80–82	22.1	22.5	22.8	23.2	23.5	23.9	24.2	24.6
83–85	22.9	23.2	23.6	23.9	24.3	24.6	25.0	25.3
86–88	23.6	24.0	24.3	24.7	25.0	25.4	25.7	26.1
89–91	24.4	24.7	25.1	25.4	25.8	26.1	26.5	26.8
92–94	25.1	25.5	25.8	26.2	26.5	26.9	27.2	27.5
95–97	25.8	26.2	26.5	26.9	27.2	27.6	27.9	28.3
98–100	26.6	26.9	27.3	27.6	27.9	28.3	28.6	29.0
101–103	27.3	27.6	28.0	28.3	28.6	29.0	29.3	29.7
104–106	27.9	28.3	28.6	29.0	29.3	29.7	30.0	30.4
107–109	28.6	29.0	29.3	29.7	30.0	30.4	30.7	31.1
110–112	29.3	29.6	30.0	30.3	30.7	31.0	31.4	31.7
113–115	30.0	30.3	30.7	31.0	31.3	31.7	32.0	32.4
116–118	30.6	31.0	31.3	31.6	32.0	32.3	32.7	33.0
119–121	31.3	31.6	32.0	32.3	32.6	33.0	33.3	33.7
122–124	31.9	32.2	32.6	32.9	33.3	33.6	34.0	34.3
125–127	32.5	32.9	33.2	33.5	33.9	34.2	34.6	34.9
128–130	33.1	33.5	33.8	34.2	34.5	34.9	35.2	35.5

Body density is calculated based on the generalized equation for predicting body density of men developed by A. S. Jackson and M. L. Pollock and published in the *British Journal of Nutrition* 40 (1978): 497–504. Percent body fat is determined from the calculated body density using the Siri formula.

rate result, but even then percent body fat may be off—typically on the higher end, by as much as 10 percentage points (or even more on some scales).

Body Mass Index

The most common technique to determine thinness and excessive fatness is the **body mass index (BMI)**. BMI incorporates height and weight to estimate critical fat values at which the risk for disease increases.

BMI is calculated by either (a) dividing the weight in kilograms by the square of the height in meters or (b) multiplying body weight in pounds by 705 and dividing this figure by the square of the height in inches. For example, the BMI for an individual who weighs 172 pounds (78 kg) and is 67 inches (1.7 m) tall would be 27: $[78 \div (1.7)^2]$ or $[172 \times 705 \div (67)^2]$. You also can look up your BMI in Table 4.6 according to your height and weight.

Table 4.3	Skinfold Thickness Technique: Percent Fat Estimates for Men Over 40 Calculated from Chest, Abdomen, and Thigh

				Age at Last Birthday				
Sum of 3 Skinfolds	41 to 43	44 to 46	47 to 49	50 to 52	53 to 55	56 to 58	59 to 61	62 and Over
8–10	3.7	4.0	4.4	4.7	5.1	5.4	5.8	6.1
11–13	4.7	5.0	5.4	5.7	6.1	6.4	6.8	7.1
14–16	5.7	6.0	6.4	6.7	7.1	7.4	7.8	8.1
17–19	6.7	7.0	7.4	7.7	8.1	8.4	8.7	9.1
20–22	7.6	8.0	8.3	8.7	9.0	9.4	9.7	10.1
23–25	8.6	8.9	9.3	9.6	10.0	10.3	10.7	11.0
26–28	9.5	9.9	10.2	10.6	10.9	11.3	11.6	12.0
29–31	10.5	10.8	11.2	11.5	11.9	12.2	12.6	12.9
32–34	11.4	11.8	12.1	12.4	12.8	13.1	13.5	13.8
35–37	12.3	12.7	13.0	13.4	13.7	14.1	14.4	14.8
38–40	13.2	13.6	13.9	14.3	14.6	15.0	15.3	15.7
41–43	14.1	14.5	14.8	15.2	15.5	15.9	16.2	16.6
44–46	15.0	15.4	15.7	16.1	16.4	16.8	17.1	17.5
47–49	15.9	16.2	16.6	16.9	17.3	17.6	18.0	18.3
50–52	16.8	17.1	17.5	17.8	18.2	18.5	18.8	19.2
53–55	17.6	18.0	18.3	18.7	19.0	19.4	19.7	20.1
56–58	18.5	18.8	19.2	19.5	19.9	20.2	20.6	20.9
59–61	19.3	19.7	20.0	20.4	20.7	21.0	21.4	21.7
62–64	20.1	20.5	20.8	21.2	21.5	21.9	22.2	22.6
65–67	21.0	21.3	21.7	22.0	22.4	22.7	23.0	23.4
68–70	21.8	22.1	22.5	22.8	23.2	23.5	23.9	24.2
71–73	22.6	22.9	23.3	23.6	24.0	24.3	24.7	25.0
74–76	23.4	23.7	24.1	24.4	24.8	25.1	25.4	25.8
77–79	24.1	24.5	24.8	25.2	25.5	25.9	26.2	26.6
80–82	24.9	25.3	25.6	26.0	26.3	26.6	27.0	27.3
83–85	25.7	26.0	26.4	26.7	27.1	27.4	27.8	28.1
86–88	26.4	26.8	27.1	27.5	27.8	28.2	28.5	28.9
89–91	27.2	27.5	27.9	28.2	28.6	28.9	29.2	29.6
92–94	27.9	28.2	28.6	28.9	29.3	29.6	30.0	30.3
95–97	28.6	29.0	29.3	29.7	30.0	30.4	30.7	31.1
98–100	29.3	29.7	30.0	30.4	30.7	31.1	31.4	31.8
101–103	30.0	30.4	30.7	31.1	31.4	31.8	32.1	32.5
104–106	30.7	31.1	31.4	31.8	32.1	32.5	32.8	33.2
107–109	31.4	31.8	32.1	32.4	32.8	33.1	33.5	33.8
110–112	32.1	32.4	32.8	33.1	33.5	33.8	34.2	34.5
113–115	32.7	33.1	33.4	33.8	34.1	34.5	34.8	35.2
116–118	33.4	33.7	34.1	34.4	34.8	35.1	35.5	35.8
119–121	34.0	34.4	34.7	35.1	35.4	35.8	36.1	36.5
122–124	34.7	35.0	35.4	35.7	36.1	36.4	36.7	37.1
125–127	35.3	35.6	36.0	36.3	36.7	37.0	37.4	37.7
128–130	35.9	36.2	36.6	36.9	37.3	37.6	38.0	38.5

Body density is calculated based on the generalized equation for predicting body density of men developed by A. S. Jackson and M. L. Pollock and published in the *British Journal of Nutrition* 40 (1978): 497–504. Percent body fat is determined from the calculated body density using the Siri formula.

Because of its simplicity and measurement consistency across populations, BMI is the most widely used method to determine overweight and obesity. Due to the various limitations of previously mentioned body composition techniques—including cost, availability to the general population, lack of consistency among technicians and laboratories, inconsistent results between techniques, and standard error of measurement of the procedures—BMI is used almost exclusively to determine health risks and mortality rates associated with excessive body weight.

Scientific evidence indicates that the risk for disease starts to increase when BMI exceeds 25.[4] Although a BMI index between 18.5 and 25 is considered normal (see Tables 4.7 and 4.9), the lowest risk for chronic disease is in the 22 to 25 range.[5] Individuals are classified as overweight if their indexes lie between 25 and 30. BMIs above 30 are defined as obese, and those below 18.5 as **underweight**. Scientific evidence has shown that even though the risk for premature illness and death is greater for those who are overweight, the risk is also increased for individuals who are underweight[6] (see Figure 4.4).

Compared with individuals with BMIs between 22 and 25, people with BMIs between 25 and 30 (overweight) exhibit mortality rates up to 25 percent higher; rates for those with BMIs above 30 (obese) are 50 to 100 percent higher.[7] Table 4.7 provides disease risk categories when

---

Figure 4.3 Procedure for body fat assessment according to girth measurements.

Girth Measurements for Women*

1. Using a regular tape measure, determine the following girth measurements in centimeters (cm):

   Upper arm: Take the measure halfway between the shoulder and the elbow.

   Hip: Measure at the point of largest circumference.

   Wrist: Take the girth in front of the bones where the wrist bends.

2. Obtain the person's age.

3. Using Table 4.4, find the subject's age and girth measurement for each site, then look up the respective constant value for each. These values will allow you to derive body density (BD) by substituting the constants in the following formula:

   $$BD = A - B - C + D$$

4. Using the derived body density, calculate percent body fat (%F) according to the following equation:

   $$\%F = (495 \div BD) - 450**$$

Example: Jane is 20 years old, and the following girth measurements were taken: biceps = 27 cm, hip = 99.5 cm, wrist = 15.4 cm

Data	Constant
Upper arm = 27 cm	A = 1.0813
Age = 20	B = .0102
Hip = 99.5 cm	C = .1206
Wrist = 15.4 cm	D = .0971

BD = A − B − C + D
BD = 1.0813 − .0102 − .1206 + .0971 = 1.0476
%F = (495 ÷ BD) − 450
%F = (495 ÷ 1.0476) − 450 = 22.5

Girth Measurements for Men***

1. Using a regular tape measure, determine the following girth measurements in inches (the men's measurements are taken in inches, as opposed to centimeters for women):

   Waist: Measure at the umbilicus (belly button).

   Wrist: Measure in front of the bones where the wrist bends.

2. Subtract the wrist from the waist measurement.

3. Obtain the weight of the subject in pounds.

4. Look up the percent body fat (%F) in Table 4.5 by using the difference obtained in number 2 above and the person's body weight.

Example: John weighs 160 pounds, and his waist and wrist girth measurements are 36.5 and 7.5 inches, respectively.

Waist girth = 36.5 inches
Wrist girth = 7.5 inches
Difference = 29.0 inches
Body weight = 160.0 lbs.
%F = 22

---

*From R. B. Lambson, "Generalized body density prediction equations for women using simple anthropometric measurements." Unpublished doctoral dissertation, Brigham Young University, Provo, UT, August 1987. Reproduced by permission.
**From W. E. Siri, Body Composition from Fluid Spaces and Density (Berkeley: University of California, Donner Laboratory of Medical Physics, March 19, 1956.)
***K. W. Penrouse, A. G. Nelson, and A. G. Fisher, "Generalized body composition equation for men using simple measurement techniques," *Medicine and Science in Sports and Exercise* 17, no. 2 (1985): 189. © American College of Sports Medicine, 1985.

© Cengage Learning 2013

BMI is used as the sole criterion to identify people at risk. More than one-fifth of the U.S. adult population has a BMI of 30 or more. Overweight and obesity trends starting in 1960 according to BMI are given in Figure 4.5.

BMI is a useful tool to screen the general population, but its one weakness is that it fails to differentiate fat from lean body mass or note where most of the fat is located (waist circumference—see discussion that follows). Using BMI, athletes with a large amount of muscle mass (such as body builders and football players) can easily fall in the moderate- or even high-risk categories.

Waist Circumference

Scientific evidence suggests that the way people store fat affects their risk for disease. The total amount of body fat by itself is not the best predictor of increased risk for disease but, rather, the location of the fat. **Android obesity** is seen in individuals who tend to store fat in the trunk or abdominal area (which produces the "apple" shape). **Gynoid obesity** is seen in people who store fat primarily around the hips and thighs (which creates the "pear" shape).

As compared with people with body fat that is stored primarily in the hips and thighs, an increasing amount of

Key Terms

Underweight Extremely low body weight.
Android obesity Obesity pattern seen in individuals who tend to store fat in the trunk or abdominal area.
Gynoid obesity Obesity pattern seen in people who store fat primarily around the hips and thighs.

Table 4.4		Girth Measurement Technique: Conversion Constants to Calculate Body Density for Women							
Upper Arm (cm)	Constant A	Age	Constant B	Hip (cm)	Constant C	Hip (cm)	Constant C	Wrist (cm)	Constant D
20.5	1.0966	17	.0086	79	.0957	114.5	.1388	13.0	.0819
21	1.0954	18	.0091	79.5	.0963	115	.1394	13.2	.0832
21.5	1.0942	19	.0096	80	.0970	115.5	.1400	13.4	.0845
22	1.0930	20	.0102	80.5	.0976	116	.1406	13.6	.0857
22.5	1.0919	21	.0107	81	.0982	116.5	.1412	13.8	.0870
23	1.0907	22	.0112	81.5	.0988	117	.1418	14.0	.0882
23.5	1.0895	23	.0117	82	.0994	117.5	.1424	14.2	.0895
24	1.0883	24	.0122	82.5	.1000	118	.1430	14.4	.0908
24.5	1.0871	25	.0127	83	.1006	118.5	.1436	14.6	.0920
25	1.0860	26	.0132	83.5	.1012	119	.1442	14.8	.0933
25.5	1.0848	27	.0137	84	.1018	119.5	.1448	15.0	.0946
26	1.0836	28	.0142	84.5	.1024	120	.1454	15.2	.0958
26.5	1.0824	29	.0147	85	.1030	120.5	.1460	15.4	.0971
27	1.0813	30	.0152	85.5	.1036	121	.1466	15.6	.0983
27.5	1.0801	31	.0157	86	.1042	121.5	.1472	15.8	.0996
28	1.0789	32	.0162	86.5	.1048	122	.1479	16.0	.1009
28.5	1.0777	33	.0168	87	.1054	122.5	.1485	16.2	.1021
29	1.0775	34	.0173	87.5	.1060	123	.1491	16.4	.1034
29.5	1.0754	35	.0178	88	.1066	123.5	.1497	16.6	.1046
30	1.0742	36	.0183	88.5	.1072	124	.1503	16.8	.1059
30.5	1.0730	37	.0188	89	.1079	124.5	.1509	17.0	.1072
31	1.0718	38	.0193	89.5	.1085	125	.1515	17.2	.1084
31.5	1.0707	39	.0198	90	.1091	125.5	.1521	17.4	.1097
32	1.0695	40	.0203	90.5	.1097	126	.1527	17.6	.1109
32.5	1.0683	41	.0208	91	.1103	126.5	.1533	17.8	.1122
33	1.0671	42	.0213	91.5	.1109	127	.1539	18.0	.1135
33.5	1.0666	43	.0218	92	.1115	127.5	.1545	18.2	.1147
34	1.0648	44	.0223	92.5	.1121	128	.1551	18.4	.1160
34.5	1.0636	45	.0228	93	.1127	128.5	.1558	18.6	.1172
35	1.0624	46	.0234	93.5	.1133	129	.1563		
35.5	1.0612	47	.0239	94	.1139	129.5	.1569		
36	1.0601	48	.0244	94.5	.1145	130	.1575		
36.5	1.0589	49	.0249	95	.1151	130.5	.1581		
37	1.0577	50	.0254	95.5	.1157	131	.1587		
37.5	1.0565	51	.0259	96	.1163	131.5	.1593		
38	1.0554	52	.0264	96.5	.1169	132	.1600		
38.5	1.0542	53	.0269	97	.1176	132.5	.1606		
39	1.0530	54	.0274	97.5	.1182	133	.1612		
39.5	1.0518	55	.0279	98	.1188	133.5	.1618		
40	1.0506	56	.0284	98.5	.1194	134	.1624		
40.5	1.0495	57	.0289	99	.1200	134.5	.1630		
41	1.0483	58	.0294	99.5	.1206	135	.1636		
41.5	1.0471	59	.0300	100	.1212	135.5	.1642		
42	1.0459	60	.0305	100.5	.1218	136	.1648		
42.5	1.0448	61	.0310	101	.1224	136.5	.1654		
43	1.0434	62	.0315	101.5	.1230	137	.1660		
43.5	1.0424	63	.0320	102	.1236	137.5	.1666		
44	1.0412	64	.0325	102.5	.1242	138	.1672		
		65	.0330	103	.1248	138.5	.1678		
		66	.0335	103.5	.1254	139	.1685		
		67	.0340	104	.1260	139.5	.1691		

| Table 4.4 | Girth Measurement Technique: Conversion Constants to Calculate Body Density for Women *(continued)* |

Upper Arm (cm)	Constant A	Age	Constant B	Hip (cm)	Constant C	Hip (cm)	Constant C	Wrist (cm)	Constant D
		68	.0345	104.5	.1266	140	.1697		
		69	.0350	105	.1272	140.5	.1703		
		70	.0355	105.5	.1278	141	.1709		
		71	.0360	106	.1285	141.5	.1715		
		72	.0366	106.5	.1291	142	.1721		
		73	.0371	107	.1297	142.5	.1728		
		74	.0376	107.5	.1303	143	.1733		
		75	.0381	108	.1309	143.5	.1739		
				108.5	.1315	144	.1745		
				109	.1321	144.5	.1751		
				109.5	.1327	145	.1757		
				110	.1333	145.5	.1763		
				110.5	.1339	146	.1769		
				111	.1345	146.5	.1775		
				111.5	.1351	147	.1781		
				112	.1357	147.5	.1787		
				112.5	.1363	148	.1794		
				113	.1369	148.5	.1800		
				113.5	.1375	149	.1806		
				114	.1382	149.5	.1812		
						150	.1818		

evidence is showing that obese individuals with abdominal fat are clearly at higher risk for heart disease, hypertension, type 2 diabetes ("non–insulin-dependent" diabetes), stroke, some types of cancer, dementia, migraines, and diminished lung function. Evidence also indicates that among individuals with a lot of abdominal fat, those whose fat deposits are located around internal organs (intra-abdominal or visceral fat) rather than subcutaneously or retroperitoneally (see Figure 4.6) have an even greater risk for disease than those with fat mainly just beneath the skin (subcutaneous fat).[5] Of even greater significance, the results of a recent study that followed more than 350,000 people over almost

| Figure 4.4 | Mortality risk versus body mass index (BMI). |

Risk of premature morbidity and mortality

15 20 25 30 35 40 45
Body mass index

- Underweight
- Recommended weight
- Overweight
- Obesity

| Figure 4.5 | Overweight and obesity trends in the United States, 1960–2010. |

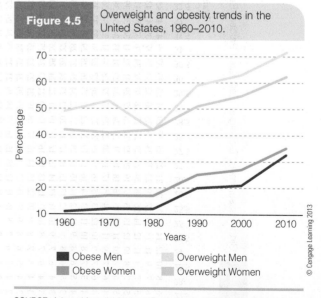

Percentage

70
60
50
40
30
20
10

1960 1970 1980 1990 2000 2010
Years

- Obese Men
- Obese Women
- Overweight Men
- Overweight Women

SOURCE: Adapted from the National Center for Health Statistics, Centers for Disease Control and Prevention, and the *Journal of the American Medical Association.*

Table 4.5   Girth Measurement Technique: Estimated Percent Body Fat for Men

Waist Minus Wrist Girth Measurement (inches)

Body Weight (pounds)	22	22.5	23	23.5	24	24.5	25	25.5	26	26.5	27	27.5	28	28.5	29	29.5	30	30.5	31	31.5	32	32.5	33	33.5	34	34.5	35	35.5	36	36.5	37	37.5	38	38.5	39	39.5	40	40.5	41	41.5	42	42.5	43	43.5	44	44.5	45	45.5	46	46.5	47	47.5	48	48.5	49	49.5	50
120	4	6	8	10	12	14	16	18	19	21	23	25	27	29	31	33	35	37	39	41	43	45	46	48	50	52	54	56	58																												
125	4	6	8	9	11	13	15	17	18	20	22	24	26	27	29	31	33	35	36	38	40	42	44	45	47	49	51	53	54	56	58																										
130	3	5	6	8	10	12	13	15	17	19	20	22	24	26	27	29	31	33	34	36	38	40	41	43	45	47	48	50	52	54	55	57																									
135	3	5	6	8	10	11	13	15	16	18	20	21	23	25	26	28	30	31	33	34	36	38	39	41	43	44	46	48	49	51	53	54	56																								
140	3	5	6	8	9	11	13	14	16	17	19	21	22	24	25	27	29	30	32	34	35	37	38	40	42	43	45	46	48	50	51	53	54	56																							
145	3	5	6	8	9	11	12	14	15	17	18	20	21	23	24	26	27	29	31	32	34	35	37	38	40	41	43	44	46	47	49	50	52	53	55																						
150	2	4	5	7	8	10	11	13	14	16	17	19	20	22	23	25	26	28	29	31	32	34	35	37	38	40	41	43	44	46	47	49	50	52	53	55																					
155	2	3	5	6	8	9	11	12	14	15	17	18	20	21	23	24	26	27	28	30	31	33	34	36	37	39	40	42	43	45	46	48	49	51	52	54	55																				
160	2	3	5	6	8	9	10	12	13	15	16	17	19	20	22	23	24	26	27	29	30	32	33	34	36	37	39	40	41	43	44	46	47	48	50	51	53	54																			
165	2	3	5	6	7	9	10	12	13	14	16	17	18	20	21	23	24	25	27	28	29	31	32	33	35	36	38	39	40	42	43	44	46	47	49	50	51	53	54																		
170	2	3	5	6	7	9	10	11	13	14	15	17	18	19	21	22	23	25	26	27	29	30	31	33	34	35	37	38	39	41	42	43	45	46	47	49	50	51	53	54																	
175	2	3	5	6	7	8	10	11	12	13	15	16	17	19	20	21	22	24	25	26	28	29	30	31	33	34	35	36	38	39	40	42	43	44	45	47	48	49	50	52	53																
180		2	3	5	6	7	8	10	11	12	13	15	16	17	19	20	21	22	24	25	26	28	29	30	31	33	34	35	36	38	39	40	42	43	44	45	47	48	49	50	52	53															
185			2	3	5	6	7	8	10	11	12	13	15	16	17	19	20	21	22	24	25	26	28	29	30	31	33	34	35	36	38	39	40	42	43	44	45	47	48	49	50	52	53														
190				2	3	4	6	7	8	10	11	12	13	15	16	17	18	20	21	22	23	25	26	27	28	30	31	32	33	35	36	37	38	40	41	42	43	45	46	47	48	50	51	52												
195					2	3	4	6	7	8	10	11	12	13	15	16	17	18	20	21	22	23	25	26	27	28	30	31	32	33	35	36	37	38	40	41	42	43	45	46	47	48	50	51	52											
200						2	3	4	6	7	8	10	11	12	13	15	16	17	18	20	21	22	23	25	26	27	28	30	31	32	33	35	36	37	38	40	41	42	43	45	46	47	48	50	51	52										
205							2	3	4	6	7	8	9	11	12	13	14	15	17	18	19	20	22	23	24	25	27	28	29	30	31	33	34	35	36	38	39	40	41	42	44	45	46	47	49	50	51									
210								2	3	4	6	7	8	9	11	12	13	14	15	17	18	19	20	22	23	24	25	27	28	29	30	31	33	34	35	36	38	39	40	41	42	44	45	46	47	49	50	51								
215									2	3	4	6	7	8	9	11	12	13	14	15	17	18	19	20	22	23	24	25	27	28	29	30	31	33	34	35	36	38	39	40	41	42	44	45	46	47	49	50	51							
220										2	3	4	6	7	8	9	11	12	13	14	15	17	18	19	20	22	23	24	25	27	28	29	30	31	33	34	35	36	38	39	40	41	42	44	45	46	47	49	50	51						
225											2	3	4	6	7	8	9	11	12	13	14	15	17	18	19	20	22	23	24	25	27	28	29	30	31	33	34	35	36	38	39	40	41	42	44	45	46	47	49	50	51					
230												2	3	4	6	7	8	9	11	12	13	14	15	17	18	19	20	22	23	24	25	27	28	29	30	31	33	34	35	36	38	39	40	41	42	44	45	46	47	49	50	51				
235													2	3	4	6	7	8	9	10	12	13	14	15	16	18	19	20	21	22	24	25	26	27	28	30	31	32	33	34	36	37	38	39	40	42	43	44	45	46	48	49	50			
240														2	3	4	6	7	8	9	10	12	13	14	15	16	18	19	20	21	22	24	25	26	27	28	30	31	32	33	34	36	37	38	39	40	42	43	44	45	46	48	49	50		
245															2	3	4	6	7	8	9	10	12	13	14	15	16	18	19	20	21	22	24	25	26	27	28	30	31	32	33	34	36	37	38	39	40	42	43	44	45	46	48	49	50	
250																2	3	4	6	7	8	9	10	12	13	14	15	16	18	19	20	21	22	24	25	26	27	28	30	31	32	33	34	36	37	38	39	40	42	43	44	45	46	48	49	50
255																	2	3	4	6	7	8	9	10	12	13	14	15	16	18	19	20	21	22	24	25	26	27	28	30	31	32	33	34	36	37	38	39	40	42	43	44	45	46	48	49	50
260																		2	3	4	6	7	8	9	10	12	13	14	15	16	18	19	20	21	22	24	25	26	27	28	30	31	32	33	34	36	37	38	39	40	42	43	44	45	46	48	49
265																			2	3	4	6	7	8	9	10	12	13	14	15	17	18	19	20	21	23	24	25	26	27	29	30	31	32	33	35	36	37	38	40	41	42	43	44	46	47	48
270																				2	3	4	6	7	8	9	11	12	13	14	15	17	18	19	20	21	23	24	25	26	28	29	30	31	32	34	35	36	37	38	40	41	42	43	45	46	47
275																					2	3	4	6	7	8	9	11	12	13	14	15	17	18	19	20	22	23	24	25	26	28	29	30	31	33	34	35	36	37	39	40	41	42	44	45	46
280																						2	3	5	6	7	8	10	11	12	13	15	16	17	18	20	21	22	23	25	26	27	28	30	31	32	33	35	36	37	38	40	41	42	43	45	46
285																							2	3	5	6	7	8	10	11	12	13	15	16	17	18	20	21	22	24	25	26	27	29	30	31	32	34	35	36	37	39	40	41	42	44	45
290																								2	3	5	6	7	8	10	11	12	13	15	16	17	19	20	21	22	24	25	26	27	29	30	31	33	34	35	36	38	39	40	41	43	44
295																									2	3	5	6	7	8	10	11	12	14	15	16	17	19	20	21	23	24	25	26	28	29	30	31	33	34	35	37	38	39	40	42	43
300																										2	3	5	6	7	9	10	11	13	14	15	17	18	19	21	22	23	24	26	27	28	30	31	32	34	35	36	38	39	40	42	43

Reproduced by permission from A. G. Fisher and P. E. Allsen, Jogging, Dubuque, IA: Wm. C. Brown, 1987.

Table 4.6	Determination of Body Mass Index (BMI)

Determine your BMI by looking up the number where your weight and height intersect on the table. According to the results, look up your disease risk in Table 4.7.

Height	\multicolumn{29}{c}{Weight}
	110	115	120	125	130	135	140	145	150	155	160	165	170	175	180	185	190	195	200	205	210	215	220	225	230	235	240	245	250
5'0"	21	22	23	24	25	26	27	28	29	30	31	32	33	34	35	36	37	38	39	40	41	42	43	44	45	46	47	48	49
5'1"	21	22	23	24	25	26	26	27	28	29	30	31	32	33	34	35	36	37	38	39	40	41	42	43	43	44	45	46	47
5'2"	20	21	22	23	24	25	26	27	27	28	29	30	31	32	33	34	35	36	37	37	38	39	40	41	42	43	44	45	46
5'3"	19	20	21	22	23	24	25	26	27	27	28	29	30	31	32	33	34	35	35	36	37	38	39	40	41	42	43	43	44
5'4"	19	20	21	21	22	23	24	25	26	27	27	28	29	30	31	32	33	33	34	35	36	37	38	39	39	40	41	42	43
5'5"	18	19	20	21	22	22	23	24	25	26	27	27	28	29	30	31	32	32	33	34	35	36	37	37	38	39	40	41	42
5'6"	18	19	19	20	21	22	23	23	24	25	26	27	27	28	29	30	31	31	32	33	34	35	36	36	37	38	39	40	40
5'7"	17	18	19	20	20	21	22	23	23	24	25	26	27	27	28	29	30	31	31	32	33	34	34	35	36	37	38	38	39
5'8"	17	17	18	19	20	21	21	22	23	24	24	25	26	27	27	28	29	30	30	31	32	33	33	34	35	36	36	37	38
5'9"	16	17	18	18	19	20	21	21	22	23	24	24	25	26	27	27	28	29	30	30	31	32	32	33	34	35	35	36	37
5'10"	16	17	17	18	19	19	20	21	22	22	23	24	24	25	26	27	27	28	29	29	30	31	32	32	33	34	34	35	36
5'11"	15	16	17	17	18	19	20	20	21	22	22	23	24	24	25	26	26	27	28	29	29	30	31	31	32	33	33	34	35
6'0"	15	16	16	17	18	18	19	20	20	21	22	22	23	24	24	25	26	26	27	28	28	29	30	31	31	32	33	33	34
6'1"	15	15	16	16	17	18	18	19	20	20	21	22	22	23	24	24	25	26	26	27	28	28	29	30	30	31	32	32	33
6'2"	14	15	15	16	17	17	18	19	19	20	21	21	22	22	23	24	24	25	26	26	27	28	28	29	30	30	31	31	32
6'3"	14	14	15	16	16	17	17	18	19	19	20	21	21	22	22	23	24	24	25	26	26	27	27	28	29	29	30	31	31
6'4"	13	14	15	15	16	16	17	18	18	19	19	20	21	21	22	23	23	24	24	25	26	26	27	27	28	29	29	30	30

© Cengage Learning 2013

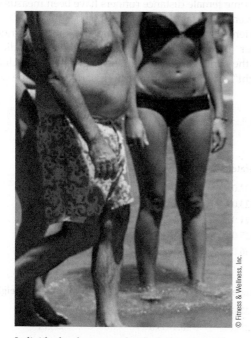

Individuals who accumulate body fat around the midsection are at greater risk for disease than those who accumulate body fat in other areas.

© Fitness & Wellness, Inc.

Table 4.7	Disease Risk According to Body Mass Index (BMI)

BMI	Disease Risk	Classification
<18.5	Increased	Underweight
18.6–21.99	Low	Acceptable
22.0–24.99	Very Low	Acceptable
25.0–29.99	Increased	Overweight
30.0–34.99	High	Obesity I
35.0–39.99	Very High	Obesity II
≥40.00	Extremely High	Obesity III

© Cengage Learning 2013

Table 4.8	Disease Risk According to Waist Circumference (WC)

Men	Women	Disease Risk
<35.5	<32.5	Low
35.5–40.0	32.5–35.0	Moderate
>40.0	>35.0	High

© Cengage Learning 2013

10 years concluded that even when body weight is viewed as "normal," individuals with a large waist circumference nearly double the risk for premature death.[6] Researchers believe that visceral fat secretes harmful inflammatory substances that contribute to chronic conditions.

Complex scanning techniques used to identify individuals at risk because of high intra-abdominal fatness are costly, so a simple **waist circumference (WC)** measure, designed by the National Heart, Lung, and Blood Institute, is used to assess this risk.[7] WC seems to predict abdominal visceral fat as accurately as the DXA technique.[8] A waist circumference of more than 40 inches in men and 35 inches in women indicates a higher risk for cardiovascular disease, hypertension, and type 2 diabetes (Table 4.8). Weight loss is encouraged when individuals exceed these measurements.

Research indicates that WC is a better predictor than BMI of the risk for disease.[9] Thus, BMI in conjunction with WC provides the best combination to identify individuals at higher risk resulting from excessive body fat. Table 4.9 provides guidelines to identify people at risk according to BMI and WC.

Determining Recommended Body Weight

After finding out your percent body fat, you can determine your current body composition classification by consulting Table 4.10, which presents percentages of fat according to both the health fitness standard and the high physical fitness standard (see discussion in Chapter 1).

For example, the recommended health fitness fat percentage for a 20-year-old female is 28 percent or less. Although there are no clearly identified percent body fat

| Table 4.9 | Disease Risk According to Body Mass Index (BMI) and Waist Circumference (WC) |

| | | Disease Risk Relative to Body Weight and WC | |
Classification	BMI (kg/m²)	Men ≤40″ (102 cm) Women ≤35″ (88 cm)	Men >40″ (102 cm) Women >35″ (88 cm)
Underweight	<18.5	Increased	Low
Normal	18.5–24.9	Very low	Increased
Overweight	25.0–29.9	Increased	High
Obesity Class I	30.0–34.9	High	Very high
Obesity Class II	35.0–39.9	Very high	Very high
Obesity Class III	≥40.0	Extremely high	Extremely high

Adapted from Expert Panel, Executive Summary of the Clinical Guidelines on the Identification, Evaluation, and Treatment of Overweight and Obesity in Adults, *Archives of Internal Medicine* 158:1855–1867, 1998.

levels at which the risk for disease definitely increases, the health fitness standard in Table 4.10 is currently the best estimate of the point at which there seems to be no harm to health.

According to Table 4.10, the high physical fitness range for this same 20-year-old woman would be between 18 and 23 percent. The high physical fitness standard does not mean that you cannot be somewhat below this number. Many highly trained male athletes are as low as 3 percent, and some female distance runners have been measured at 6 percent body fat (which may not be healthy).

Scientists generally agree that the mortality rate is higher for obese people, and some evidence indicates that the same is true for underweight people. "Underweight" and "thin" do not necessarily mean the same

| Table 4.10 | Body Composition Classification According to Percent Body Fat |

MEN

Age	Underweight	Excellent	Good	Moderate	Overweight	Obese
≤19	<3	12.0	12.1–17.0	17.1–22.0	22.1–27.0	≥27.1
20–29	<3	13.0	13.1–18.0	18.1–23.0	23.1–28.0	≥28.1
30–39	<3	14.0	14.1–19.0	19.1–24.0	24.1–29.0	≥29.1
40–49	<3	15.0	15.1–20.0	20.1–25.0	25.1–30.0	≥30.1
≥50	<3	16.0	16.1–21.0	21.1–26.0	26.1–31.0	≥31.1

WOMEN

Age	Underweight	Excellent	Good	Moderate	Overweight	Significantly Overweight
≤19	<12	17.0	17.1–22.0	22.1–27.0	27.1–32.0	≥32.1
20–29	<12	18.0	18.1–23.0	23.1–28.0	28.1–33.0	≥33.1
30–39	<12	19.0	19.1–24.0	24.1–29.0	29.1–34.0	≥34.1
40–49	<12	20.0	20.1–25.0	25.1–30.0	30.1–35.0	≥35.1
≥50	<12	21.0	21.1–26.0	26.1–31.0	31.1–36.0	≥36.1

■ High physical fitness standard   Health fitness standard

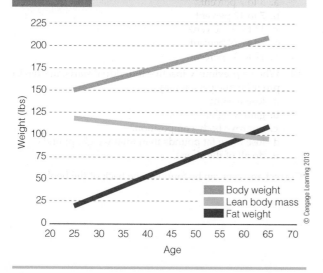

Figure 4.7 Typical body composition changes for adults in the United States.

Body weight
Lean body mass
Fat weight

© Cengage Learning 2013

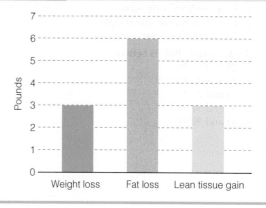

Figure 4.8 Effects of a 6-week aerobics exercise program on body composition.

Weight loss   Fat loss   Lean tissue gain

SOURCE: Hoeger, W.W.K., data collected at the University of Texas of the Permain Basin, 1985.

Assess Your Behavior

Log on to www.cengagebrain.com to access CengageNOW and the Behavior Change Planner where you can assess the behaviors that might benefit most from healthy change.

1. Do you know what your percent body fat is according to a reliable body composition assessment technique administered by a qualified technician?

2. Do you know your disease risk according to BMI and WC parameters?

3. Have you been able to maintain your body weight at a stable level during the past 12 months?

Assess Your Knowledge

Evaluate how well you understand the concepts presented in this chapter using the chapter-specific quizzing available in the online materials at www.cengagebrain.com.

1. Body composition incorporates
    a. a fat component.
    b. a non-fat component.
    c. percent body fat.
    d. lean body mass.
    e. all of the four components above.

2. Recommended body weight can be determined through
    a. body mass index.
    b. body composition analysis.
    c. BMI and waist circumference.
    d. waist circumference.
    e. all of the above.

3. Essential fat in women is
    a. 3 percent.
    b. 5 percent.
    c. 8 percent.
    d. 12 percent.
    e. 17 percent.

4. Which of the following is *not* a technique to assess body fat?
    a. body mass index
    b. skinfold thickness
    c. hydrostatic weighing
    d. circumference measurements
    e. air displacement

5. Which of the following sites is used to assess percent body fat according to skinfold thickness in men?
    a. suprailium
    b. chest
    c. scapular
    d. triceps
    e. All four sites are used.

6. Which variable is *not* used to assess percent body fat in women according to girth measurements?
    a. age
    b. hip
    c. wrist
    d. upper arm
    e. height

7. Waist circumference can be used to
   a. determine percent body fat.
   b. assess risk for disease.
   c. measure lean body mass.
   d. identify underweight people.
   e. All of the above are correct.

8. An acceptable BMI is between
   a. 15 and 18.49.
   b. 18.5 and 24.99.
   c. 25 and 29.99.
   d. 30 and 34.99.
   e. 35 and 39.99.

9. The health fitness percent body fat for women of various ages is in the range of
   a. 3 to 7 percent.
   b. 7 to 12 percent.
   c. 12 to 20 percent.
   d. 20 to 27 percent.
   e. 27 to 31 percent.

10. When a previously inactive individual starts an exercise program, the person may
    a. lose weight.
    b. gain weight.
    c. improve body composition.
    d. lose more fat pounds than total weight pounds.
    e. do all of the above.

Correct answers can be found at the back of the book.

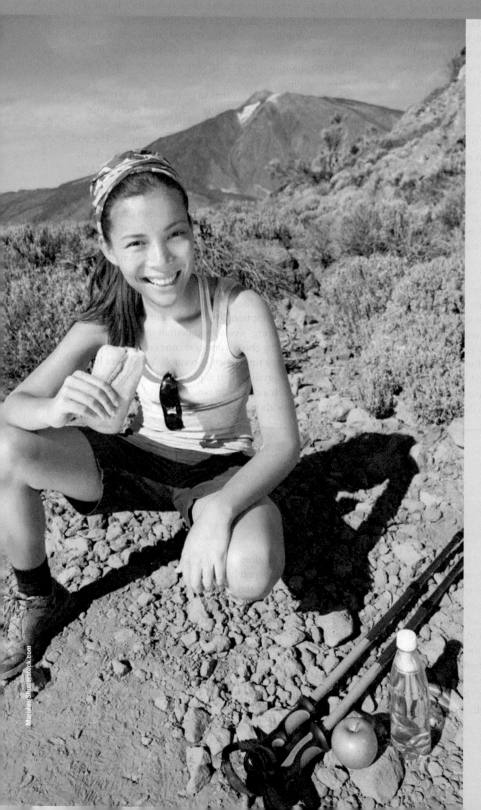

Weight Management

"Physical activity is the cornerstone of any sound weight management program. If you are unwilling to increase daily physical activity, do not attempt to lose weight because most likely you won't be able to keep it off."

Objectives

▶ **Describe** the health consequences of obesity.

▶ **Expose** some popular fad diets and myths and fallacies regarding weight control.

▶ **Describe** eating disorders and their associated medical problems and behavior patterns, and outline the need for professional help in treating these conditions.

▶ **Explain** the physiology of weight loss, including setpoint theory and the effects of diet on basal metabolic rate.

▶ **Explain** the role of a lifetime exercise program as the key to a successful weight loss and weight maintenance program.

▶ **Be able** to implement a physiologically sound weight reduction and weight maintenance program.

▶ **Describe** behavior modification techniques that help support adherence to a lifetime weight maintenance program.

CENGAGEbrain

On your exercise log, check your progress.

Visit www.cengagebrain.com to access course materials and companion resources for this text including quiz questions designed to check your understanding of the chapter contents. See the preface on page xv for more information.

What is more important for weight loss: a negative caloric balance (diet) or increasing physical activity? Most of the research shows that weight loss is more effective when you cut back on calories (dieting), as opposed to only increasing physical activity or exercise. Weight loss is more effective, nonetheless, when 150 or more minutes of physical activity per week are added to dieting. Body composition changes are also much more effective when dieting and exercise are combined while attempting to lose body weight. Most of the weight loss when dieting with exercise comes in the form of body fat and not lean body tissue, a desirable outcome. Weight loss maintenance, however, in most cases is possible only with 60 to 90 minutes of sustained daily physical activity or exercise.

Does the time of day when calories are consumed matter in a weight loss program? The time of day when a person eats food appears to play a part in weight reduction. When attempting to lose weight, intake should consist of a minimum of 25 percent of the total daily calories for breakfast, 50 percent for lunch, and 25 percent or less at dinner. Also, try not to eat within three hours of going to bed. This is the time of day when your metabolism is slowest. Your caloric intake is less likely to be used for energy and more likely to be stored as fat.

Are some diet plans more effective than others? The term *diet* implies a negative caloric balance. A negative caloric balance means that you are consuming fewer calories than those required to maintain your current weight. When energy output surpasses energy intake, weight loss will occur. Popular diets differ widely in the food choices that you are allowed to have. The more limited the choices, the lower the chances to overeat, and thus you will have a lower caloric intake. And the fewer the calories that you consume, the greater the weight loss. For health reasons, to obtain the variety of nutrients the body needs, even during weight loss periods, you should not consume fewer than 1,500 calories per day (except very small individuals). These calories should be distributed over a wide range of foods, emphasizing grains, fruits, vegetables, and small amounts of low-fat animal products or fish.

Why is it so difficult to change dietary habits? In most developed countries, there is an overabundance of food and practically an unlimited number of food choices. With unlimited supply and choices, most people do not have the willpower, stemming from their core values, to avoid overconsumption.

Our bodies were not created to go hungry or to overeat. We are uncomfortable overeating and we feel even worse when we have to go hungry. Our health values, however, are not strong enough to prevent overconsumption. The end result: weight gain. Next, we restrict calories (go on a diet), we feel hungry, and we have a difficult time adhering to the diet. Stated quite simply, going hungry is an uncomfortable and unpleasant experience.

To avoid this vicious cycle, our dietary habits (and most likely physical activity habits) must change. A question you need to ask yourself is: Do you value health and quality of life more than food overindulgence? If you do not, then the achievement and maintenance of recommended body weight and good health is a moot point. If you desire to avoid disease and increase quality of life, you have to value health more than food overconsumption. If we have spent the past 20 years tasting and "devouring" every food item in sight, it is now time to make healthy choices and consume only moderate amounts of food at a time (portion control). You do not have to taste and eat everything that is placed before your eyes. If you can make such a change in your eating habits, you may not have to worry about another diet for the rest of your life.

Real Life Story David's Experience

I played high school football and I knew I was in real good shape and had a lot of muscle. After high school, my football days were over. My freshman year in college took some adjustment, even more so being away from home and all my buddies. I wasn't exercising and gained 12 pounds that year. At 192 pounds, I still thought I was in pretty good shape. My sophomore year I stopped at the school's annual health and fitness fair during the fall semester. There I had my body fat checked. It turned out to be 26.5 percent. I always thought I was pretty fit and I wasn't happy to be rated "overweight." That one body fat test motivated me to enroll in the fitness and wellness course. In class, I learned how to set up a good aerobic and strength-training exercise program, eat better, and the value of increasing daily physical activity. At the end of the semester I had only lost eight pounds, but I was 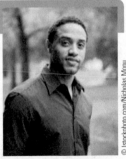 pleasantly surprised to find out that I had also gained seven pounds of lean body mass (in essence I lost 15 pounds of body fat) and my body fat decreased to 19.6 percent.

© istockphoto.com/Nicholas Monu

Personal Lifetime Weight Management Program

I. **Do you understand the concept of recommended body weight and do you consider yourself to be at this weight?**
_____ Yes _____ No

II. **What type of exercise program do you consider most effective for weight management: aerobic exercise or strength training?**

III. **Have you gained weight since you started college? If so, what do you attribute this weight gain to?**

IV. **What can you learn from David's experience and what strategies can you use to help you properly manage your body weight?**

V. **Do you understand the concept of long-term gratification derived through a lifetime exercise program and the required process to do so?**

Obesity is a health hazard of epidemic proportions in most developed countries around the world. According to the World Health Organization, an estimated 35 percent of the adult population in industrialized nations is obese. Obesity has been defined as a body mass index (BMI) of 30 or higher. The obesity level is the point at which excess body fat can lead to serious health problems.

The number of people who are obese and overweight in the United States has increased dramatically, a direct result of physical inactivity and poor dietary habits. The average weight of American adults between the ages of 20 and 74 has increased by 25 pounds or more since 1965. More than one-half of all adults in the United States do not achieve the minimum recommended amount of physical activity (see Figure 1.8, page 11). In 2004, American women consumed 335 more calories daily than they had 20 years earlier, and men an additional 170 calories per day.[1]

About 68 percent of U.S. adults age 20 and older are overweight (have a BMI greater than 25), and 34 percent are obese (see Figure 5.1).[2] More than 120 million people are overweight and 30 million are obese. Between 1960 and 2002, the overall (men and women combined) prevalence of adult obesity increased from about 13 percent to 30 percent. Most of this increase occurred in the 1990s.

As illustrated in Figure 5.2, the obesity epidemic continues to escalate. Before 1990, not a single state reported an obesity rate above 15 percent of the state's total population (includes both adults and children). By the year 2009, only Colorado and the District of Columbia had an obesity rate below 20 percent, and 33 states had an obesity rate equal to or greater than 25 percent, including nine states with a rate above 30 percent.

In the past decade alone, the average weight of American adults increased by about 15 pounds. The prevalence of obesity is even higher in certain ethnic groups, especially African Americans and Hispanic Americans.

Further, as the nation continues to evolve into a more mechanized and automated society (relying on escalators, elevators, remote controls, computers, e-mail, cell phones, and automatic-sensor doors), the amount of required daily physical activity continues to decrease. We are being lulled into a high-risk sedentary lifestyle.

More than a third of the population is on a diet at any given moment. People spend about $40 billion yearly attempting to lose weight, with more than $10 billion going to memberships in weight reduction centers and another $30 billion to diet food sales. Furthermore, the total cost attributable to treating obesity-related diseases is estimated at $117 billion per year.[3]

Excessive body weight combined with physical inactivity is the second leading cause of preventable death in the United States, causing more than 112,000 deaths each year.[4] Furthermore, obesity is more prevalent than

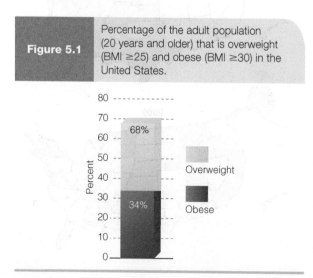

Figure 5.1 Percentage of the adult population (20 years and older) that is overweight (BMI ≥25) and obese (BMI ≥30) in the United States.

SOURCE: Centers for Disease Control and Prevention, 2010.

Figure 5.2   Obesity trends in the United States, 1985–2010, based on BMI ≥30 or 30 pounds overweight.

Percentages of the total number of people in the respective state who are obese.

○ No data   ○ <10%   ○ 10–14%   ○ 15–19%   ● 20–24%   ● 25–29%   ● ≥30%

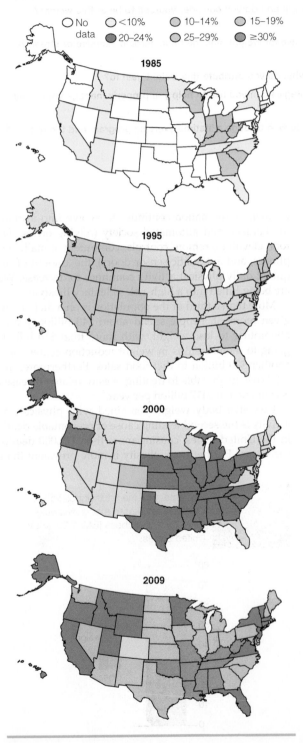

1985

1995

2000

2009

SOURCE: *Obesity Trends Among U.S. Adults Between 1985 and 2006* (Atlanta: Centers for Disease Control and Prevention, 2010).

smoking (19 percent), poverty (14 percent), and problem drinking (6 percent).[5] Obesity and unhealthy lifestyle habits are the most critical public health problems we face in the 21st century.

Excessive body weight and obesity are associated with poor health status and are risk factors for many physical ailments, including cardiovascular disease, type 2 diabetes, and some types of cancer. Evidence indicates that health risks associated with increased body weight start at a BMI over 25 and are enhanced greatly at a BMI over 30.

The American Heart Association has identified obesity as one of the six major risk factors for coronary heart disease. Estimates also indicate that 14 percent of all cancer deaths in men and 20 percent in women are related to current overweight and obesity patterns in the United States.[6] Excessive body weight also is implicated in psychological maladjustment and a higher accidental death rate. Extremely obese people have a lower mental health–related quality of life.

Health Consequences of Excessive Body Weight

Being overweight or obese increases the risk for

- high blood pressure
- elevated blood lipids (high blood cholesterol and triglycerides)
- type 2 (non–insulin-dependent) diabetes
- insulin resistance, glucose intolerance
- coronary heart disease
- angina pectoris
- congestive heart failure
- stroke
- gallbladder disease
- gout
- osteoarthritis
- obstructive sleep apnea and respiratory problems
- some types of cancer (endometrial, breast, prostate, and colon)
- complications of pregnancy (gestational diabetes, gestational hypertension, preeclampsia, and complications during C-sections)
- poor female reproductive health (menstrual irregularities, infertility, irregular ovulation)
- bladder control problems (stress incontinence)
- psychological disorders (depression, eating disorders, distorted body image, discrimination, and low self-esteem)
- shortened life expectancy
- decreased quality of life

SOURCE: Centers for Disease Control and Prevention, downloaded March 30, 2011.

Overweight versus Obesity

Overweight and obesity are not the same thing. Many overweight people (who weigh about 10 to 20 pounds over the recommended weight) are not obese. Although a few pounds of excess weight may not be harmful to most people, this is not always the case. People with excessive body fat who have type 2 diabetes and other cardiovascular risk factors (elevated blood lipids, high blood pressure, physical inactivity, and poor eating habits) benefit from losing weight. People who have a few extra pounds of weight but are otherwise healthy and physically active, exercise regularly, and eat a healthy diet may not be at higher risk for early death. Such is not the case, however, with obese individuals.

Research indicates that individuals who are 30 or more pounds overweight during middle age (30 to 49 years of age) lose about seven years of life, whereas being 10 to 30 pounds overweight decreases the lifespan by about three years.[7] These decreases are similar to those seen with tobacco use. Severe obesity (BMI greater than 45) at a young age, nonetheless, may cut up to 20 years off one's life.[8]

Although the loss of years of life is significant, the decreased life expectancy doesn't even begin to address the loss in quality of life and increase in illness and disability throughout the years. Even a modest reduction of two to three percent can reduce the risk for chronic diseases, including heart disease, high blood pressure, high cholesterol, and diabetes.[9]

A primary objective to achieve overall physical fitness and enhanced quality of life is to attain recommended body composition. Individuals at recommended body weight are able to participate in a wide variety of moderate to vigorous activities without functional limitations. These people have the freedom to enjoy most of life's recreational activities to their fullest potential. Excessive body weight does not afford an individual the fitness

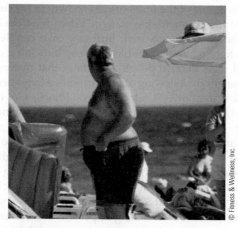

Obesity is a health hazard of epidemic proportions in industrialized nations.

© Fitness & Wellness, Inc.

level to enjoy many lifetime activities such as basketball, soccer, racquetball, surfing, mountain cycling, or mountain climbing. Maintaining high fitness and recommended body weight gives a person a degree of independence throughout life that most people in developed nations no longer enjoy.

Scientific evidence also recognizes problems with being underweight. Although the social pressure to be thin has declined slightly in recent years, the pressure to attain model-like thinness is still with us and contributes to the gradual increase in the number of people who develop eating disorders (anorexia nervosa and bulimia, discussed under "Eating Disorders" on pages 151–153).

Extreme weight loss can lead to medical conditions such as heart damage, gastrointestinal problems, shrinkage of internal organs, abnormalities of the immune system, disorders of the reproductive system, loss of muscle tissue, damage to the nervous system, and even death. About 14 percent of people in the United States are underweight.

> **Critical Thinking**
>
> Do you consider yourself overweight? • If so, how long have you had a weight problem, what attempts have you made to lose weight, and what has worked best for you?

Tolerable Weight

Many people want to lose weight so they will look better. That's a worthy goal. The problem, however, is that they have a distorted image of what they would really look like if they were to reduce to what they think is their ideal weight. Hereditary factors play a big role, and only a small fraction of the population has the genes for a "perfect body."

The media have the greatest influence on people's perception of what constitutes "ideal" body weight. Most people consult fashion, fitness, and beauty magazines to determine what they should look like. The "ideal" body shapes, physiques, and proportions illustrated in these magazines are rare and are achieved mainly through airbrushing and medical reconstruction.[10] Many individuals, primarily young women, go to extremes in attempts to achieve these unrealistic figures. Failure to attain a "perfect body" may lead to eating disorders in some individuals.

When people set their own target weight, they should be realistic. Attaining the "Excellent" percent of body fat shown in Table 4.10 (page 134) is extremely difficult for some. It is even more difficult to maintain over time, unless the person makes a commitment to a vigorous lifetime exercise program and permanent dietary changes. Few people are willing to do that. The "Moderate" percent body fat category may be more realistic for many people.

The question you should ask yourself is: Am I happy with my weight? Part of enjoying a higher quality of life is being happy with yourself. If you are not, you need to either do something about it or learn to live with it.

If your percent of body fat is higher than those in the Moderate category of Table 4.10 in Chapter 4, you should try to reduce it and stay in this category for health reasons. This is the category that seems to pose no detriment to health.

If you are in the Moderate category but would like to reduce your percent of body fat further, you need to ask yourself a second question: How badly do I want it? Do I want it badly enough to implement lifetime exercise and dietary changes? If you are not willing to change, you should stop worrying about your weight and deem the Moderate category "tolerable" for you.

The Weight Loss Dilemma

Yo-yo dieting carries as great a health risk as being overweight and remaining overweight in the first place. Epidemiological data show that frequent fluctuations in weight (up or down) markedly increase the risk for dying from cardiovascular disease. Based on the findings that constant losses and regains can be hazardous to health, quick-fix diets should be replaced by a slow but permanent weight loss program (as described under "Losing Weight the Sound and Sensible Way," page 165). Individuals reap the benefits of recommended body weight when they get to that weight and stay there throughout life.

Unfortunately, only about 10 percent of all people who begin a traditional weight loss program without exercise are able to lose the desired weight. Worse, only 5 in 100 are able to keep the weight off. The body is highly resistant to permanent weight changes through caloric restrictions alone.

Traditional diets have failed because few of them incorporate permanent behavioral changes in food selection and an overall increase in physical activity and exercise as fundamental to successful weight loss and weight maintenance. When the diet stops, weight gain begins. The $40 billion diet industry tries to capitalize on the false idea that a person can lose weight quickly without considering the consequences of fast weight loss or the importance of lifetime behavioral changes to ensure proper weight loss and maintenance.

In addition, various studies indicate that most people, especially obese people, underestimate their energy intake. Those who try to lose weight but apparently fail to do so are often described as "diet resistant." One study found that while on a "diet," a group of obese individuals with a self-reported history of diet resistance underreported their average daily caloric intake by almost 50 percent (1,028 self-reported versus 2,081 actual calories) (see Figure 5.3).[11] These individuals also over-

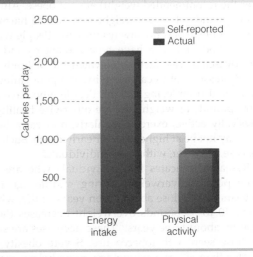

Figure 5.3 Differences between self-reported and actual daily caloric intake and exercise in obese individuals attempting to lose weight.

SOURCE: Lichtman, S. W., et al. "Discrepancy Between Self-Reported and Actual Caloric Intake and Exercise in Obese Subjects," *New England Journal of Medicine* 327 (1992): 1893–1898.

estimated their amount of daily physical activity by about 25 percent (1,022 self-reported versus 771 actual calories). These differences represent an additional 1,304 calories of energy per day unaccounted for by the subjects in the study. The findings indicate that failing to lose weight often is related to misreports of actual food intake and level of physical activity.

Diet Crazes

Capitalizing on hopes that the latest diet to hit the market will really work this time, fad diets continue to appeal to people of all shapes and sizes. These diets may work for a while, but their success is usually short-lived. Regarding the effectiveness of these diets, Dr. Kelly Brownell, one of the foremost researchers in the field of weight management, has stated: "When I get the latest diet fad, I imagine a trick birthday cake candle that keeps lighting up and we have to keep blowing it out."

Fad diets deceive people and claim that dieters will lose weight by following all instructions. Many diets are very low in calories. Under these conditions, a lot of the weight lost is in the form of water and protein, and not fat.

On average, a 150-pound person stores about 1.3 pounds of glycogen (carbohydrate or glucose storage) in the body. This amount of glycogen is higher in aerobically trained individuals, as intense training (elite athletes) can more than double the body's capacity to store glycogen. About 80 percent of the glycogen is stored in muscles and the remaining 20 percent in the liver. Water, however, is required to store glycogen. A 2.6-to-1 water to glycogen ratio is necessary to store **glycogen**.[12]

Thus, our 150-pound person stores about 3.4 pounds of water (1.3 × 2.6), along with the 1.3 pounds of glycogen, accounting for a total of 4.7 pounds of the person's normal body weight.

When fasting or on a crash diet (typically defined as less than 800 calories per day), glycogen storage can be completely depleted in just a few days. This loss of weight is not in the form of body fat and is typically used to promote and guarantee rapid weight loss with many fad diets on the market today. When the person resumes a normal eating plan, the body will again store its glycogen, along with the water required to do so, and subsequent weight gain.

Furthermore, on a crash diet, close to half the weight loss is in lean (protein) tissue. When the body uses protein instead of a combination of fats and carbohydrates as a source of energy, weight is lost as much as 10 times faster. This is because a gram of protein produces half the amount of energy that fat does. In the case of muscle protein, one-fifth of protein is mixed with four-fifths water. Therefore, each pound of muscle yields only one-tenth the amount of energy of a pound of fat. As a result, most of the weight lost is in the form of water, which on the scale, of course, looks good.

Long-term crash dieting also increases the risk of heart attacks because low calorie intake eventually leads to heart muscle (protein) loss. Limiting potassium, magnesium, and cooper intake as a result of very low calorie diets may induce fatal cardiac arrhythmias. Furthermore, sodium depletion may cause a dangerous drop in blood pressure. Very low calorie diets should always be followed under a physician's supervision. Unfortunately, most crash dieters simply consult a friend rather than seek a physician's advice.

Diet books are frequently found on best-seller lists. The market is flooded with these books. Examples include the Volumetrics Eating Plan, the Ornish Diet, the Atkins Diet, the Zone Diet, the South Beach Diet, the Best Life Diet, the Abs Diet, and You on a Diet. Some of these popular diets are becoming more nutritionally balanced and encourage consumption of fruits and vegetables, whole grains, some lean meat and fish, and low-fat milk and dairy products. Such plans reduce the risk for chronic diseases, including cardiovascular diseases and cancer.

While it is clear that some diets are healthier than others, strictly from a weight loss point of view, it doesn't matter what diet plan you follow, if caloric intake is lower than your caloric output, weight will come off. Dropout rates for many popular diets, however, are high because of the difficulty in long-term adherence to limited dietary plans.

Low-Carb Diets

Among the most popular diets on the market in recent years were the low-carbohydrate/high-protein (LCHP) diet plans. Although they vary slightly, low-carb diets, in general, limit the intake of carbohydrate-rich foods—bread, potatoes, rice, pasta, cereals, crackers, juices, sodas, sweets (candy, cake, cookies), and even fruits and vegetables. Dieters are allowed to eat all the protein-rich foods they desire, including steak, ham, chicken, fish, bacon, eggs, nuts, cheese, tofu, high-fat salad dressings, butter, and small amounts of a few fruits and vegetables. Typically, these diets also are high in fat content. Examples of these diets are the Atkins Diet, the Zone, Protein Power, the Scarsdale Diet, the Carb Addict's Diet, the South Beach Diet, and Sugar Busters.

During digestion, carbohydrates are converted into glucose, a basic fuel used by every cell in the body. As blood glucose rises, the pancreas releases insulin. Insulin is a hormone that facilitates the entry of glucose into the cells, thereby lowering the glucose level in the bloodstream. A rapid rise in glucose also causes a rapid spike in insulin, which is followed by a rapid removal and drop in blood glucose that leaves you hungry again. A slower rise in blood glucose is desirable because the level is kept constant longer, delaying the onset of hunger. If the cells don't need the glucose for normal cell functions or to fuel physical activity, and if cellular glucose stores are already full, glucose is converted to, and stored as, body fat.

Not all carbohydrates cause a similar rise in blood glucose. The rise in glucose is based on the speed of digestion, which depends on a number of factors, including the size of the food particles. Small-particle carbohydrates break down rapidly and cause a quick, sharp rise in blood glucose. Thus, to gauge a food's effect on blood glucose, carbohydrates are classified by their **glycemic index**.

A high glycemic index signifies a food that causes a quick rise in blood glucose. At the top of the 100-point scale is glucose itself. This index is not directly related to simple and complex carbohydrates, and the glycemic values are not always what one might expect. Rather, the index is based on the actual laboratory-measured speed of absorption. Processed foods generally have a high glycemic index, whereas high-fiber foods tend to have a lower index (see Table 5.1). Other factors that affect the index are the amount of carbohydrate, fat, and protein in the food; how refined the ingredients are; and whether the food was cooked.

The body functions best when blood sugar remains at a constant level. Although this is best accomplished by

Glycogen Manner in which carbohydrates (glucose molecules) are stored in the human body, predominantly in the liver and muscles.

Glycemic index A measure that is used to rate the plasma glucose response of carbohydrate-containing foods with the response produced by the same amount of carbohydrate from a standard source, usually glucose or white bread.

Popular Diets

The Volumetrics Eating Plan

Diet plan that focuses on maximizing the volume of food and limiting calories by emphasizing high-water-content/ low-fat foods (lower energy density), low-fat cooking techniques, and extensive use of vegetables. The average daily caloric intake is reduced by 500–1,000 calories, with a macronutrient composition of approximately 55% carbohydrates, less than 20–30% fat, and more than 20% protein.

The Best Life Diet

The initial phase of the diet plan encourages exercise and a recommended eating schedule. The second phase requires a reduction in caloric intake through consumption of healthful foods to satisfy hunger. The plan deals extensively with "emotional eating." Caloric intake averages about 1,700 with maintenance of daily moderate physical activity. The diet composition is about 50% carbohydrates, 30% fat, and 20% protein.

Ornish Diet

Very low fat, vegetarian-type diet. Dieters are not allowed to drink alcohol or eat meat, fish, oils, sugar, or white flour. Data indicate that strict adherence to the Ornish Diet can prevent and reverse heart disease. An average daily caloric intake is about 1,500, composed of approximately 75% carbohydrates, 15% protein, and less than 10% fat.

The Zone Diet

The diet proposes that proper macronutrient (carbohydrate/ fat/protein) distribution is critical to keep blood sugar and hormones in balance to prevent weight gain and disease. All meals need to provide 40% carbohydrate calories, 30% fat calories, and 30% protein calories. Daily caloric allowance is about 1,100 for women and 1,400 for men.

Atkins Diet

A low-carbohydrate/high-protein diet. Practically all carbohydrates are eliminated the first two weeks of the diet. Thereafter, very small amounts of carbohydrates are allowed, primarily in the form of limited fruits, vegetables, and wine. No caloric guidelines are given, but a typical daily diet plan is about 1,500 calories, extremely high in fat (about 60% of calories), followed by protein (about 30% of calories), and limited carbohydrates (about 10% of calories). Dieters may not be as hungry on the Atkins Diet, but they tend to find it too restrictive for long-term adherence.

The South Beach Diet

Also a low-carbohydrate/high-protein diet, but not as restrictive as the Atkins Diet. Emphasizes low-glycemic foods thought to decrease cravings for sugar and refined carbohydrates. Sugar, fruits, and grains are initially eliminated. In phase 2, some high-fiber grains, fruit, and dark chocolate are permitted. No caloric guidelines are given, but a typical dietary plan provides about 1,400 calories per day composed of 40% fat, 40% carbohydrate, and 20% protein.

consuming foods with a low glycemic index (nuts, apples, oranges, low-fat yogurt), a person does not have to eliminate all high-glycemic index foods (sugar, potatoes, bread, white rice, soda drinks) from the diet. Foods with a high glycemic index along with some protein are useful to replenish depleted glycogen stores following prolonged or exhaustive aerobic exercise. Combining high- with low-glycemic index items or with some fat and protein brings down the average index.

Regular consumption of high-glycemic foods by themselves may increase the risk for cardiovascular disease, especially in people at risk for diabetes. A person does not need to plan the diet around the index itself, as many popular diet programs indicate. The glycemic index deals with single foods eaten alone. Most people eat high-glycemic index foods in combination with other foods as part of a meal. In combination, these foods have a lower effect on blood sugar. Even people at risk for diabetes or who have the disease can eat high-glycemic foods in moderation.

Low-glycemic foods may also aid in weight loss and weight maintenance. As blood sugar levels drop between snacks and meals, hunger increases. Keeping

blood sugar levels constant by including low-glycemic foods in the diet helps stave off hunger, appetite, and overeating (see Figure 5.4).

Proponents of LCHP diets claim that if a person eats fewer carbohydrates and more protein, the pancreas will produce less insulin, and as insulin drops, the body will turn to its own fat deposits for energy. There is no scientific proof, however, that high levels of insulin lead to weight gain. None of the authors of these diets published any studies validating their claims. Yet, these authors base their diets on the faulty premise that high insulin leads to obesity. We know the opposite to be true: Excessive body fat causes insulin levels to rise, thereby increasing the risk for developing diabetes.

The reason for rapid weight loss in LCHP dieting is that a low carbohydrate intake forces the liver to produce glucose. The source for most of this glucose is body proteins— your lean body mass, including muscle. As indicated earlier, protein is mostly water; thus, weight is lost rapidly. When a person terminates the diet, the body rebuilds some of the protein tissue and quickly regains some weight.

Research studies indicated that individuals on an LCHP (Atkins) diet lost slightly more weight in the first

Table 5.1		Glycemic Index of Selected Foods	
Item	**Index**	**Item**	**Index**
All-Bran cereal	38	Milk, chocolate	43
Apples	40	Milk, chocolate, low-fat	34
Bagel, white	72	Milk, skim	32
Banana	56	Milk, whole	40
Bread, French	95	Jelly beans	80
Bread, wheat	73	Oatmeal	75
Bread, white	70	Oranges	48
Carrots, boiled (Australia)	41	Pasta, white	50
Carrots, boiled (Canada)	92	Pasta, wheat	32
Carrots, raw	47	Peanuts	20
Cherries	20	Peas	50
Colas	65	Pizza, cheese	60
Corn, sweet	60	Potato, baked	56–100
Corn Flakes	92	Potato, French fries	75
Doughnut	76	Potato, sweet	51
Frosted Flakes	55	Rice, white	56
Fruit cocktail	55	Sugar, table	65
Gatorade	78	Watermelon	72
Glucose	100	Yogurt, low-fat	32
Honey	58		

© Cengage Learning 2013

few months than those on a low-fat diet.[13] The effectiveness of the diet, however, seemed to dwindle over time. In one of the studies, at 12 months into the diet, participants in the LCHP diet had regained more weight than those on the low-fat diet plan.

Years of research will be required to determine the extent to which adhering over the long term to LCHP diets increases the risk for heart disease, cancer, and kid-

Are Low-Carb/High Protein Diets More Effective?

A few studies suggest that, at least over the short-term, low-carb/high-protein (LCHP) diets are more effective in producing weight loss then carbohydrate-based diets. These results are preliminary and controversial. In LCHP diets:

- A large amount of weight loss is water and muscle protein, not body fat. Some of this weight is quickly regained when regular dietary habits are resumed.
- Few people are able to stay with LCHP diets for more than a few weeks at a time. The majority stop dieting before the targeted program completion.
- LCHP dieters are rarely found in a national weight loss registry of people who have lost 30 pounds and kept them off for a minimum of 6 years.
- Food choices are severely restricted in LCHP diets. With less variety, individuals tend to eat less (800 to 1,200 calories/day) and thus lose more weight.
- LCHP diets may promote heart disease, cancer, and increase the risk for osteoporosis.
- LCHP diets are fundamentally high in fat (about 60 percent fat calories).
- LCHP diets are not recommended for people with diabetes, high blood pressure, heart disease, or kidney disease.
- LCHP diets do not promote long-term healthy eating patterns.

ney or bone damage. Low-carb diets are contrary to the nutrition advice of most national leading health organizations (which recommend a diet lower in saturated fat and trans fats and high in complex carbohydrates). Without fruits, vegetables, and whole grains, high-protein

Figure 5.4	Effects of high- and low-glycemic carbohydrate intake on blood glucose levels.

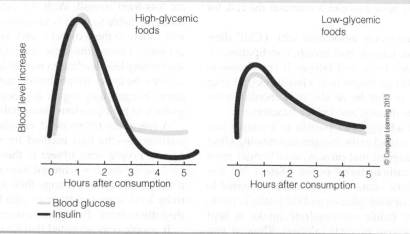

© Cengage Learning 2013

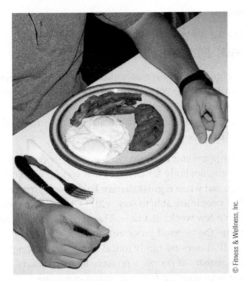

Long-term adherence to a low-carbohydrate/high-protein diet creates nutritional deficiencies and contributes to the development of cardiovascular disease, cancer, and osteoporosis.

diets lack many vitamins, minerals, antioxidants, phytonutrients, and fiber—all dietary factors that protect against an array of ailments and diseases.

The major risk associated with long-term adherence to LCHP diets could be the increased risk for heart disease, because high-protein foods are also high in fat content (see Chapter 10). Short-term (a few weeks or months) adherence to LCHP diets does not appear to increase heart disease risk. The long-term (years) effects of these types of diet, nonetheless, have not been evaluated by scientific research (very few people would be willing to adhere to such a diet for several years). A possible long-term adverse effect of adherence to an LCHP diet is a potential increase in cancer risk. Phytonutrients found in fruits, vegetables, and whole grains protect against certain types of cancer. A low-carbohydrate intake also produces a loss of vitamin B, calcium, and potassium. Potential bone loss can accentuate the risk for osteoporosis.

Side effects commonly associated with LCHP diets include weakness, nausea, bad breath, constipation, irritability, lightheadedness, and fatigue. If you choose to go on an LCHP diet for longer than a few weeks, let your physician know so that he or she may monitor your blood lipids, bone density, and kidney function.

The benefit of adding extra protein to a weight loss program may be related to the hunger-suppressing effect of protein. Data suggest that protein curbs hunger more effectively than carbohydrates or fat. Dieters feel less hungry when caloric intake from protein is increased to about 30 percent of total calories and fat intake is cut to about 20 percent (while carbohydrate intake is kept constant at 50 percent of total calories). Thus, if you struggle with frequent hunger pangs, try to include 10 to

How to Recognize Fad Diets

Fad diets have characteristics in common. These diets typically

- are nutritionally unbalanced.
- rely primarily on a single food (for example, grapefruit).
- are based on testimonials.
- were developed according to "confidential research."
- are based on a "scientific breakthrough."
- promote rapid and "painless" weight loss.
- promise miraculous results.
- restrict food selection.
- are based on pseudo claims that excessive weight is related to a specific condition such as insulin resistance, combinations or timing of nutrient intake, food allergies, hormone imbalances, certain foods (fruits, for example).
- require the use of selected products.
- use liquid formulas instead of foods.
- misrepresent salespeople as individuals qualified to provide nutrition counseling.
- fail to provide information on risks associated with weight loss and of the diet use.
- do not involve physical activity.
- do not encourage healthy behavioral changes.
- are not supported by the scientific community or national health organizations.
- fail to provide information for weight maintenance upon completion of the diet phase.

15 grams of lean protein with each meal. This amount of protein is the equivalent of one and a half ounces of lean meat (beef, fowl, or fish), two tablespoons of natural peanut butter, or eight ounces of plain low-fat yogurt.

The reason why many of these diets succeed is because they restrict a large number of foods. Thus, people tend to eat less food overall. With the extraordinary variety of foods available to us, it is unrealistic to think that people will adhere to these diets for very long. People eventually get tired of eating the same thing day in and day out and start eating less, leading to weight loss. If they happen to achieve the lower weight but do not make permanent dietary changes, they regain the weight quickly once they go back to their previous eating habits.

A few diets recommend exercise along with caloric restrictions—the best method for weight reduction, of course. People who adhere to these programs will succeed, so the diet has achieved its purpose. Unfortunately, if the people do not change their food selection and activity level permanently, they gain back the weight once they discontinue dieting and exercise.

If people only accepted that no magic foods will provide all of the necessary nutrients and that a person has to eat a variety of foods to be well nourished, dieters would be more successful and the diet industry would go broke. Also, let's not forget that we eat for pleasure and for health. Two of the most essential components of a wellness lifestyle are healthy eating and regular physical activity, and they provide the best weight management program available today.

Eating Disorders

Eating disorders are medical illnesses that involve crucial disturbances in eating behaviors thought to stem from some combination of environmental pressures. These disorders are characterized by an intense fear of becoming fat, which does not disappear even when the person is losing weight in extreme amounts. The three most common types of eating disorders are **anorexia nervosa**, **bulimia nervosa**, and **binge-eating disorder**. A fourth disorder, **emotional eating**, can also be listed under disordered eating.

Most people who have eating disorders are afflicted by significant family and social problems. They may lack fulfillment in many areas of their lives. The eating disorder then becomes the coping mechanism to avoid dealing with these problems. Taking control over their own body weight helps them believe that they are restoring some sense of control over their lives.

Anorexia nervosa and bulimia nervosa are common in industrialized nations where society encourages low calorie diets and thinness. The female role in society has changed rapidly, which makes women more susceptible to eating disorders. Although frequently seen in young women, eating disorders are most prevalent among individuals between the ages of 25 and 50. Surveys, nonetheless, indicate that as many as 40 percent of college-age women are struggling with an eating disorder.

Eating disorders are not limited to women. Every 1 in 10 cases occurs in men. But because men's role and body image are viewed differently in our society, these cases often go unreported.

Although genetics may play a role in the development of eating disorders, most cases are environmentally related. Individuals who have clinical depression and obsessive-compulsive behavior are more susceptible. About half of all people with eating disorders have some sort of chemical dependency (alcohol and drugs), and most of them come from families with alcohol- and drug-related problems. Of reported cases of eating disorders, a large number are individuals who are, or have been, victims of sexual molestation.

Eating disorders develop in stages. Typically, individuals who are already dealing with significant issues in life start a diet. At first they feel in control and are happy about the weight loss, even if they are not overweight. Encouraged by the prospect of weight loss and the control they can exert over their own weight, the dieting becomes

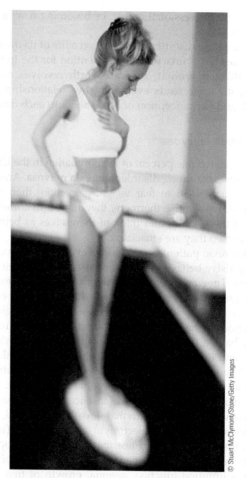

Society's unrealistic view of what constitutes recommended weight and "ideal" body image contributes to the development of eating disorders.

extreme and often is combined with exhaustive exercise and the overuse of laxatives and diuretics.

The syndrome typically emerges following emotional issues or a stressful life event and the uncertainty about one's ability to cope efficiently. Life experiences that can trigger the syndrome might be gaining weight, starting the menstrual period, beginning college, losing a boyfriend, having poor self-esteem, being socially rejected,

Key Terms

Anorexia nervosa An eating disorder characterized by self-imposed starvation to lose and maintain very low body weight.

Bulimia nervosa An eating disorder characterized by a pattern of binge eating and purging in an attempt to lose weight and maintain low body weight.

Binge-eating disorder An eating disorder characterized by uncontrollable episodes of eating excessive amounts of food within a relatively short time.

Emotional eating The consumption of large quantities of food to suppress negative emotions.

starting a professional career, or becoming a wife or a mother.

The eating disorder then takes on a life of its own and becomes the primary focus of attention for the individual afflicted with it. Her self-worth revolves around what the scale reads every day, her relationship with food, and her perception of how she looks each day.

Anorexia Nervosa

An estimated one percent of the population in the United States has the eating disorder **anorexia nervosa**. Anorexic individuals seem to fear weight gain more than death from starvation. Furthermore, they have a distorted image of their bodies and think of themselves as being fat even when they are emaciated.

Anorexic patients commonly develop obsessive and compulsive behaviors and emphatically deny their condition. They are preoccupied with food, meal planning, and grocery shopping, and they have unusual eating habits. As they lose weight and their health begins to deteriorate, they feel weak and tired. They might realize they have a problem, but they will not stop the starvation, and refuse to consider the behavior abnormal.

Once they have lost a lot of weight and malnutrition sets in, the physical changes become more visible. Typical changes are amenorrhea (absence of menstruation), digestive problems, extreme sensitivity to cold, hair problems, fluid and electrolyte abnormalities (which may lead to an irregular heartbeat and sudden stopping of the heart), injuries to nerves and tendons, abnormalities of immune function, anemia, growth of fine body hair, mental confusion, inability to concentrate, lethargy, depression, dry skin, lower skin and body temperature, and osteoporosis.

Diagnostic criteria for anorexia nervosa are[14]:

- Refusal to maintain body weight over a minimal normal weight for age and height (weight loss leading to maintenance of body weight less than 85 percent of that expected, or failure to make expected weight gain during periods of growth, leading to body weight less than 85 percent of that expected)
- Intense fear of gaining weight or becoming fat, even though underweight
- Disturbance in the way in which one's body weight, size, or shape is perceived, undue influences of body weight or shape on self-evaluation, or denial of the seriousness of the current low body weight
- In postmenarcheal females, amenorrhea (absence of at least three consecutive menstrual cycles) (A woman is considered to have amenorrhea if her periods occur only following estrogen therapy.)

Many of the changes induced by anorexia nervosa can be reversed. Individuals with this condition can get better with professional therapy, or they sometimes turn to bulimia nervosa, or they die from the disorder. Anorexia nervosa has the highest mortality rate of all psychosomatic illnesses today—20 percent of anorexic individuals die as a result of their condition. The disorder is 100 percent curable, but treatment almost always requires professional help. The sooner it is started, the better are the chances for reversibility and cure. Therapy consists of a combination of medical and psychological techniques to restore proper nutrition, prevent medical complications, and modify the environment or events that triggered the syndrome.

Seldom can anorexia sufferers overcome the problem by themselves. They strongly deny their condition. They are able to hide it and deceive friends and relatives. Based on their behavior, many of them meet all of the characteristics of anorexia nervosa, but it goes undetected because both thinness and dieting are socially acceptable. Only a well-trained clinician is able to diagnose anorexia nervosa.

Bulimia Nervosa

Bulimia nervosa is more prevalent than anorexia nervosa. As many as one in five women on college campuses may be bulimic, according to some estimates. Bulimia nervosa also is more prevalent than anorexia nervosa in males, although bulimia is still much more prevalent in females.

People with bulimia usually are healthy looking, well educated, and near recommended body weight. They seem to enjoy food and often socialize around it. In actuality, they are emotionally insecure, rely on others, and lack self-confidence and self-esteem. Recommended weight and food are important to them.

The binge–purge cycle usually occurs in stages. As a result of stressful life events or the simple compulsion to eat, bulimic individuals engage periodically in binge eating that may last an hour or longer. With some apprehension, bulimics anticipate and plan the cycle. Next they feel an urgency to begin, followed by large and uncontrollable food consumption, during which time they may eat several thousand calories (up to 10,000 calories in extreme cases). After a short period of relief and satisfaction, feelings of deep guilt and shame and intense fear of gaining weight emerge. Purging seems to be an easy answer, as the bingeing cycle can continue without fear of gaining weight.

The diagnostic criteria for bulimia nervosa follow[15]:

- Recurrent episodes of binge eating. An episode of binge eating is characterized by both of the following: (a) eating in a discrete period of time (e.g., within any two-hour period) an amount of food that is definitely more than most people would eat during a similar period and under similar circumstances; (b) a sense of lack of control over eating during the episode (a feeling that one cannot stop eating or control what or how much one is eating)

- Recurring inappropriate compensatory behaviors to prevent weight gain, such as self-induced vomiting; misuse of laxatives, diuretics, other medications, or enemas; fasting; or excessive exercise
- Occurrence of the binge eating and inappropriate compensatory behaviors both occur, on average, at least twice a week for three months
- Undue influence of body shape and weight on self-evaluation

The most typical form of purging is self-induced vomiting. Bulimics also frequently ingest strong laxatives and emetics. Near-fasting diets and strenuous bouts of exercise are common. Medical problems associated with bulimia nervosa include cardiac arrhythmias, amenorrhea, kidney and bladder damage, ulcers, colitis, tearing of the esophagus or stomach, tooth erosion, gum damage, and general muscular weakness.

Unlike anorexics, bulimia sufferers realize that their behavior is abnormal and feel shame about it. Fearing social rejection, they pursue the binge–purge cycle in secrecy and at unusual hours of the day.

Bulimia nervosa can be treated successfully when the person realizes that this destructive behavior is not the solution to life's problems. A change in attitude can prevent permanent damage or death.

Binge-Eating Disorder

Binge-eating disorder is probably the most common of the three main eating disorders. About two percent of American adults are afflicted with binge-eating disorder in any six-month period. Although most people overeat from time to time, eating more than one should now and then does not mean the individual has a binge-eating disorder. The disorder is slightly more common in women than in men; three women for every two men have the disorder.

Binge-eating disorder is characterized by uncontrollable episodes of eating excessive amounts of food within a relatively short time. The causes of binge-eating disorder are unknown, although depression, anger, sadness, boredom, and worry can trigger an episode. Unlike bulimic sufferers, binge eaters do not purge; thus, most people with this disorder are either overweight or obese.

Typical symptoms of binge-eating disorder include:

- Eating what most people think is an unusually large amount of food
- Eating until uncomfortably full
- Eating out of control
- Eating much faster than usual during binge episodes
- Eating alone because of embarrassment of how much food one is consuming
- Feeling disgusted, depressed, or guilty after overeating

Emotional Eating

In addition to physiological purposes, eating also fulfills psychological, social, and cultural purposes. We eat to sustain our daily energy requirements, but we also eat at family celebrations, national holidays, social gatherings, sporting events (as spectators), and even when we become very emotional (some people stop eating when emotional). **Emotional eating** involves the consumption of large quantities of food, mostly "comfort" and junk food, to suppress negative emotions. Such emotions include stress, anxiety, uncertainty, guilt, anger, pain, depression, loneliness, sadness, or boredom. In such circumstances, people eat for comfort when they are at their weakest point emotionally. Comfort foods often include calorie-dense, sweet, salty, and fatty foods. Excessive emotional eating hinders proper weight management.

Some palatable foods, such as chocolate, cause the body to release small amounts of mood-elevating opiates, helping to offset negative emotions. A preference for certain foods is also present when one experiences specific feelings (loneliness, anxiety, fear). Eating helps to divert the stressor away for a while, but the distraction is only temporary. The emotions return and may be compounded by a feeling of guilt from overeating.

If you are an emotional overeater, you can always seek help from a therapist at the school's counseling center. The following list of suggestions may also help:

1. Learn to differentiate between emotional and physical hunger.
2. Avoid storing and snacking on unhealthy foods.
3. Keep healthy snacks handy.
4. Use countering techniques (going for a walk instead of reaching for the ice cream, listening to music instead of eating the candy bar).
5. Keep a "trigger log" and get to know what triggers your emotional food consumption.
6. Work it out with exercise instead of food.

Treatment

Treatment for eating disorders is available on most school campuses through the school's counseling center or health center. Local hospitals also offer treatment for these conditions. Many communities have support groups, frequently led by professional personnel and often free of charge. All information and the individual's identity are kept confidential, so the person need not fear embarrassment or repercussions when seeking professional help.

Physiology of Weight Loss

Traditional concepts related to weight control have centered on three assumptions:

1. Balancing food intake against output allows a person to achieve recommended weight.
2. All fat people simply eat too much.
3. The human body doesn't care how much (or little) fat it stores.

Although these statements contain some truth, they are open to much debate and research. We now know that the causes of obesity are complex, involving a combination of genetics, behavior, and lifestyle factors.

Energy-Balancing Equation

The principle embodied in the **energy-balancing equation** is simple: As long as caloric input equals caloric output, the person will not gain or lose weight. If caloric intake exceeds output, the person gains weight; when output exceeds input, the person loses weight. If daily energy requirements could be determined accurately, caloric intake could be balanced against output. This is not always the case, though, because genetic and lifestyle-related individual differences determine the number of calories required to maintain or lose body weight.

Table 5.3 (page 167) offers general guidelines to determine the **estimated energy requirement (EER)** in calories per day. This is an estimated figure and (as discussed under "Losing Weight the Sound and Sensible Way," page 165) serves only as a starting point from which individual adjustments have to be made.

The total daily energy requirement has three basic components (see Figure 5.5):

1. Resting metabolic rate
2. Thermic effect of food
3. Physical activity

The **resting metabolic rate (RMR)**—the energy requirement to maintain the body's vital processes in the resting state—accounts for approximately 60 to 70 percent of the total daily energy requirement. The thermic effect of food—the energy required to digest, absorb, and store food—accounts for about 5 to 10 percent of the total daily requirement. Physical activity accounts for 15 to 30 percent of the total daily requirement.

One pound of fat is the equivalent of 3,500 calories. If a person's EER is 2,500 calories and that person were to decrease intake by 500 calories per day, it should result in a loss of one pound of fat in seven days ($500 \times 7 = 3,500$). But research has shown—and many people have experienced—that even when dieters carefully balance caloric input against caloric output, weight loss does not always result as predicted. Furthermore, two people with similar measured caloric intake and output seldom lose weight at the same rate.

The most common explanation for individual differences in weight loss and weight gain has been variation in human metabolism from one person to another. We are all familiar with people who can eat "all day long" and not gain an ounce of weight, while others cannot even "dream about food" without gaining weight. Because experts did not believe that human metabolism alone could account for such extreme differences, they developed other theories that might better explain these individual variations.

Setpoint Theory

Results of research studies point toward a **weight-regulating mechanism (WRM)** in the human body that has a **setpoint** for controlling both appetite and the amount of fat stored. Setpoint is hypothesized to work like a thermostat for body fat, maintaining fairly constant body weight, because it "knows" at all times the exact amount of adipose tissue stored in the fat cells. Some people have high settings; others have low settings.

If body weight decreases (as in dieting), the setpoint senses this change and triggers the WRM to increase the person's appetite or make the body conserve energy to maintain the "set" weight. The opposite also may be true. Some people have a hard time gaining weight. In this case, the WRM decreases appetite or causes the body to waste energy to maintain the lower weight.

Every person has his or her own certain body fat percentage (as established by the setpoint) that the body attempts to maintain. The genetic instinct to survive tells the body that fat storage is vital, and therefore it sets an acceptable fat level. This level may remain somewhat constant or may climb gradually because of poor lifestyle habits.

For instance, under strict calorie reduction, the body may make extreme metabolic adjustments in an effort to maintain its setpoint for fat. The **basal metabolic rate (BMR)**, the lowest level of caloric intake necessary to sustain life, may drop dramatically when operating under a consistent negative caloric balance, and that person's weight loss may plateau for days or even weeks. A

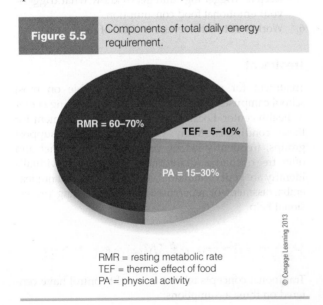

| Figure 5.5 | Components of total daily energy requirement. |

RMR = 60–70%
TEF = 5–10%
PA = 15–30%

RMR = resting metabolic rate
TEF = thermic effect of food
PA = physical activity

© Cengage Learning 2013

low metabolic rate compounds a person's problems in maintaining recommended body weight.

These findings were substantiated by research conducted at Rockefeller University in New York.[16] The authors showed that the body resists maintaining altered weight. Obese and lifetime nonobese individuals were used in the investigation. Following a 10-percent weight loss, the body, in an attempt to regain the lost weight, compensated by burning up to 15 percent fewer calories than expected for the new reduced weight (after accounting for the 10 percent loss). The effects were similar in the obese and nonobese participants. These results imply that after a 10-percent weight loss, a person would have to eat even less or exercise even more to compensate for the estimated 15-percent slowdown (a difference of about 200 to 300 calories).

In this same study, when the participants were allowed to increase their weight to 10 percent above their "normal" body (before weight loss) weight, the body burned 10 to 15 percent *more* calories than expected—attempting to waste energy and maintain the preset weight. This is another indication that the body is highly resistant to weight changes unless additional lifestyle changes are incorporated to ensure successful weight management. (These methods are discussed under "Losing Weight the Sound and Sensible Way," page 165.)

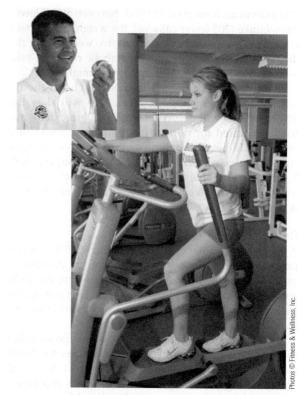

Achieving and maintaining a high physical fitness percent body fat standard requires a lifetime commitment to regular physical activity and proper nutrition.

Critical Thinking

Do you see a difference in the amount of food that you are now able to eat compared with the amount that you ate in your mid- to late-teen years? • If so, to what do you attribute this difference? • What actions are you taking to account for the difference?

Dietary restriction alone will not lower the setpoint, even though the person may lose weight and fat. When the dieter goes back to the normal or even below-normal caloric intake (at which the weight may have been stable for a long time), he or she quickly regains the lost fat as the body strives to regain a comfortable fat store.

An Example

Let's use a practical illustration. A person would like to lose some body fat and assumes that his or her current stable body weight has been reached at an average daily caloric intake of 1,800 calories (no weight gain or loss occurs at this daily intake). In an attempt to lose weight rapidly, this person now goes on a **very low calorie diet** (defined as 800 calories per day or less), or, even worse, a near-fasting diet. This immediately activates the body's survival mechanism and readjusts the metabolism to a lower caloric balance. After a few weeks of dieting at the 800-calories-per-day level, the body now can maintain its normal functions at 1,300 calories per day. This new figure (1,300) represents a drop of 500 calories per day in the metabolic rate.

Having lost the desired weight, the person terminates the diet but realizes that the original intake of 1,800 calories per day will have to be lower to maintain the new lower weight. To adjust to the new lower body weight, the person restricts intake to about 1,600 calories per day.

Key Terms

Energy-balancing equation A principle holding that as long as caloric input equals caloric output, the person will not gain or lose weight. If caloric intake exceeds output, the person gains weight; when output exceeds input, the person loses weight.

Estimated energy requirement (EER) The average dietary energy (caloric) intake that is predicted to maintain energy balance in a healthy adult of defined age, gender, weight, height, and level of physical activity, consistent with good health.

Resting metabolic rate (RMR) The energy requirement to maintain the body's vital processes in the resting state.

Weight-regulating mechanism (WRM) A feature of the hypothalamus of the brain that controls how much the body should weigh.

Setpoint Weight control theory that the body has an established weight and strongly attempts to maintain that weight.

Basal metabolic rate (BMR) The lowest level of oxygen consumption (and energy requirement) necessary to sustain life.

Very low calorie diet A diet that allows an energy intake (consumption) of only 800 calories or less per day.

The individual is surprised to find that even at this lower daily intake (200 fewer calories), the weight comes back at a rate of one pound every one to two weeks. After the diet is over, this new lowered metabolic rate may take several months to kick back up to its normal level.

Based on this explanation, individuals clearly should not go on very low calorie diets. This will slow the RMR and also will deprive the body of basic daily nutrients required for normal function. Very low calorie diets should be used only in conjunction with dietary supplements and under proper medical supervision. Furthermore, people who use very low calorie diets are not as effective in keeping the weight off once the diet is terminated.

Recommendation

A daily caloric intake of approximately 1,500 calories provides the necessary nutrients if they are distributed properly over the basic food groups (meeting the daily recommended amounts from each group). Of course, the individual will have to learn which foods meet the requirements and yet are low in fat and sugar.

Under no circumstances should a person go on a diet that calls for a level of 1,200 calories or less for petite women or 1,500 calories or less for most men and women. Weight (fat) is gained over months and years, not overnight. Likewise, weight loss should be gradual, not abrupt. At 1,200 calories per day you may require a multivitamin supplement. Your health care professional should be consulted regarding such supplement.

A second way in which the setpoint may work is by keeping track of the nutrients and calories consumed daily. It is thought that the body, like a cash register, records the daily food intake, and that the brain will not feel satisfied until the calories and nutrients have been "registered."

This setpoint for calories and nutrients seems to operate even when people participate in moderately intense exercise. Some evidence suggests that people do not become hungrier with moderate physical activity. Therefore, people can choose to lose weight either by going hungry or by combining a sensible calorie-restricted diet with an increase in daily physical activity.

Lowering the Setpoint

The most common question regarding the setpoint is how to lower it so that the body will feel comfortable at a reduced fat percentage. The following factors seem to affect the setpoint directly by lowering the fat thermostat:

- Exercise
- A diet high in complex carbohydrates
- Nicotine
- Amphetamines

The last two are more destructive than the extra fat weight, so they are not reasonable alternatives (as far as the extra strain on the heart is concerned, smoking one

---

Behavior Modification Planning

Eating Right When on the Run

Current lifestyles often require people to be on the run. We don't seem to have time to eat right, but fortunately it doesn't have to be that way. If you are on the run, it is even more critical to make healthy choices to keep up with a challenging schedule. Look at the following food choices for eating on the run:

Water
Whole-grain cereal and skim milk
Whole-grain bread and bagels
Whole-grain bread with peanut butter
Non-fat or low-fat yogurt
Fresh fruits
Frozen fresh fruit (grapes, cherries, banana slices)
Dried fruits
Raw vegetables (carrots, red peppers, cucumbers, radishes, cauliflower, asparagus)
Crackers
Pretzels
Bread sticks
Low-fat cheese sticks
Granola bars
Snack-size cereal boxes
Nuts
Trail mix
Plain popcorn
Vegetable soups

Try It In your Online Journal or class notebook, plan your fast-meal menus for the upcoming week. It may require extra shopping and some food preparation (for instance, cutting vegetables to place in snack-size plastic bags). At the end of the week, evaluate how many days you had a "healthy eating on the run day." What did you learn from the experience?

---

pack of cigarettes per day is said to be the equivalent of carrying 50 to 75 pounds of excess body fat). A diet high in fats and refined carbohydrates, near-fasting diets, and perhaps even artificial sweeteners seem to raise the setpoint. Therefore, the only practical and sensible way to lower the setpoint and lose fat weight is a combination of exercise and a diet high in complex carbohydrates and only moderate amounts of fat.

Because of the effects of proper food management on the body's setpoint, most of the successful dieter's effort should be spent in reforming eating habits, increasing the intake of complex carbohydrates and high-fiber foods, and decreasing the consumption of processed foods that are high in refined carbohydrates (sugars) and fats. This change in eating habits will bring about a decrease in total daily caloric intake. Because one gram of carbohydrates provides only four calories, as opposed to nine calories per gram of fat, you could eat twice the volume of food (by weight) when substituting carbohydrates for fat. Some fat, however, is recommended in the diet—preferably polyunsaturated and monounsaturated fats. These so-called good fats do more than help protect the heart; they help delay hunger pangs.

A "diet" should not be viewed as a temporary tool to aid in weight loss but, instead, as a permanent change in eating behaviors to ensure weight management and better health. The role of increased physical activity also must be considered, because successful weight loss, maintenance, and recommended body composition are seldom attained without a moderate reduction in caloric intake combined with a regular exercise program.

Diet and Metabolism

Fat can be lost by selecting the proper foods, exercising, or restricting calories. However, when dieters try to lose weight by dietary restrictions alone, they also lose lean body mass (muscle protein, along with vital organ protein). The amount of lean body mass lost depends entirely on caloric limitation. When people go on a near-fasting diet, up to half of the weight loss is lean body mass and the other half is actual fat loss (see Figure 5.6).[17] When diet is combined with exercise, close to 100 percent of the weight loss is in the form of fat, and lean tissue actually may increase. Loss of lean body mass is never good, because it weakens the organs and muscles and slows metabolism. Large losses in lean tissue can cause disturbances in heart function and damage to other organs. Equally important is not to overindulge (binge) following a very low calorie diet, as this may cause changes in metabolic rate and electrolyte balance, which could trigger fatal cardiac arrhythmias.

Contrary to some beliefs, aging is not the main reason for the lower metabolic rate. It is not so much that metabolism slows down as that people slow down. As people age, they tend to rely more on the amenities of life (remote controls, cell phones, intercoms, single-level homes, riding lawnmowers) that lull a person into sedentary living.

Basal metabolism also is related to lean body weight. More lean tissue yields a higher metabolic rate. As a consequence of sedentary living and less physical activity, the lean component decreases and fat tissue increases. The human body requires a certain amount of oxygen per pound of lean body mass. Given that fat is considered metabolically inert from the point of view of caloric use, the lean tissue uses most of the oxygen, even at rest. As muscle and organ mass (lean body mass) decrease, so do the energy requirements at rest.

Diets with caloric intakes below 1,500 calories cannot guarantee the retention of lean body mass. Even at this intake level, some loss is inevitable unless the diet is combined with exercise. Despite the claims of many diets that they do not alter the lean component, the simple truth is that regardless of what nutrients may be added to the diet, severe caloric restrictions *always* prompt the loss of lean tissue. Sadly, many people go on very low calorie diets constantly. Every time they do, their metabolic rate slows as more lean tissue is lost.

People in their 40s and older who weigh the same as they did when they were 20 tend to think they are at recommended body weight. During this span of 20 years or more, though, they may have dieted many times without participating in an exercise program. After they terminate each diet, they regain the weight, and much of that gain is additional body fat. Maybe at age 20 they weighed 150 pounds, of which only 15 percent was fat. Now at age 40, even though they still weigh 150 pounds, they might be 30 percent fat (see Figure 5.7). At "recommended" body weight, they wonder why they are eating very little and still having trouble staying at that weight.

Hormonal Regulation of Appetite

Ghrelin and leptin are two hormones currently being extensively researched because they appear to play a role in appetite. Ghrelin, produced primarily in the stomach, stimulates appetite: that is, the more ghrelin the body produces, the more you want to eat. Leptin, produced by fat cells, on the other hand, lets the brain know when you are full; the more leptin you produce, the less you want to eat. Similar to insulin resistance (leading to type 2 diabetes), research is beginning to show that a lack of physical activity also leads to leptin resistance, setting up a vicious cycle that leads to excessive eating. Scientists are now looking into the role these hormones play in weight gain and weight loss, as

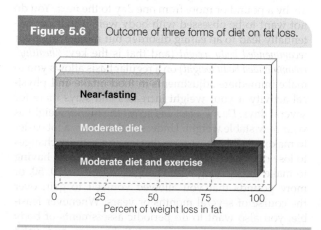

Figure 5.6 Outcome of three forms of diet on fat loss.

Near-fasting
Moderate diet
Moderate diet and exercise

0   25   50   75   100
Percent of weight loss in fat

SOURCE: Adapted from Shephard, R.J. *Alive Man: The Physiology of Physical Activity* (Springfield, IL: Charles C. Thomas, 1975): 484–488.

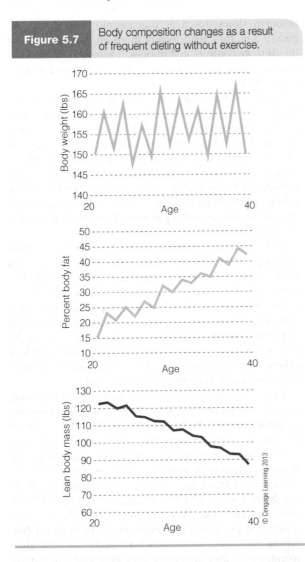

Figure 5.7   Body composition changes as a result of frequent dieting without exercise.

U.S. population is overweight or obese, and according to the National Sleep Foundation, 63 percent of Americans report that they do not get eight hours of sleep per night. The question must be raised: Is there a connection? Let's examine some of the data.

One of the most recent studies examining this issue showed that individuals who get less than six hours of sleep per night have a higher average BMI (28.3) compared with those who average eight hours per night (24.5).[18] Another study on more than 68,000 women between the ages of 30 and 55 found that those who got five or less hours of sleep per night were 30 percent more likely to gain 30 or more pounds compared with women who got eight hours per night.[19]

Researchers believe that lack of sleep disrupts normal body hormonal balances. Sleep deprivation has now been shown to elevate ghrelin levels and decrease leptin levels, potentially leading to weight gain or keeping you from losing weight.[20] Data comparing these hormone levels in five-hour versus eight-hour sleepers found that the short sleepers had a 14.9 percent increase in ghrelin levels and a 15.5-percent decrease in leptin levels. The short sleepers also had a 3.6 percent higher BMI than the regular sleepers.[21]

Based on all these studies, the data appear to indicate that sleep deprivation has a negative impact on weight loss or maintenance. Thus, an important component to a well-designed weight management program should include a good night's rest (eight hours of sleep).

Monitoring Body Weight

A most critical component to lifetime weight management is to regularly monitor your body weight. Get into the habit of weighing yourself, preferably at the same time of day and under the same conditions; for instance, in the morning just as you get out of bed. Depending on your body size, activity patterns, rehydration level, and dietary intake on any given day, your weight will fluctuate by a pound or more from one day to the next. You do not want to be obsessed with body weight that can potentially lead to an eating disorder, but monitoring your *recommended body weight* (and that is the key: *"healthy" recommended body weight*) on a regular basis allows you to make immediate adjustments in food intake and physical activity if your weight increases and stays there for several days. *Do not adapt and accept* the higher weight as your new stable weight. Understand that it is a lot easier to make sensible short-term dietary and activity changes to lose one or two pounds of weight, rather than having to make drastic long term changes to lose 10, 20, 50, or more pounds that you allowed yourself to gain over the course of several months or years. Whenever feasible, you also want to do periodic assessments of body composition using experienced technicians and valid techniques.

well as at the effects of sleep deprivation and exercise dose on these hormones and subsequent appetite regulation.

Sleep and Weight Management

As presented under the Healthy Lifestyle Habits box in Chapter 1 (see page 27), adequate sleep is one of the 12 key components that enhance health and extend life. New evidence shows that sleep is also important to adequate weight management. Sleep deprivation appears to be conducive to weight gain and may interfere with the body's capability to lose weight.

Current obesity and sleep deprivation data point toward a possible correlation between excessive body weight and sleep deprivation. About 68 percent of the

Exercise and Weight Management

To tilt the energy-balancing equation in your favor, you need to burn more calories through physical activity. Research indicates that exercise accentuates weight loss while on a negative caloric balance (diet) as long as you do not replenish the calories expended during exercise. The debate, however, centers on what amount of exercise is best for individuals who are trying to lose weight and those who are trying to maintain weight. The data is clear, nonetheless, that exercise is the best predictor of long-term maintenance of weight loss.[22]

Regular exercise seems to exert control over how much a person weighs. On average, the typical adult American gains one to two pounds of weight per year. A one-pound weight gain represents a simple energy surplus of under 10 calories per day (10×365 days $= 3,650$ calories and one pound of fat represents 3,500 calories). This simple surplus of under 10 calories per day is the equivalent of less than one teaspoon of sugar. Weight gain is clearly related to a decrease in physical activity and an increase in caloric intake. Physical inactivity, however, might very well be the primary cause leading to excessive weight and obesity. The human body was meant to be physically active and *a minimal level of activity* appears to be necessary to accurately balance caloric intake to caloric expenditure. In sedentary individuals, the body seems to lose control over this fine energy balance.

Most people understand that exercise enhances the rate of weight loss, enhances body composition, and is vital in maintaining the lost weight. Not only will exercise maintain lean tissue, but advocates of the setpoint theory say that exercise resets the fat thermostat to a new, lower level.

Most people who struggle with weight management need 60 to 90 minutes of daily physical activity to effectively manage body weight. While accumulating 30 minutes of moderate-intensity activity per day provides substantial health benefits (the minimum daily recommended amount of activity), from a weight management point of view, however, the Institute of Medicine of the National Academy of Sciences recommends that people accumulate 60 minutes of moderate-intensity physical activity most days of the week.[23] The evidence shows that people who maintain recommended weight typically accumulate an hour or more of daily physical activity.

According to the American College of Sports Medicine position stand on strategies for weight loss and prevention of weight regain for adults (see Figure 5.8), greater weight loss is achieved by increasing the amount of weekly physical activity. Of even greater significance, physical activity is required for weight maintenance following weight loss. People who exercise regain less

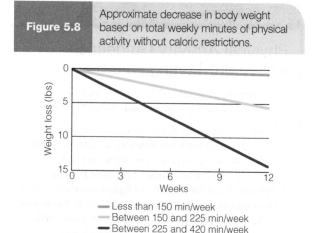

Figure 5.8 Approximate decrease in body weight based on total weekly minutes of physical activity without caloric restrictions.

— Less than 150 min/week
— Between 150 and 225 min/week
— Between 225 and 420 min/week

SOURCE: Adapted from American College of Sports Medicine, "Position Stand: Appropriate Physical Activity Intervention Strategies for Weight Loss and Prevention of Weight Regain for Adults," *Medicine and Science in Sports and Exercise* 41 (2009): 459–471.

weight than those who do not. And those who exercise the most regain the least amount of weight. Individuals who remain physically active for 60 or more minutes per day are able to keep the weight off.

Further, data from the National Weight Control Registry (http://www.nwcr.ws) on more than 6,000 individuals who have lost at least 30 pounds and have kept them off for a minimum of five years indicates that they typically expend about 300 calories through daily moderate-intensity exercise.[24] Three hundred calories represents about three miles jogging in 30 minutes or walking briskly the same distance in 60 minutes. Individuals who completely stop physical activity regain almost 100 percent of the weight within 18 months of discontinuing the weight loss program. Most of the successful "weight maintainers" also show greater dietary restraint and follow a low-fat diet, consuming less than 30 percent of the total daily calories from fat.

Most experts and leading organizations now recognize that if weight management is not a consideration, 30 minutes of daily activity five days per week provides substantial health benefits. To prevent weight gain, nonetheless, 60 minutes of daily activity is recommended; to maintain substantial weight loss, 90 minutes may be required.

The most important reason why physical activity and exercise are so vital for weight loss maintenance is because sedentary living expends no additional energy (calories) over the resting metabolic rate. With limited physical activity throughout the day, sedentary people cannot afford to eat very many calories, perhaps only 1,000 to 1,200 calories per day. And such a low level of energy intake is not sufficient to keep the person from constantly feeling hungry. The only choice they now have is to go hungry every day, an impossible task to

Physical Activity Guidelines for Weight Management

The following physical activity guidelines are recommended to effectively manage body weight:

- 30 minutes of physical activity on most days of the week if you do not have difficulty maintaining body weight (more minutes and/or higher intensity if you choose to reach a high level of physical fitness).
- Between 30 and 60 minutes of light-to-moderate exercise on most days of the week if you are trying to lose weight. Incorporate as many light ambulatory activities as possible during the course of each day.
- 60 minutes of daily activity if you want to prevent weight gain.
- Between 60 and 90 minutes each day if you want to keep weight off following extensive weight loss (30 pounds of weight loss or more). Be sure to include some high-intensity/low impact activities at least twice a week in your program.

Try It In your Behavior Change Planner Progress Tracker, Online Journal, or class notebook, record how many minutes of daily physical activity you accumulate on a regular basis and record your thoughts on how effectively your activity has helped you manage your body weight. Is there one thing you could do today to increase your physical activity?

Weight Maintenance Benefits of a Lifetime Exercise Program

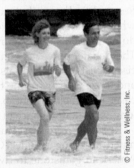

The authors of this book have been jogging together a minimum of 15 miles per week (3 miles/5 times per week) for the past 35 years. Without considering the additional energy expenditure from their regular strength-training program and their many other sport and recreational activities, the energy cost of this regular jogging program over 35 years has been approximately 2,730,000 calories (15 miles × 100 calories/mile × 52 weeks × 35 years) or the equivalent of 780 pounds of fat (2,730,000 ÷ 3,500). In essence, without this 30-minute jogging workout 5 times per week, the authors would weigh 922 and 896 pounds respectively. Such is the long-term gratification (reward) of a lifetime exercise program—not to mention the myriad of health benefits, joy, and quality of life derived through this program.

Try It Ask yourself whether a regular aerobic exercise program is part of your long-term gratification and health enhancement program. If the answer is no, are you ready to change your behavior? Use the Behavior Change Planner to help you answer the question.

sustain. After terminating the diet, in just a few short days, energy intake climbs with an end result of weight regain. Thus, the only logical way to increase caloric intake and maintain weight loss is by burning more calories through exercise and incorporating physical activity throughout daily living.

If a person is trying to lose weight, a combination of aerobic and strength-training exercises works best. Aerobic exercise is the best exercise modality to offset the setpoint, and the continuity and duration of these types of activities cause many calories to be burned in the process. The role of aerobic exercise in successful lifetime weight management cannot be overestimated.

Strength training is critical in helping maintain and increase lean body mass. The number of calories burned during a typical hour-long strength-training session is much less than during an hour of aerobic exercise. Because of the high intensity of strength training, the person needs frequent rest intervals to recover from each set of exercises. In the long run, however, the person enjoys the benefits of gains in lean tissue. Guidelines for developing aerobic and strength-training programs are given in Chapters 6 and 7.

Although the increase in BMR through increased muscle mass is being debated in the literature and merits further research, data indicate that each additional pound of muscle tissue raises the BMR in the range of 6 to 35 calories per day.[25] The latter figure is based on calculations that an increase of 3 to 3.5 pounds of lean tissue through strength training increased BMR by about 105 to 120 calories per day.[26]

Most likely, the benefit of strength training goes beyond the new muscle tissue itself. Maybe a pound of muscle tissue requires only six calories per day to sustain itself, but as all muscles undergo strength training, they undergo increased protein synthesis to build and repair themselves, resulting in increased energy expenditure of 1 to 1.5 calories per pound in all trained muscle tissue. Such an increase would explain the 105- to 120-calorie BMR increase in this research study.

To examine the effects of a small increase in BMR on long-term body weight, let's use a very conservative estimate of an additional 50 calories per day as a result of a regular strength-training program. An increase of 50 calories represents an additional 18,250 calories per year (50 × 365), or the equivalent of 5.2 pounds of fat (18,250 ÷ 3,500). This increase in BMR would more than offset the typical adult weight gain of one to two pounds per year.

This figure of 18,250 calories per year does not include the actual energy cost of the strength-training workout. If we use an energy expenditure of only 150 calories per strength-training session, done twice per week, over a year's time it would represent 15,600 calories (150 × 2 × 52), or the equivalent of another 4.5 pounds of fat (15,600 ÷ 3,500).

In addition, although the amounts seem small, the previous calculations do not account for the increase in metabolic rate following the strength-training workout (the time it takes the body to return to its preworkout resting rate—about two hours). Depending on the training volume (see Chapter 7, page 237), this recovery energy expenditure ranges from 20 to 100 calories following each strength-training workout. All these "apparently small" changes make a big difference in the long run.

Although size (inches) and percent body fat both decrease when sedentary individuals begin an exercise program, body weight often remains the same or may even increase during the first couple of weeks of the program. Exercise helps to increase muscle tissue, connective tissue, blood volume (as much as 500 mL, or the equivalent of one pound, following the first week of aerobic exercise), enzymes and other structures within the cell, and glycogen (which binds water). All of these changes lead to a higher functional capacity of the human body. With exercise, most of the weight loss becomes apparent after a few weeks of training, when the lean component has stabilized.

We know that a negative caloric balance of 3,500 calories does not always result in a loss of exactly one pound of fat, but the role of exercise in achieving a negative balance by burning additional calories is significant in weight reduction and maintenance programs. Sadly, some individuals claim that the number of calories burned during exercise is hardly worth the effort. They think that cutting their daily intake by 300 calories is easier than participating in some sort of exercise that would burn the same amount of calories. The problem is that the willpower to cut those 300 calories lasts only a few weeks, and then the person goes back to the old eating patterns.

If a person gets into the habit of exercising regularly, say three times a week, jogging three miles per exercise session (about 300 calories burned), this represents 900 calories in one week, about 3,600 calories in one month, or 46,800 calories per year. This minimal amount of exercise represents as many as 13.5 extra pounds of fat in one year, 27 in two, and so on.

We tend to forget that our weight creeps up gradually over the years, not just overnight. Hardly worth the effort? And we have not even taken into consideration the increase in lean tissue, possible resetting of the setpoint, benefits to the cardiovascular system, and, most impor-

"Alli" Weight Loss Drug

"Alli" is an over-the-counter weight loss drug that promises 50 percent greater weight loss than achieved through diet and exercise alone. Alli is not a miracle weight loss pill but may enhance the rate of weight loss.

Alli contains orlistat, the same active ingredient found in the prescription weight loss drug Xenical, but only at half the dose of Xenical. Alli is recommended for overweight people who are not obese and who are willing to commit to a rigorous online diet and exercise program. Orlistat works by preventing the absorption of about 25 percent of all fat in the diet. Along with unhealthy fat, the drug also blocks essential fatty acids (omega-3) and fat-soluble nutrients (such as vitamins A, E, and D) needed for good health. A daily multivitamin is encouraged to offset the loss of fat-soluble nutrients. Alli is not recommended for people with an organ transplant (it interferes with antirejection drugs) or those with health problems that prevent nutrient absorption.

Unpleasant and uncomfortable side effects include gas with oily spotting, loose stools, more frequent stools, and urgent, uncontrollable bowel movements. The magnitude of the side effects increases with increased fat intake. To reduce side effects, the manufacturer recommends consumption of less than 15 grams of fat per meal. At 15 grams of fat per meal, one consumes 45 grams of fat per day, for a total of 405 fat calories, or 20 percent fat calories based on a 2,000-calorie daily diet (405 ÷ 2000). Such a low-fat diet, in and of itself (without the drug), combined with exercise, leads to healthy weight loss in most individuals.

Alli is marketed under the slogan "If you have the will, we have the power." Alli costs about $2 per day. If you have the will to commit to a "rigorous diet and exercise program," lifetime weight management will be accomplished without the need of expensive drugs with undesirable and potentially embarrassing side effects.

tant, the improved quality of life. Fundamental reasons for excessive weight and obesity, few could argue, are sedentary living and lack of a regular exercise program.

In terms of preventing disease, many of the health benefits that people seek by losing weight are reaped through exercise alone, even without weight loss. Exercise offers protection against premature morbidity and mortality for everyone, including people who are overweight or already have risk factors for disease.

The Role of Exercise Intensity and Duration in Weight Management

A hotly debated and controversial current topic is the exercise volume required for adequate weight management. Depending on the degree of the initial weight

Table 5.2	Comparison of Approximate Energy Expenditure Between 30–40 Minutes of Exercise at Three Different Intensity Levels						
Exercise Intensity	Total Energy Expenditure (Calories)	Percent Calories from Fat	Total Fat Calories	Percent Calories from CHO*	Total CHO* Calories	Calories Burned per Minute	Calories per Pound per Minute
Light Intensity	200	50%	100	50%	100	6.67	0.045
Moderate Intensity	280	40%	112	60%	168	9.45	0.063
Vigorous Intensity	400	30%	120	70%	280	13.50	0.090

*CHO = Carbohydrates
© Cengage Learning 2013

problem and the person's fitness level, there appears to be a difference in the volume of exercise that is most conducive toward adequate weight loss, weight loss maintenance, and weight management.

We have known for years that compared with vigorous intensity, a greater proportion of calories burned during light-intensity exercise are derived from fat. The lower the intensity of exercise, the higher the percentage of fat utilization as an energy source. During light-intensity exercise, up to 50 percent of the calories burned may be derived from fat (the other 50 percent from glucose [carbohydrates]). With vigorous exercise, only 30 to 40 percent of the caloric expenditure comes from fat. Overall, however, you can burn twice as many calories during vigorous-intensity exercise and, subsequently, more fat as well.

Let's look at a practical illustration (also see Table 5.2). If you exercised for 30 to 40 minutes at light intensity and burned 200 calories, about 100 of those calories (50 percent) would come from fat. If you exercised at a vigorous intensity during those same 30 to 40 minutes, you could burn 400 calories, with 120 to 160 of the calories (30 to 40 percent) coming from fat. Thus, even though it is true that the percentage of fat used is greater during light-intensity exercise, the overall amount of fat used is still less during light-intensity exercise. Plus, if you were to exercise at a light intensity, you would have to do so twice as long to burn the same amount of calories. Another benefit is that the metabolic rate remains at a slightly higher level longer after vigorous-intensity exercise, so you continue to burn a few extra calories following exercise.

The previous discussion does not mean that light-intensity exercise is ineffective. Light-intensity exercise provides substantial health benefits, including a decrease in premature morbidity among overweight individuals. Additionally, beginners are more willing to participate and stay with light-intensity programs. The risk of injury when starting out is quite low with this type of program. Light-intensity exercise does promote weight loss.

In terms of overall weight loss, there is controversy regarding the optimal exercise dose. Initial research indicated that vigorous-intensity exercise triggered more fat loss than light- to moderate-intensity exercise. Research conducted in the 1990s at Laval University in Quebec,

Canada, using both men and women participants, showed that subjects who performed a high-intensity intermittent-training (HIIT) program lost more body fat than participants in a low- to moderate-intensity continuous aerobic endurance group.[27] Even more surprisingly, this finding occurred despite the fact that the vigorous-intensity group burned fewer total calories per exercise session. The researchers concluded that the "results reinforce the notion that for a given level of energy expenditure, vigorous exercise favors negative energy and lipid balance to a greater extent than exercise of low- to moderate-intensity. Moreover, the metabolic adaptations taking place in the skeletal muscle in response to the HIIT program appear to favor the process of lipid oxidation." If time constrains do not allow much time for exercise, to increase energy expenditure, a vigorous 20- to 30-minute exercise programs is recommended.

Recently, it has been suggested that *when attempting to lose weight*, particularly for women, lengthy exercise sessions may not be helpful because they actually trigger greater food consumption following exercise; whereas shorter exercise sessions do not lead to a greater caloric intake. Thus, some people think that the potential weight reduction effect of lengthy exercise sessions may be attenuated because people end up eating more food when they exercise.

A recent 2009 study had postmenopausal women exercise at 50 percent of their maximal aerobic capacity for about 20 minutes, 40 minutes, or 60 minutes three to four times per week.[28] On average, the groups lost 3, 4.6, and 3.3 pounds of weight, respectively. The data indicated that the 20- and 40-minute groups lost weight closely to what had been predicted, whereas the 60 minute group lost significantly less than predicted. The researchers concluded that 60 minutes of exercise led this group of women to compensate with greater food intake, possibly triggered by an increase in ghrelin levels. All three groups, nonetheless, exhibited a significant decrease in waist circumference, independent of total weight lost. Researchers theorize that the biological mechanism to maintain fat stores in women is stronger than in men.

On the other hand, a 2010 study of more than 34,000 women who were followed for 13 years, starting at an average age of 54, found that on average the women gained six pounds of weight; but a small group of them who reported 60 minutes of almost daily exercise at a moderate intensity closely maintained their body weight.[29] The exercise routine of the latter group was not something new to them, but rather exercise that they had been doing for years. While the best exercise dose for optimal weight loss may not be a precise science, the research is quite clear that regular exercise is the best predictor of long-term weight maintenance. The data also indicate that even as little as 80 weekly minutes of aerobic or strength training exercise prevents regain of the harmful visceral fat (also see page 130 in Chapter 4).

The take-home message from these studies is that when trying to lose weight, initial lengthy exercise sessions (longer than 60 minutes) may not be the best approach to weight loss, *unless* you carefully monitor daily caloric intake and avoid caloric compensation. The data show that people who carefully monitor caloric intake, instead of "guesstimating" energy intake, are by far more successful with weight loss.

Caloric compensation in response to extensive exercise in overweight individuals may be related to a low initial fitness level and the already low caloric intake. Overall, inactive people tend to eat fewer calories, and a lengthy exercise session may very well trigger a greater appetite due to the large negative caloric balance. Research confirms that energy deficit, and not exercise, is the most significant regulator of the hormonal responses seen in previously inactive individuals who begin an exercise program.[30] In active/fit individuals, lengthy exercise sessions are not at all counterproductive. If such was the case, health clubs and jogging trails would be full of overweight and obese people.

New research is beginning to look into the role of increasing light-intensity ambulation (walking) and standing activities (doing some of the work on your feet instead of sitting the entire time) on weight loss. In essence, the individual will increase light-intensity physical activity throughout the day. Light-intensity activities do not seem to trigger the increase in ghrelin levels seen in previously inactive individuals who undertake long moderate- or vigorous-intensity exercise sessions. The difference in energy expenditure by increasing light-intensity activities throughout the day can represent several hundred calories. As you achieve a higher fitness level, you can combine light-intensity activities performed throughout the day with moderate- and/or vigorous-intensity exercise. A graphic illustration of such lifestyle patterns and the effects on the metabolic rate and overall energy expenditure is provided in Figure 5.9.

If you wish to engage in vigorous-intensity exercise to either maintain lost weight or for adequate weight management, a word of caution is in order: Be sure that it is medically safe for you to participate in such activities and that you build up gradually to that level. If you are cleared to participate in vigorous-intensity exercise, do not attempt to do too much too quickly, because you may incur injuries and become discouraged. You must allow your body a proper conditioning period of 8 to 12 weeks or even longer.

Also keep in mind that vigorous intensity does not mean high impact. High-impact activities are the most common cause of exercise-related injuries. Additional information on proper exercise prescription is presented in Chapter 6. And remember, when on a weight loss program, *always* carefully monitor your daily caloric intake to avoid food overconsumption.

Healthy Weight Gain

"Skinny" people, too, should realize that the only healthy way to gain weight is through exercise (mainly strength-training exercises) and a slight increase in caloric intake. Attempting to gain weight by overeating alone will raise the fat component and not the lean component—which is not the path to better health. Exercise is the best solution to weight (fat) reduction and weight (lean) gain alike.

A strength-training program such as explained in Chapter 7 is the best approach to add body weight. The training program should include at least two exercises of one to three sets for each major body part. Each set should consist of about 8 to 12 repetitions maximum.

Even though the metabolic cost of synthesizing a pound of muscle tissue is still unclear, consuming an estimated 500 additional calories per day is recommended to gain lean tissue. Your diet should include a daily total intake of about 1.5 grams of protein per kilogram of body weight. If your daily protein intake already exceeds 1.5 grams per day, the extra 500 calories should be primarily in the form of complex carbohydrates. The higher caloric intake must be accompanied by a strength-training program; otherwise, the increase in body weight will be in the form of fat, not muscle tissue (Activity 5.4 can be used to monitor your caloric intake for healthy weight gain). Additional information on nutrition to optimize muscle growth and strength development is provided in Chapter 7 in the section "Dietary Guidelines for Strength Development," page 244.

Weight Loss Myths

Cellulite and **spot reducing** are mythical concepts. **Cellulite** is caused by the herniation of subcutaneous fat within fibrous connective tissue, giving it a padded-like appearance.

Key Terms

Spot reducing Fallacious theory proposing that exercising a specific body part will result in significant fat reduction in that area.

Cellulite Term frequently used in reference to fat deposits that "bulge out"; caused by the herniation of subcutaneous fat within fibrous connective tissue, giving it a padded-like appearance.

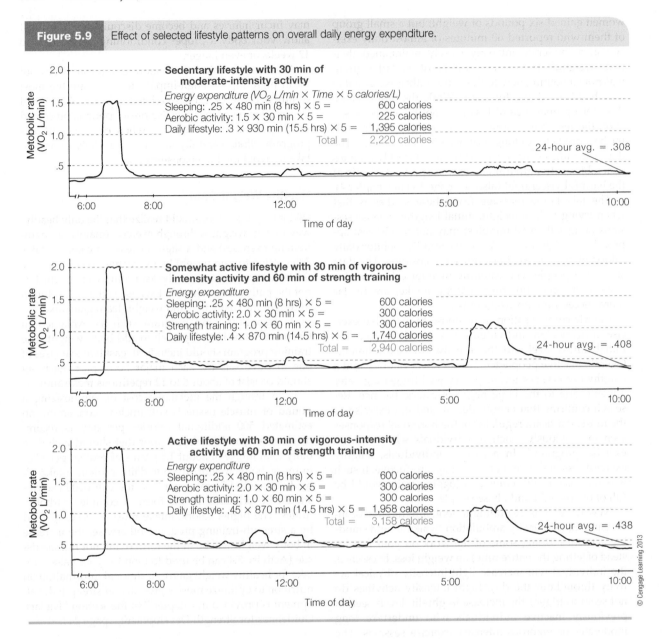

Figure 5.9   Effect of selected lifestyle patterns on overall daily energy expenditure.

Doing several sets of daily sit-ups will not get rid of fat in the midsection of the body. When fat comes off, it does so throughout the entire body, not just the exercised area. The greatest proportion of fat may come off the biggest fat deposits, but the caloric output of a few sets of sit-ups has practically no effect on reducing total body fat. A person has to exercise much longer to see results.

Other touted means toward quick weight loss, such as rubberized sweat suits, steam baths, and mechanical vibrators, are misleading. When a person wears a sweat suit or steps into a sauna, the weight lost is not fat but merely a significant amount of water. Sure, it looks nice when you step on the scale immediately afterward, but

this represents a false loss of weight. As soon as you replace body fluids, you gain back the weight quickly.

Wearing rubberized sweat suits hastens the rate of body fluid that is lost—fluid that is vital during prolonged exercise—and raises core temperature at the same time. This combination puts a person in danger of dehydration, which impairs cellular function and, in extreme cases, can even cause death.

Similarly, mechanical vibrators are worthless in a weight-control program. Vibrating belts and turning rollers may feel good, but they require no effort whatsoever. Fat cannot be shaken off. It is lost primarily by burning it in muscle tissue.

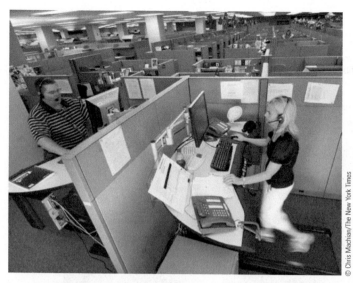

© Chris Machian/The New York Times

Increasing ambulatory activities throughout the day enhances fitness and is an excellent weight management strategy. These employees at Mutual of Omaha, working at Walkstations, typically walk 5 miles at a light-intensity level during the course of most days.

Losing Weight the Sound and Sensible Way

Dieting never has been fun and never will be. People who are overweight and are serious about losing weight, however, have to include regular physical activity and exercise in their lives, along with proper food management and a sensible reduction in caloric intake.

Because excessive body fat is a risk factor for cardiovascular disease, some precautions are in order. Depending on the extent of the weight problem, a medical examination may be a good idea before undertaking the exercise program. Consult a physician in this regard.

Significantly overweight individuals need to choose activities in which they will not have to support their own body weight but that still will be effective in burning calories. Injuries to joints and muscles are common in excessively overweight individuals who participate in weight-bearing exercises such as walking, jogging, and aerobics.

Swimming may not be a good weight loss exercise modality for some people. More body fat makes a person more buoyant, and many people are not at the skill level required to swim fast enough to get a good training effect, thus limiting the number of calories burned as well as the benefits to the cardiorespiratory system. During the initial stages of exercise, better alternatives include riding a bicycle (either road or stationary), walking in a shallow pool, doing water aerobics, or running in place in deep water (treading water). The latter forms of water exercise aid with weight loss without fear of injuries.

How long should each exercise session last? The amount of exercise needed to lose weight and maintain the weight loss is different from the amount of exercise needed to improve fitness. For health fitness, accumulating 30 minutes of physical activity a minimum of five days per week is recommended. To develop and maintain cardiorespiratory fitness, 20 to 60 minutes of vigorous-intensity exercise, three to five times per week, is suggested (see Chapter 6). For successful weight loss, however, 30 to 60 minutes of light to moderate exercise on most days of the week are recommended. Additional light-intensity ambulation and standing throughout the day are also strongly encouraged. To maintain substantial weight loss, 60 to 90 minutes of physical activity on a nearly daily basis is recommended.

A person should not try to do too much too fast. Unconditioned beginners should start with about 15 minutes of aerobic exercise three times a week, and during the next 3 to 4 weeks gradually increase the duration by approximately 5 minutes per week and the frequency by one day per week.

In addition to exercise and food management, a sensible reduction in caloric intake and careful monitoring of this intake are recommended. Research indicates that a negative caloric balance is required to lose weight because:

1. People tend to underestimate their caloric intake and are eating more than they should be eating.
2. Developing new behaviors takes time, and most people have trouble changing and adjusting to new eating habits.
3. Many individuals are in such poor physical condition that they take a long time to increase their activity level enough to offset the setpoint and burn enough calories to aid in losing body fat.
4. Most successful dieters carefully monitor their daily caloric intake.
5. A few people simply will not alter their food selection. For those who will not (which will increase their risk for chronic diseases), the only solution to lose weight successfully is a large increase in physical activity, a negative caloric balance, or a combination of the two.

Perhaps the only exception to a decrease in caloric intake for weight loss purposes is in people who already are eating too few calories. A nutrient analysis (see Chapter 3) often reveals that long-term dieters are not consuming enough calories. These people actually need to increase their daily caloric intake and combine it with an exercise program to get their metabolism to kick back up to a normal level.

You also must learn to make wise food choices. Think in terms of long-term benefits (weight management) instead of instant gratification (unhealthy eating and subsequent weight gain). Making healthful choices allows you to eat more food, eat more nutritious food, and in-

Figure 5.10	Making wise food choices.

These illustrations provide a comparison of how much more food you can eat when you make healthy choices. You also get more vitamins, minerals, phytochemicals, antioxidants, and fiber by making healthy choices.

Breakfast

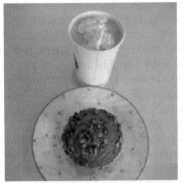

1 banana nut muffin, 1 cafe mocha
Calories: 940
Percent fat calories: 48%

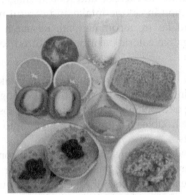

1 cup oatmeal, 1 English muffin with jelly,
1 slice whole wheat bread with honey,
½ cup peaches, 1 kiwi fruit, 1 orange,
1 apple, 1 cup skim milk
Calories: 900
Percent fat calories: 5%

Lunch

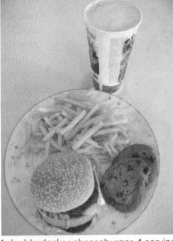

1 double-decker cheeseburger, 1 serving
medium French fries, 2 chocolate chip
cookies, 1 medium strawberry milkshake
Calories: 1,790
Percent fat calories: 37%

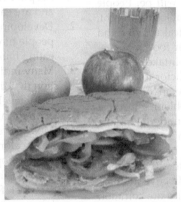

6-inch turkey breast/vegetable sandwich,
1 apple, 1 orange,
1 cup sweetened green tea
Calories: 500
Percent fat calories: 10%

Dinner

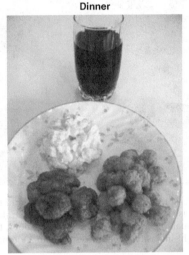

6 oz. popcorn chicken, 3 oz. barbecue
chicken wings, 1 cup potato salad,
1 12-oz. cola drink
Calories: 1,250
Percent fat calories: 42%

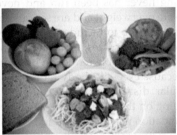

2 cups spaghetti with tomato sauce
and vegetables, a 2-cup salad bowl
with 2 tablespoons Italian dressing,
2 slices whole wheat bread, 1 cup
grapes, 3 large strawberries, 1 kiwi fruit,
1 peach, 1 12-oz. fruit juice drink
Calories: 1,240
Percent fat calories: 14%

gest fewer calories. For example, instead of eating a high-fat, 700-calorie scone, you could eat as much as one orange, one cup of grapes, a hard-boiled egg, two slices of whole-wheat toast, two teaspoons of jam, one-half cup of honey-sweetened oatmeal, and one glass of skim milk (see Figure 5.10).

You can estimate your daily energy (caloric) requirement by consulting Tables 5.3 and 5.4 and completing Activity 5.1. Given that this is only an estimated value,

individual adjustments related to many of the factors discussed in this chapter may be necessary to establish a more precise value. Nevertheless, the estimated value does offer beginning guidelines for weight control or reduction.

The EER without additional planned activity and exercise is based on age, total body weight, height, and gender. Individuals who hold jobs that require a lot of walking or heavy manual labor burn more calories during

Table 5.3	Estimated Energy Requirement (EER) Based on Age, Body Weight, and Height
Men	EER = 662 − (9.53 × Age) + (15.91 × BW) + (539 × HT)
Women	EER = 354 − (6.91 × Age) + (9.36 × BW) + (726 × HT)

Note: Includes activities of independent living only and no moderate physical activity or exercise.
BW = body weight in kilograms (divide BW in pounds by 2.2046),
HT = height in meters (multiply HT in inches by .0254).
© Cengage Learning 2013

the day than those who have sedentary jobs (such as working behind a desk). To estimate your EER, refer to Table 5.3. For example, the EER computation for a 20-year-old man, 71 inches tall, who weighs 160 pounds, would be as follows:

1. Body weight (BW) in kilograms = 72.6 kg
   (160 lb ÷ 2.2046)
   Height (Ht) in meters = 1.8 m (71 × 0.0254)
2. EER = 662 − (9.53 × Age) + (15.91 × BW) + (539 × Ht)
   EER = 662 − (9.53 × 20) + (15.91 × 72.6) + (539 × 1.8)
   EER = 662 − 190.6 + 1155 + 970
   EER = 2,596 calories/day

Thus, the EER to maintain body weight for this individual would be 2,596 calories per day.

To determine the average number of calories you burn daily as a result of exercise, figure out the total number of minutes you exercise weekly, then figure the daily average exercise time. For instance, a person cycling at 10 miles per hour five times a week, 60 minutes each time, exercises 300 minutes per week (5 × 60). The average daily exercise time, therefore, is 42 minutes (300 ÷ 7, rounded off to the lowest unit).

Next, from Table 5.4, find the energy expenditure for the activity (or activities) chosen for the exercise program. In the case of cycling (10 miles per hour), the expenditure is .05 calories per pound of body weight per minute of activity (cal/lb/min). With a body weight of 160 pounds, this man would burn eight calories each minute (body weight × .05, or 160 × .05). In 42 minutes he would burn approximately 336 calories (42 × 8).

Now you can obtain the daily energy requirement, with exercise, needed to maintain body weight. To do this, add the EER obtained from Table 5.3 and the average calories burned through exercise. In our example, it is 2,932 calories (2,596 + 336).

If a negative caloric balance is recommended to lose weight, this person has to consume fewer than 2,932 calories daily to achieve the objective. Because of the many factors that play a role in weight control, this 2,932-calorie value is only an estimated daily requirement. Furthermore, we cannot predict that you will lose exactly one pound of fat in one week if you cut your daily intake by

Table 5.4	Caloric Expenditure of Selected Physical Activities

Activity*	Cal/lb/min	Activity*	Cal/lb/min
Aerobics		Running (on a level surface)	
Moderate	0.065	8.5 min/mile	0.090
Vigorous	0.095	7.0 min/mile	0.102
Step aerobics	0.070	6.0 min/mile	0.114
Archery	0.030	Deep water**	0.100
Badminton		Skating (moderate)	0.038
Recreation	0.038	Skiing	
Competition	0.065	Downhill	0.060
Baseball	0.031	Level (5 mph)	0.078
Basketball		Soccer	0.059
Moderate	0.046	Stairmaster	
Competition	0.063	Moderate	0.070
Bowling	0.030	Vigorous	0.090
Calisthenics	0.033	Stationary Cycling	
Cycling (on a level surface)		Moderate	0.055
5.5 mph	0.033	Vigorous	0.070
10.0 mph	0.050	Strength Training	0.050
13.0 mph	0.071	Swimming (crawl)	
Dance		20 yds/min	0.031
Moderate	0.030	25 yds/min	0.040
Vigorous	0.055	45 yds/min	0.057
Golf	0.030	50 yds/min	0.070
Gymnastics		Table Tennis	0.030
Light	0.030	Tennis	
Heavy	0.056	Moderate	0.045
Handball	0.064	Competition	0.064
Hiking	0.040	Volleyball	0.030
Judo/Karate	0.086	Walking	
Racquetball	0.065	4.5 mph	0.045
Rope Jumping	0.060	Shallow pool	0.090
Rowing (vigorous)	0.090	Water Aerobics	
Running (on a level surface)		Moderate	0.050
11.0 min/mile	0.070	Vigorous	0.070
		Wrestling	0.085

*Values are for actual time engaged in the activity.
**Treading water.
Adapted from:

P. E. Allsen, J. M. Harrison, and B. Vance, *Fitness for Life: An Individualized Approach* (Dubuque, IA: Wm. C. Brown, 1989);

C. A. Bucher and W. E. Prentice, *Fitness for College and Life* (St. Louis: Times Mirror/Mosby College Publishing, 1989);

C. F. Consolazio, R. E. Johnson, and L. J. Pecora, *Physiological Measurements of Metabolic Functions in Man* (New York: McGraw-Hill, 1963);

R. V. Hockey, *Physical Fitness: The Pathway to Healthful Living* (St. Louis: Times Mirror/Mosby College Publishing, 1989);

W. W. K. Hoeger et al., Research conducted at Boise State University, 1986–1993.

500 calories (500 × 7 = 3,500 calories, or the equivalent of one pound of fat).

The daily energy requirement figure is only a target guideline for weight control. Periodic readjustments are necessary because individuals differ, and the daily requirement changes as you lose weight and modify your exercise habits.

To determine the target caloric intake to lose weight, multiply your current weight by 5 and subtract this amount from the total daily energy requirement (2,932 in our example) with exercise. For our example, this would mean 2,132 calories per day to lose weight (160 × 5 = 800 and 2,932 − 800 = 2,132 calories).

This final caloric intake to lose weight should not be below 1,500 daily calories for most people. If distributed properly over the various food groups, 1,500 calories appears to be the lowest caloric intake that still provides the necessary nutrients the body needs. A multivitamin complex is recommended for diets that call for less than 1,500 calories. In terms of percentages of total calories, the daily distribution should be approximately 60 percent carbohydrates (mostly complex carbohydrates), less than 30 percent fat, and about 12 percent protein.

Many experts believe that a person can take off weight more efficiently by reducing the amount of daily fat intake to about 20 percent of the total daily caloric intake. Because 1 gram of fat supplies more than twice the amount of calories that carbohydrates and protein do, the tendency when someone eats less fat is to consume fewer calories. With fat intake at 20 percent of total calories, the individual will have sufficient fat in the diet to feel satisfied and avoid frequent hunger pangs.

Further, it takes only three to five percent of ingested calories to store fat as fat, whereas it takes approximately 25 percent of ingested calories to convert carbohydrates to fat. Some evidence indicates that if people eat the same number of calories as carbohydrate or as fat, those on the fat diet will store more fat. Long-term successful weight loss and weight management programs are low in fat content.

Many people have trouble adhering to a low fat calorie diet. During times of weight loss, however, you are strongly encouraged to do so. Refer to Table 5.5 to aid you in determining the grams of fat at 20 percent of the total calories for selected energy intakes. Also, use the form provided in Activity 3.2 (Chapter 3, page 90) to monitor your daily fat intake. For weight maintenance, individuals who have been successful in maintaining an average weight loss of 30 pounds for more than six years are consuming about 24 percent of calories from fat, 56 percent from carbohydrates, and 20 percent from protein.[31]

Breakfast is a critical meal while on a weight loss program. Many people skip breakfast because it's the easiest meal to skip. Evidence indicates that people who skip breakfast are hungrier later in the day and end up con-

Table 5.5	Grams of Fat at 10%, 20%, and 30% of Total Calories for Selected Energy Intakes		
	Grams of Fat		
Caloric Intake	**10%**	**20%**	**30%**
1,200	13	27	40
1,300	14	29	43
1,400	16	31	47
1,500	17	33	50
1,600	18	36	53
1,700	19	38	57
1,800	20	40	60
1,900	21	42	63
2,000	22	44	67
2,100	23	47	70
2,200	24	49	73
2,300	26	51	77
2,400	27	53	80
2,500	28	56	83
2,600	29	58	87
2,700	30	60	90
2,800	31	62	93
2,900	32	64	97
3,000	33	67	100

© Cengage Learning 2013

Behavior Modification Planning

Healthy Breakfast Choices

Breakfast is the most important meal of the day. Skipping breakfast makes you hungrier later in the day and leads to overconsumption and greater caloric intake throughout the rest of the day. Regular breakfast eaters have less of a weight problem, lose weight more effectively, have less difficulty maintaining lost weight, and live longer. Skipping breakfast also temporarily raises LDL (bad) cholesterol and lowers insulin sensitivity, changes that may increase the risk for heart disease and diabetes. Here are some healthy breakfast food choices:

Fresh fruit
Low-fat or skim milk
Low-fat yogurt
Whole-grain cereal
Whole-grain bread or bagel with fat-free cream cheese and slices of red or green pepper
Hummus over a whole-grain bagel
Peanut butter with whole-grain bread or bagel
Low-fat cottage cheese with fruit
Oatmeal
Reduced-fat cheese
Egg Beaters with salsa
An occasional egg

Try It Select a healthy breakfast choice each day for the next 7 days. Evaluate how you feel the rest of the morning. What effect did eating breakfast have on your activities of daily living and daily caloric intake? Be sure to record your food choices, how you felt, and what activities you engaged in.

suming more total daily calories than those who eat breakfast. Furthermore, regular breakfast eaters have less of a weight problem, lose weight more effectively, and have less difficulty maintaining the weight loss.

If most of the daily calories are consumed during one meal (as in the typical evening meal), the body may perceive that something is wrong and will slow the metabolism so that it can store more calories in the form of fat. Also, eating most of the calories during one meal causes a person to go hungry the rest of the day, making it more difficult to adhere to the diet.

Consuming most of the calories earlier in the day seems helpful in losing weight and also in managing atherosclerosis. The time of day when most of the fats and cholesterol are consumed can influence blood lipids and coronary heart disease. Peak digestion time following a heavy meal is about seven hours after that meal. If most lipids are consumed during the evening meal, digestion peaks while the person is sound asleep, when the metabolism is at its lowest rate. Consequently, the body may not metabolize fats and cholesterol as well, leading to a higher blood lipid count and increasing the risk for atherosclerosis and coronary heart disease.

Before you proceed to develop a thorough weight-loss program, take a moment to identify, in Activity 5.2, your current stage of change as it pertains to your recommended body weight. If applicable—that is, if you are not at recommended weight—list also the processes and techniques for change that you will use to accomplish your goal. In Activity 5.2 you also outline your exercise program for weight management.

Monitoring Your Diet with Daily Food Logs

To help you monitor and adhere to a weight loss program, use the daily food logs provided in Activity 5.3. If the goal is to maintain or increase body weight, use Activity 5.4.

Evidence indicates that people who monitor daily caloric intake are more successful at weight loss than those who don't self-monitor. Before using the forms in Activity 5.3, make a master copy for your files so you can make future copies as needed. Guidelines are provided for 1,200-, 1,500-, 1,800-, and 2,000-calorie diet plans. These plans have been developed based on the MyPlate and the Dietary Guidelines for Americans to meet the Recommended Dietary Allowances.[32] The objective is to meet (not exceed) the number of servings allowed for each diet plan. Each time you eat a serving of a certain food, record it in the appropriate box.

To lose weight, you should use the diet plan that most closely approximates your target caloric intake. The plan is based on the following caloric allowances for these food groups:

- Grains: 80 calories per serving.
- Fruits: 60 calories per serving.

- Vegetables: 25 calories per serving.
- Dairy (use low-fat products): 120 calories per serving.
- Protein: Use low-fat (300 calories per serving) frozen entrees or an equivalent amount if you prepare your own main dish (see the following discussion).

As you start your diet plan, pay particular attention to food serving sizes. Take care with cup and glass sizes. A standard cup is 8 ounces, but most glasses nowadays contain between 12 and 16 ounces. If you drink 12 ounces of fruit juice, in essence you are getting two servings of fruit because a standard serving is three-fourths cup of juice.

Read food labels carefully to compare the caloric value of the serving listed on the label with the caloric guidelines provided above. Here are some examples:

- One slice of standard whole-wheat bread has about 80 calories. A plain bagel may have 200 to 350 calories. Although it is low in fat, a 350-calorie bagel is equivalent to almost four servings in the grains group.
- The standard serving size listed on the food label for most cereals is one cup. As you read the nutrition information, however, you will find that for the same cup of cereal, one type of cereal has 120 calories and another cereal has 200 calories. Because a standard serving in the grains group is 80 calories, the first cereal would be 1.5 servings and the second one 2.5 servings.
- A medium-size fruit is usually considered to be one serving. A large fruit provides more than one serving.
- In the dairy group, one serving represents 120 calories. A cup of whole milk has about 160 calories, compared with a cup of skim milk, which contains 88 calories. A cup of whole milk, therefore, would provide 1.33 servings in this food group.

Low-Fat Entrees

To be more accurate with caloric intake and to simplify meal preparation, use commercially prepared low-fat frozen entrees as the main dish for lunch and dinner meals (only one entree per meal for the 1,200-calorie diet plan; see Activity 5.3). Look for entrees that provide about 300 calories and no more than six grams of fat per entree. These two entrees can be used as selections for the protein group and will provide most of your daily requirement. Along with each entree, supplement the meal with some of your servings from the other food groups. This diet plan has been used successfully in weight loss research programs.[33] If you choose not to use these low-fat entrees, prepare a similar meal using three ounces (cooked) of lean meat, poultry, or fish with additional vegetables, rice, or pasta that will provide 300 calories with fewer than six grams of fat per dish.

In your daily logs, be sure to record the precise amount in each serving. You also can run a computerized nutrient analysis to verify your caloric intake and

Computing Your Daily Caloric Requirement

Name: _____ Date: _____

Course: _____ Section: _____ Gender: _____ Age: _____

A. Current body weight (BW) in kilograms (body weight in pounds ÷ 2.2046) .... ☐

B. Current height (HT) in meters (HT in inches × .0254) .... ☐

C. Estimated energy requirement (EER) (Table 5.3, page 167)

   Men: EER = 663 − (9.53 × Age) + (15.91 × BW) + (539.6 × HT)

   Women: EER = 354 − (6.91 × Age) + (9.36 × BW) + (726 × HT)

   EER = ☐ − (☐ × ☐) + (☐ × ☐) + (☐ × ☐)

   EER = ☐ − ☐ + ☐ + ☐

   EER = ☐ − ☐ + ☐ = ☐ calories

D. Selected physical activity (e.g., jogging)[a] .... ☐

E. Number of exercise sessions per week .... ☐

F. Duration of exercise session (in minutes) .... ☐

G. Total weekly exercise time in minutes (E × F) .... ☐

H. Average daily exercise time in minutes (G ÷ 7) .... ☐

I. Caloric expenditure per pound per minute (cal/lb/min) of physical activity (use Table 5.4, page 167) ... ☐

J. Body weight in pounds .... ☐

K. Total calories burned per minute of physical activity (I × J) .... ☐

L. Average daily calories burned as a result of the exercise program (H × K) .... ☐

M. Total daily energy requirement with exercise to maintain body weight (C + L) .... ☐

Stop here if no weight loss is required; otherwise proceed to items N and O.

N. Number of calories to subtract from daily requirement to achieve a negative caloric balance (J × 5) ... ☐

O. Target caloric intake to lose weight (M − N)[b] .... ☐

[a]If more than one physical activity is selected, you will need to estimate the average daily calories burned as a result of each additional activity (steps D through L) and add all of these figures to M above.

[b]This figure should never be fewer than 1,200 calories for small women or 1,500 calories for everyone else. See Activity 5.3 for the 1,200, 1,500, 1,800, and 2,000 calorie diet plans.

Weight Loss Behavior Modification Plan

Name: _____ Date: _____

Course: _____ Section: _____ Gender: _____ Age: _____

1. Using Figure 2.5 (page 61) and Table 2.3 (page 60), identify your current stage of change regarding **recommended body weight:** [_____]

2. How much weight do you want to lose? [_____] Is it a realistic goal? [_____]

3. Target caloric intake to lose weight (diet plan—see Activity 5.1, item O) [_____]

4. Based on the processes and techniques of change discussed in Chapter 2, indicate what you can do to help yourself implement a weight management program.

_____

_____

5. How much effort are you willing to put into reaching your weight loss goal?

_____

Indicate your feelings about participating in an exercise program.

_____

6. Will you commit to participate in a combined aerobic and strength-training program?* Yes [____] No [____]

If your answer is "Yes," proceed to the next question; if you answered "No," please review Chapters 3–5 again and read Chapters 6–9.

7. Select one or two aerobic activities in which you will participate regularly.

[_____] [_____]

List facilities available to you where you can carry out the aerobic and strength-training programs.

_____

_____

8. Indicate days and times you will set aside for your aerobic and strength-training programs (5 or 6 days per week should be devoted to aerobic exercise and 1 to 3 nonconsecutive days per week to strength training).

Monday: [_____]

Tuesday: [_____]

Wednesday: [_____]

Thursday: [_____]

Friday: [_____]

Saturday: [_____]

Sunday: A complete day of rest once a week is recommended to allow your body to fully recover from exercise.

Behavior Modification

Briefly describe whether you think you can meet the goals of your aerobic and strength-training programs. What obstacles will you have to overcome, and how will you overcome them?

_____

_____

*Flexibility programs are necessary for adequate fitness, possible injury prevention, and good health but do not help with weight loss. Stretching exercises can be conducted regularly during the cool-down phase of your aerobic and strength-training programs (see Chapter 8).

Weight Loss Strategies

1. *Make a commitment to change.* The first necessary ingredient is the desire to modify your behavior. You have to stop precontemplating or contemplating change and get going! You must accept that you have a problem and decide by yourself whether you really want to change. Sincere commitment increases your chances for success.

2. *Set realistic goals.* The weight problem developed over several years. Similarly, new lifetime eating and exercise habits take time to develop. A realistic long-term goal also will include short-term objectives that allow for regular evaluation and help maintain motivation and renewed commitment to attain the long-term goal.

3. *Weigh yourself regularly,* preferably at the same time of day and under the same conditions. Do not adapt and accept a higher body weight as a new stable weight. Make dietary and physical activity adjustments accordingly.

4. *Incorporate exercise into the program.* Choosing enjoyable activities, places, times, equipment, and people to work out with will help you adhere to an exercise program. (See Chapters 6–9.)

5. *Differentiate hunger and appetite.* Hunger is the actual physical need for food. Appetite is a desire for food, usually triggered by factors such as stress, habit, boredom, depression, availability of food, or just the thought of food itself. Developing and sticking to a regular meal pattern will help control hunger.

6. *Eat less fat.* Each gram of fat provides 9 calories, and protein and carbohydrates provide only 4. In essence, you can eat more food on a low-fat diet because you consume fewer calories with each meal. Most of your fat intake should come from unsaturated sources.

7. *Pay attention to calories.* Just because food is labeled "low-fat" does not mean you can eat as much as you want. When reading food labels—and when eating—don't just look at the fat content. Pay attention to calories as well. Many low-fat foods are high in calories.

8. *Cut unnecessary items from your diet.* Substituting water for a daily can of soda would cut 51,100 (140 × 365) calories yearly from the diet—the equivalent of 14.6 (51,000 ÷ 3,500) pounds of fat.

9. *Maintain a daily intake of calcium-rich foods,* especially low-fat or non-fat dairy products.

10. *Add foods to your diet that reduce cravings,* such as eggs; small amounts of red meat, fish, poultry, tofu, oils, fats; and nonstarchy vegetables such as lettuce, green beans, peppers, asparagus, broccoli, mushrooms, and Brussels sprouts. Also increasing the intake of low-glycemic carbohydrates with your meals helps you go longer before you feel hungry again.

11. *Avoid automatic eating.* Many people associate certain daily activities with eating, for example, cooking, watching television, or reading. Most foods consumed in these situations lack nutritional value or are high in sugar and fat.

12. *Stay busy.* People tend to eat more when they sit around and do nothing. Occupying the mind and body with activities not associated with eating helps take away the desire to eat. Some options are walking; cycling; playing sports; gardening; sewing; or visiting a library, a museum, or a park. You also might develop other skills and interests not associated with food.

13. *Plan meals and shop sensibly.* Always shop on a full stomach, because hungry shoppers tend to buy unhealthy foods impulsively—and then snack on the way home. Always use a shopping list, which should include whole-grain breads and cereals, fruits and vegetables, low-fat milk and dairy products, lean meats, fish, and poultry.

14. *Cook wisely:*
    • Use less fat and fewer refined foods in food preparation.
    • Trim all visible fat from meats and remove skin from poultry before cooking.
    • Skim the fat off gravies and soups.
    • Bake, broil, boil, or steam instead of frying.
    • Sparingly use butter, cream, mayonnaise, and salad dressings.
    • Avoid coconut oil, palm oil, and cocoa butter.
    • Prepare plenty of foods that contain fiber.

food distribution pattern (percent of total calories from carbohydrate, fat, and protein).

Effect of Food Choices on Long-Term Weight Gain

Although still in its infancy, research published in 2011 on more than 120,000 people who were evaluated every four years over a 20-year period showed that food choices have a significant effect on weight gain.[34] On average, study participants gained 17 pounds over the course of 20 years. Regardless of other lifestyle habits, individuals who consumed unhealthy foods gained the most weight, whereas those who made healthy food choices gained the least amount of weight. Although more research is needed, in this study, four-year weight change was most strongly associated with the consumption of potato chips, potatoes, sugar-sweetened beverages, unprocessed and processed red meats and inversely associated with the consumption of vegetables, whole grains, fruits, nuts, and yogurt. The take-home message: Consume more fruits, vegetables, whole grains,

- Include whole-grain breads and cereals, vegetables, and legumes in most meals.
- Eat fruits for dessert.
- Stay away from soda pop, fruit juices, and fruit-flavored drinks.
- Use less sugar, and cut down on other refined carbohydrates, such as corn syrup, malt sugar, dextrose, and fructose.
- Drink plenty of water—at least six glasses a day.

15. *Do not serve more food than you should eat.* Measure the food in portions and keep serving dishes away from the table. Do not force yourself or anyone else to "clean the plate" after they are satisfied (including children after they already have had a healthy, nutritious serving).

16. *Try "junior size" instead of "super size."* People who are served larger portions eat more, whether they are hungry or not. Use smaller plates, bowls, cups, and glasses. Try eating half as much food as you commonly eat. Watch for portion sizes at restaurants as well: Supersized foods create supersized people.

17. *Eat out infrequently.* The more often people eat out, the more body fat they have. People who eat out six or more times per week consume an average of about 300 extra calories per day and 30 percent more fat than those who eat out less often.

18. *Eat slowly and at the table only.* Eating on the run promotes overeating because the body doesn't have enough time to "register" consumption and people overeat before the body perceives the fullness signal. Eating at the table encourages people to take time out to eat and deters snacking between meals. After eating, do not sit around the table but, rather, clean up and put away the food to avoid snacking.

19. *Avoid social binges.* Social gatherings tend to entice self-defeating behavior. Use visual imagery to plan ahead. Do not feel pressured to eat or drink and don't rationalize in these situations. Choose low-calorie foods and entertain yourself with other activities, such as dancing and talking.

20. *Do not place unhealthy foods within easy reach.* Ideally, avoid bringing high-calorie, high-sugar, or high-fat foods into the house. If they are there already, store them where they are hard to get to or see—perhaps the garage or basement.

21. *Avoid evening food raids.* Most people do really well during the day but then "lose it" at night. Take control. Stop and think. To avoid excessive nighttime snacking, stay busy after your evening meal. Go for a short walk; floss and brush your teeth, and get to bed earlier. Even better, close the kitchen after dinner and try not to eat anything 3 hours prior to going to sleep.

22. *Practice stress management techniques* (discussed in Chapter 12). Many people snack and increase their food consumption in stressful situations.

23. *Get support.* People who receive support from friends, relatives, and formal support groups are much more likely to lose and maintain weight loss than those without such support. The more support you receive, the better off you will be.

24. *Monitor changes and reward accomplishments.* Being able to exercise without interruption for 15, 20, 30, or 60 minutes; swimming a certain distance; running a mile—all these accomplishments deserve recognition. Create rewards that are not related to eating: new clothing, a tennis racquet, a bicycle, exercise shoes, or something else that is special and you would not have acquired otherwise.

25. *Prepare for slip-ups.* Most people will slip and occasionally splurge. Do not despair and give up. Reevaluate and continue with your efforts. An occasional slip won't make much difference in the long run.

26. *Think positive.* Avoid negative thoughts about how difficult changing past behaviors might be. Instead, think of the benefits you will reap, such as feeling, looking, and functioning better, plus enjoying better health and improving the quality of life. Avoid negative environments and unsupportive people.

Try It In your Online Journal or class notebook, answer the following questions: How many of the above strategies do you use to help you maintain recommended body weight? Do you feel that any of these strategies specifically help you manage body weight more effectively? If so, explain why.

low-fat dairy products, and nuts (the last in moderation because of their high caloric content).

Behavior Modification and Adherence to a Weight Management Program

Achieving and maintaining recommended body composition is certainly possible, but it does require desire and commitment. If weight management is to become a priority, people must realize that they have to transform their behavior to some extent.

Modifying old habits and developing new, positive behaviors takes time. Individuals who apply the management techniques provided in the Behavior Modification Planning box (pages 172–173) are more successful at changing detrimental behavior and adhering to a positive lifetime weight-control program. In developing a retraining program, you are not expected to incorporate all of the strategies given but should note the ones that apply to you. The form provided in Activity 5.5 will allow you to evaluate and monitor your own weight-management behaviors.

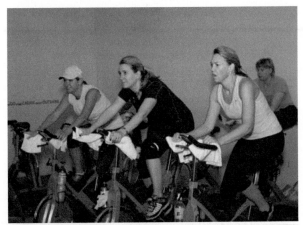

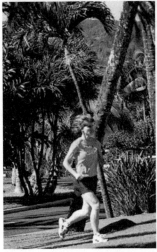

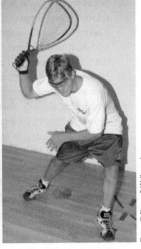

Photos © Fitness & Wellness, Inc.

Exercising with other people and in different places helps people maintain exercise regularity.

Critical Thinking

What behavioral strategies have you used to properly manage your body weight? • How do you think those strategies would work for others?

During the weight loss process, surround yourself with people who have the same goals as you do (weight loss). Data released in 2007 showed that obesity can spread through "social networks."[35] That is, if your friends, siblings, or spouse gain weight, you are more likely to gain weight as well. People tend to accept a higher weight standard if someone they are close to or care about gains weight.

In the study, the social ties of more than 12,000 were examined over 32 years. The findings revealed that if a close friend becomes obese, your risk of becoming obese during the next two to four years increases 171 percent. The risk also increases 57 percent for casual friends, 40 percent for siblings, and 37 percent for the person's spouse. The reverse was also found to be true. When a person loses weight, the likelihood of friends, siblings, or spouse to lose weight is also enhanced.

Furthermore, the research found that gender plays a role in social networks. A male's weight has a greater effect on the weight of male friends and brothers than on female friends or sisters. Similarly, a woman's weight has a far greater influence on sisters and girlfriends than on brothers or male friends. Thus, if you are trying to lose weight, choose your friendships carefully: Do not surround yourself with people who either have a weight problem or are still gaining weight.

The Simple Truth

There is no quick and easy way to take off excess body fat and keep it off for good. Weight management is accomplished by making a lifetime commitment to physical activity and proper food selection. When taking part in a weight (fat) reduction program, people also have to decrease their caloric intake moderately, use portion control, be physically active, and implement strategies to modify unhealthy eating behaviors.

During the process, relapses into past negative behaviors are almost inevitable. The three most common reasons for relapse are:

1. Stress-related factors (such as major life changes, depression, job changes, illness)
2. Social reasons (entertaining, eating out, business travel)
3. Self-enticing behaviors (placing yourself in a situation to see how much you can get away with: "One small taste won't hurt" leads to "I'll eat just one slice" and finally to "I haven't done well, so I might as well eat some more").

Making mistakes is human and does not necessarily mean failure. Failure comes to those who give up and do not build on previous experiences and thereby develop skills that will prevent self-defeating behaviors in the future. Where there's a will, there's a way, and those who persist will reap the rewards.

Daily Food Intake Record: 1,200 Calorie Diet Plan

Name: _____ Date: _____

Course: _____ Section: _____ Gender: _____ Age: _____

Instructions:

The objective of the diet plan is to meet (not exceed) the number of servings allowed for the food groups listed. Each time you eat a specific food, record it in the space provided for each group, along with the amount you ate. Refer to the number of calories below to find out what counts as one serving for each group listed. Instead of the meat and beans group, you are allowed to have a commercially available low-fat frozen entree for your main meal (this entree should provide no more than 300 calories and fewer than 6 grams of fat). You can make additional copies of this form as needed.

Dairy: 2 servings
Grains: 6 servings
Fruits: 2 servings
Veggies: 3 servings
Protein: 1 low-fat frozen entree

Choose**MyPlate**.gov

Grains (80 calories/serving): 6 servings

1	
2	
3	
4	
5	
6	

Vegetables (25 calories/serving): 3 servings

1	
2	
3	

Fruits (60 calories/serving): 2 servings

| 1 | |
| 2 | |

Dairy (120 calories/serving, use low-fat milk and milk products): 2 servings

| 1 | |
| 2 | |

Low-Fat Frozen Entree (300 calories and fewer than 6 grams of fat): 1 serving

| 1 | |

Today's physical activity: _____ Intensity: _____ Duration: _____ min Number of steps: _____

Daily Food Intake Record: 1,500 Calorie Diet Plan

Instructions:

The objective of the diet plan is to meet (not exceed) the number of servings allowed for the food groups listed. Each time you eat a specific food, record it in the space provided for each group, along with the amount you ate. Refer to the number of calories below to find out what counts as one serving for each group listed. Instead of the meat and beans group, you are allowed to have 2 commercially available low-fat frozen entrees for your main meal (these entrees should provide no more than 300 calories each and fewer than 6 grams of fat). You can make additional copies of this form as needed.

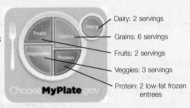

Dairy: 2 servings
Grains: 6 servings
Fruits: 2 servings
Veggies: 3 servings
Protein: 2 low-fat frozen entrees

MyPlate

Grains (80 calories/serving): 6 servings

1	
2	
3	
4	
5	
6	

Vegetables (25 calories/serving): 3 servings

1	
2	
3	

Fruits (60 calories/serving): 2 servings

1	
2	

Dairy (120 calories/serving, use low-fat milk and milk products): 2 servings

1	
2	

Two Low-Fat Frozen Entrees (300 calories and fewer than 6 grams of fat): 2 servings

1	
2	

Today's physical activity: _____ Intensity: _____ Duration: _____ min Number of steps: _____

Daily Food Intake Record: 1,800 Calorie Diet Plan

Instructions:

The objective of the diet plan is to meet (not exceed) the number of servings allowed for the food groups listed. Each time you eat a specific food, record it in the space provided for each group, along with the amount you ate. Refer to the number of calories below to find out what counts as one serving for each group listed. Instead of the meat and beans group, you are allowed to have 2 commercially available low-fat frozen entrees for your main meal (these entrees should provide no more than 300 calories each and fewer than 6 grams of fat). You can make additional copies of this form as needed.

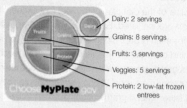

Dairy: 2 servings
Grains: 8 servings
Fruits: 3 servings
Veggies: 5 servings
Protein: 2 low-fat frozen entrees

Grains (80 calories/serving): 8 servings

1	
2	
3	
4	
5	
6	
7	
8	

Vegetables (25 calories/serving): 5 servings

1	
2	
3	
4	
5	

Fruits (60 calories/serving): 3 servings

1	
2	
3	

Dairy (120 calories/serving, use low-fat milk and milk products): 2 servings

1	
2	

Two Low-Fat Frozen Entrees (300 calories and fewer than 6 grams of fat): 2 servings

1	
2	

Today's physical activity: _____ Intensity: _____ Duration: _____ min Number of steps: _____

Daily Food Intake Record: 2,000 Calorie Diet Plan

Instructions:

The objective of the diet plan is to meet (not exceed) the number of servings allowed for the food groups listed. Each time you eat a specific food, record it in the space provided for each group, along with the amount you ate. Refer to the number of calories below to find out what counts as one serving for each group listed. Instead of the meat and beans group, you are allowed to have 2 commercially available low-fat frozen entrees for your main meal (these entrees should provide no more than 300 calories each and fewer than 6 grams of fat). You can make additional copies of this form as needed.

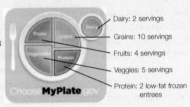

Dairy: 2 servings
Grains: 10 servings
Fruits: 4 servings
Veggies: 5 servings
Protein: 2 low-fat frozen entrees

Grains (80 calories/serving): 10 servings

1	
2	
3	
4	
5	
6	
7	
8	
9	
10	

Vegetables (25 calories/serving): 5 servings

1	
2	
3	
4	
5	

Fruits (60 calories/serving): 4 servings

1	
2	
3	
4	

Dairy (120 calories/serving, use low-fat milk and milk products): 2 servings

1	
2	

Two Low-Fat Frozen Entrees (300 calories and fewer than 6 grams of fat): 2 servings

1	
2	

Today's physical activity: _____ Intensity: _____ Duration: _____ min Number of steps: _____

Healthy Dietary Plan for Weight Maintenance or Weight Gain

Name: _____ Date: _____

Course: _____ Section: _____ Gender: _____ Age: _____

I. Daily Caloric Requirement

A. Current body weight in pounds .... [ ]

B. Current percent body fat .... [ ]

C. Current body composition classification (Table 4.10, page 134) .... [ ]

D. Total daily energy requirement with exercise to maintain body weight (use item M from Activity 5.1). Use this figure and stop further computations if the goal is to maintain body weight .... [ ]

E. Target body weight (if your goal is to increase body weight) .... [ ]

F. Number of additional daily calories to increase body weight (combine this increased caloric intake with a strength-training program, see Chapter 7) .... [500]

G. Total daily energy (caloric) requirement with exercise to increase body weight (D + 500) .... [ ]

II. Strength-Training Program

For weight gain purposes, indicate three days during the week and the time when you will engage in a strength-training program.

_____

_____

III. Healthy Diet Plan

Design a sample healthy daily diet plan according to the total daily energy requirement computed in D (maintenance) or G (weight gain) above. Using Appendix B, list all individual food items that you can consume on that day, along with their caloric, carbohydrate, fat, and protein content. Be sure that the diet meets your recommended MyPlate number of servings from the various food groups.

Breakfast

	Food item	Amount	Calories	Carbohydrates (gr)	Fat (gr)	Protein (gr)
1.						
2.						
3.						
4.						
5.						
6.						
7.						
8.						

Healthy Dietary Plan for Weight Maintenance or Weight Gain (continued)

Lunch

	Food item	Amount	Calories	Carbohydrates (gr)	Fat (gr)	Protein (gr)
1.						
2.						
3.						
4.						
5.						
6.						
7.						
8.						

Snack

	Food item	Amount	Calories	Carbohydrates (gr)	Fat (gr)	Protein (gr)
1.						

Dinner

	Food item	Amount	Calories	Carbohydrates (gr)	Fat (gr)	Protein (gr)
1.						
2.						
3.						
4.						
5.						
6.						
7.						
8.						
	Totals:					

IV. Percent of Macronutrients

Determine the percent of total calories that are derived from carbohydrates, fat, and protein.

A. Total calories = [ ]

B. Grams of carbohydrates [ ] × 4 ÷ [ ] (total calories) = [ ] %

C. Grams of fat [ ] × 9 ÷ [ ] (total calories) = [ ] %

D. Grams of protein [ ] × 4 ÷ [ ] (total calories) = [ ] %

E. Body weight (BW) in kilograms (BW in pounds divided by 2.2046) = [ ] kg

F. Grams of protein per kilogram of body weight [ ] (grams of protein) ÷ [ ] (BW in kg) = [ ] gr/kg

G. Please summarize your diet and protein intake to either maintain or gain weight.

_____

_____

Weight Management: Measuring Progress

Name: _____ Date: _____

Course: _____ Section: _____ Gender: _____ Age: _____

I. Please answer all of the following:

1. State your feelings regarding your current body weight, your target body composition, and a completion date for this goal.

_____

_____

_____

_____

_____

_____

2. Do you have an eating disorder? If so, express your feelings about it. Can your instructor help you find professional advice so that you can work toward resolving this problem?

_____

_____

_____

_____

_____

_____

_____

3. Is your present diet adequate according to the nutrient analysis?   Yes   No

4. State dietary changes necessary to achieve a balanced diet and/or to lose weight (increase or decrease caloric intake, decrease fat intake, increase intake of complex carbohydrates, and so on). List specific foods that will help you improve in areas in which you may have deficiencies and food items to avoid or consume in moderation to help you achieve better nutrition.

Changes to make: _____

_____

_____

Foods that will help: _____

_____

Foods to avoid: _____

_____

Weight Management: Measuring Progress (continued)

II. Behavior Modification Progress Form

Instructions: On a weekly or bi-weekly basis, go through the list of strategies in the box on pages 172–173 and provide a "Yes" or "No" answer to each statement. If you are able to answer "Yes" to most questions, you have been successful in implementing positive weight management behaviors. (Make additional copies of this page as needed.)

Strategy	Date						
1. I have made a commitment to change.							
2. I set realistic goals.							
3. I monitor body weight on a regular basis.							
4. I exercise regularly.							
5. I exercise control over my appetite.							
6. I am consuming less fat in my diet.							
7. I pay attention to the number of calories in food.							
8. I have eliminated unnecessary food items from my diet.							
9. I include calcium-rich food in my diet.							
10. I use craving-reducing foods in my diet.							
11. I avoid automatic eating.							
12. I stay busy.							
13. I plan meals ahead of time and shop sensibly.							
14. I cook wisely.							
15. I do not serve more food than I should eat.							
16. I use portion control in my diet and when dining out.							
17. I do not eat out more than once per week. When I do, I eat low-fat meals.							
18. I eat slowly and at the table only.							
19. I avoid social binges.							
20. I avoid temptation by relocating or removing unhealthy foods.							
21. I avoid evening food raids.							
22. I practice stress management.							
23. I have a strong support group.							
24. I monitor changes and reward my accomplishments.							
25. I prepare for lapses/relapses.							
26. I think positive.							
27. I make sensible adjustments in caloric intake and physical activity if my weight increases and stabilizes there for several days.							

Assess Your Behavior

Log on to www.cengagebrain.com to access CengageNOW where you can update your pedometer log if you are tracking your steps.

1. Are you satisfied with your current body composition (including body weight) and quality of life? If not, are you willing to do something about it to properly resolve the problem?

2. Are physical activity, aerobic exercise, and strength training a regular part of your lifetime weight management program?

3. Do you weigh yourself regularly and make adjustments in energy intake and physical activity habits if your weight starts to slip upward?

4. Do you exercise portion control, watch your overall fat intake, and plan ahead before you eat out or attend social functions that entice overeating?

Assess Your Knowledge

Evaluate how well you understand the concepts presented in this chapter using the chapter-specific quizzing available in the online materials at www.cengagebrain.com.

1. During the last decade, the rate of obesity in the United States has
   a. been on the decline.
   b. increased at an alarming rate.
   c. increased slightly.
   d. remained steady.
   e. increased in men and decreased in women.

2. Obesity is defined as a body mass index (BMI) equal to or above
   a. 10.
   b. 25.
   c. 30.
   d. 45.
   e. 50.

3. Obesity increases the risk for
   a. hypertension.
   b. congestive heart failure.
   c. atherosclerosis.
   d. type 2 diabetes.
   e. all of the above.

4. Tolerable weight is a body weight
   a. that is not ideal but one that you can live with.
   b. that will tolerate the increased risk for chronic diseases.
   c. with a BMI range between 25 and 30.
   d. that meets both ideal values for percent body weight and BMI.
   e. All are correct choices.

5. When the body uses protein instead of a combination of fats and carbohydrates as a source of energy,
   a. weight loss is very slow.
   b. a large amount of weight loss is in the form of water.
   c. muscle turns into fat.
   d. fat is lost very rapidly.
   e. fat cannot be lost.

6. Eating disorders
   a. are characterized by an intense fear of becoming fat.
   b. are physical and emotional conditions.
   c. almost always require professional help for successful treatment of the disease.
   d. are common in societies that encourage thinness.
   e. All are correct choices.

7. The mechanism that seems to regulate how much a person weighs is known as
   a. setpoint.
   b. weight factor.
   c. basal metabolic rate.
   d. metabolism.
   e. energy-balancing equation.

8. The key to maintaining weight loss successfully is
   a. frequent dieting.
   b. very low calorie diets when "normal" dieting doesn't work.
   c. a lifetime physical activity program.
   d. regular high-protein/low-carbohydrate meals.
   e. All are correct choices.

9. The daily amount of physical activity recommended for weight loss purposes is
   a. 15 to 20 minutes.
   b. 20 to 30 minutes.
   c. 30 to 60 minutes.
   d. 60 to 90 minutes.
   e. Any amount is sufficient as long as it is done daily.

10. A daily energy expenditure of 300 calories through physical activity is the equivalent of approximately _____ pounds of fat per year.
    a. 12
    b. 15
    c. 22
    d. 27
    e. 31

Correct answers can be found at the back of the book.

Cardiorespiratory Endurance

6

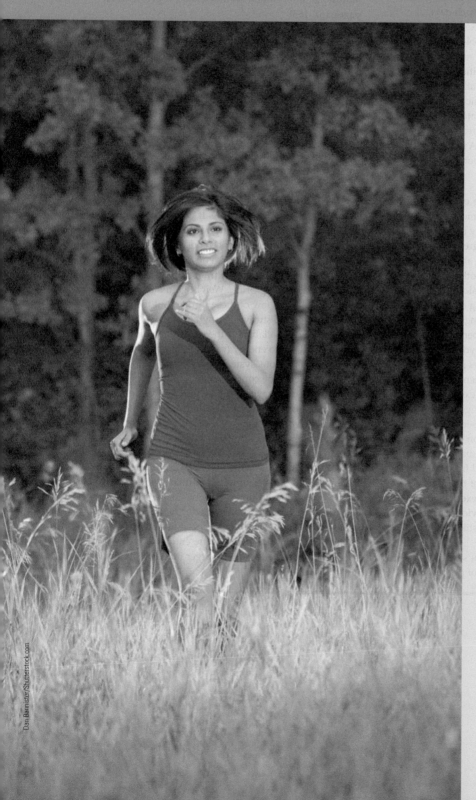

Dan Bannister/Shutterstock.com

"Daily physical activity is the miracle medication that people are looking for. It makes you look and feel younger, boosts energy, provides lifetime weight management, improves self-confidence and self-esteem, and enhances independent living, health, and quality of life. It further allows you to enjoy a longer life by decreasing the risk of many chronic conditions, including heart disease, high blood pressure, stroke, diabetes, some cancers, and osteoporosis."

Objectives

▶ **Define** cardiorespiratory endurance and describe the benefits of cardiorespiratory endurance training in maintaining health and well-being.

▶ **Define** aerobic and anaerobic exercise, and give examples.

▶ **Be able** to assess cardiorespiratory fitness through five different test protocols: 1.5-Mile Run Test, 1.0-Mile Walk Test, Step Test, Astrand-Ryhming Test, and 12-Minute Swim Test.

▶ **Be able** to interpret the results of cardiorespiratory endurance assessments according to health fitness and physical fitness standards.

▶ **Determine** your readiness to start an exercise program.

▶ **Explain** the principles that govern cardiorespiratory exercise prescription: intensity, mode, duration, frequency, and rate of progression.

▶ **Learn** some ways to foster adherence to exercise.

CENGAGEbrain.com

Assess your cardiorespiratory endurance. Maintain a log of all your fitness activities.

Visit www.cengagebrain.com to access course materials and companion resources for this text including quiz questions designed to check your understanding of the chapter contents. See the preface on page xv for more information.

Does aerobic exercise make a person immune to heart and blood vessel disease? Although aerobically fit individuals as a whole have a lower incidence of cardiovascular disease, a regular aerobic exercise program by itself does not offer an absolute guarantee against cardiovascular disease. The best way to minimize the risk for cardiovascular disease is to manage the risk factors. Many factors, including a genetic predisposition, can increase the risk. Research data, however, indicate that a regular aerobic exercise program will delay the onset of cardiovascular problems and will improve the chances of surviving a heart attack. Even moderate increases in aerobic fitness significantly lower the incidence of premature cardiovascular deaths. Data from the research study on death rates by physical fitness groups (illustrated in Figure 1.11, page 19) indicate that the decrease in cardiovascular mortality is greatest between the unfit and the moderately fit groups. A further decrease in cardiovascular mortality is observed between the moderately fit and the highly fit groups.

Is light-intensity aerobic exercise more effective in burning fat? During light-intensity and moderate-intensity exercise a greater percentage of the energy is derived from fat. It is also true, however, that an even greater percentage of the energy comes from fat when doing absolutely nothing (resting/sleeping). And when one does nothing, as in a sedentary lifestyle, one doesn't burn many calories.

Let's examine this issue. During resting conditions, the human body is a very efficient "fat-burning machine." That is, most of the energy, approximately 70 percent, is derived from fat and only 30 percent from carbohydrates. But we burn few calories at rest, about 1.5 calories per minute compared with 3 to 4 calories during light-intensity exercise, 5 to 7 calories during moderate-intensity exercise, and 8 to 10 (or more) calories per minute during vigorous-intensity exercise. As we begin to exercise and subsequently increase its intensity, we progressively rely more on carbohydrates and less on fat for energy, until we reach maximal intensity, when 100 percent of the energy is derived from carbohydrates. Even though a lower percentage of the energy is derived from fat during vigorous-intensity exercise, the total caloric expenditure is so much greater (twice as high or more) that overall the total fat burned is still higher than during moderate intensity.

A word of caution, nonetheless: Do not start vigorous-intensity exercise without several weeks of proper and gradual conditioning. Even worse is if such exercise is a weight-bearing activity. If you do such exercise from the outset, you increase the risk of injury and may have to stop exercising altogether. Also, people with an initial low level of fitness often compensate with greater caloric intake following vigorous-intensity exercise, thus defeating the added energy expenditure obtained through exercise (additional information on this subject is provided on pages 161–163).

Do energy drinks enhance performance? People associate energy with work. If an energy drink can enhance work capacity, the benefits of such drinks would surpass plain thirst-quenching drinks. Energy drinks typically contain sugar (discussed in Chapter 3), herbal extracts, large amounts of caffeine, and water-soluble vitamins. Consumers are led to believe that these ingredients increase energy metabolism, provide an energy boost, improve endurance, and aid in weight loss. These purported benefits are yet to be proven through scientific research.

The energy content of many of these drinks is around 60 grams of sugar and 240 calories in a 16-ounce drink, with little additional nutritive value. If you are going to participate in an intense and lengthy workout, the carbohydrate content can boost performance and help you get through the workout. If, however, you are concerned with weight management, 240 calories is an extraordinarily large amount of calories in a two-cup drink. Weight gain may be the end result if you drink a few of these throughout the day to give you a boost while studying or while at work. Sugar-free energy drinks, available for the weight-conscious consumer, provide little or no energy (calories), although they are packed with nervous system stimulants.

The high caffeine content can also have adverse health effects. Caffeine intake above 400 mg can precipitate cardiac arrhythmias, nervousness, irritability, and gastrointestinal discomfort. Many of the popular energy drinks (Red Bull, Sobe Adrenaline Rush, Full Throttle, Rip It Energy Fuel) contain about 80 mg of caffeine per 8-ounce cup. If you drink two 16-ounce cans, you'll end up with upward of 300 mg of caffeine through these drinks alone. You may also have to consider additional caffeine intake from other beverages that you routinely consume during the day (coffee, tea, sodas). As with most addictive substances, invariably a sugar and caffeine rush is likely to end up in a physiological crash, requiring a subsequent larger intake to obtain a similar "physical high."

Real Life Story   Kaleo's Experience

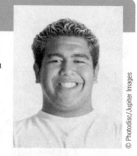

When I first started exercising, I really dreaded doing it. I was 50 pounds overweight, and I would run out of breath just trying to walk to the end of the block. But I was determined to stop being a couch potato and get moving; so I began walking every day. I started really slow, and worked my way up. I walked just a couple blocks and back and slowly I increased it by a block each time. Eventually I was able to walk a mile a day. I was really proud of that. To other people in my class, that was nothing, but I couldn't compare myself to other people. I just had to focus on what I was able to do and be happy that I was improving. That was a couple years ago and I am still exercising. Eventually I combined walking and jogging, until I was able to jog a full

mile, and then some more. I first set my goals on a 5-K run, which I accomplished without much difficulty. Then last March my buddy and I ran a half marathon! It wasn't easy, but we jogged the entire 13.1 miles. Although I have lost 35 pounds and I am still overweight, I know I am much healthier than I was before. I know that having good cardiorespiratory fitness puts me at less of a health risk. Also, running makes me feel really good. I have never regretted the time and effort I have put into my exercise program.

PERSONAL PROFILE

Personal Cardiorespiratory Fitness Profile

I. Have you ever experienced the feeling of being aerobically fit? If so, can you describe that feeling?

II. Do you understand the concept of oxygen uptake and the difference between absolute and relative oxygen uptake? What are the applications of the latter two?

III. At 70-percent training intensity, your exercise prescription requires a heart rate of 156 beats per minute. Is there a difference between jogging and doing zumba when exercising at this same heart rate? Please expound on your response.

IV. Can you identify and relate to the factors that motivated Kaleo to become aerobically fit and what helped him stay with the exercise program? What factors do you think can help you start or stay with aerobic exercise?

V. Your cardiorespiratory fitness test indicates that your VO_{2max} is 48 mL/kg/min. If you chose to exercise at 50 percent of your VO_{2max} (moderate intensity, as most people like to do during aerobic exercise), can you compute how many calories you burn per minute at this intensity level and the total minutes that you'd have to exercise to burn the equivalent of one pound of fat?

Cardiorespiratory endurance is the single most important component of health-related physical fitness. The exception occurs among older adults, for whom muscular strength is particularly important. In any case, people can get by without high levels of strength and flexibility, but we cannot do without a good cardiorespiratory (CR) system, facilitated by aerobic exercise.

Aerobic exercise is especially important in preventing cardiovascular disease. A poorly conditioned heart, which has to pump more often just to keep a person alive, is subject to more wear and tear than a well-conditioned heart. In situations that place strenuous demands on the heart, such as doing yard work, lifting heavy objects or weights, or running to catch a bus, the unconditioned heart may not be able to sustain the strain. Regular participation in CR endurance activities also helps a person achieve and maintain recommended

body weight—the fourth component of health-related physical fitness.

Physical activity, unfortunately, is no longer a natural part of our existence. Technological developments have driven most people in developed countries into sedentary lifestyles. For instance, when many people go to a store only a couple of blocks away, they drive their automobiles and then spend a couple of minutes driving around the parking lot to find a spot 20 yards closer to the store's entrance. At times, they don't even have to

Key Terms

Cardiorespiratory endurance The ability of the lungs, heart, and blood vessels to deliver adequate amounts of oxygen to the cells to meet the demands of prolonged physical activity.

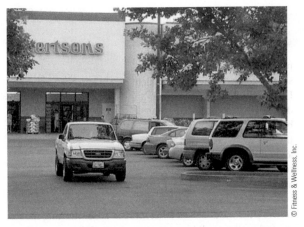

The epitome of physical inactivity: driving around a parking lot for several minutes in search of a parking spot 20 yards closer to the store's entrance.

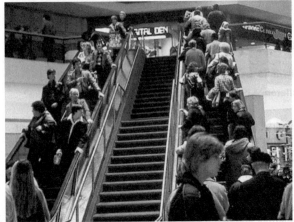

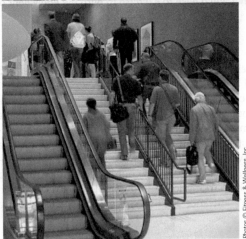

Advances in modern technology have almost completely eliminated the need for physical activity, but you can choose to be physically active and greatly decrease the risk for premature mortality.

carry the groceries to the car, as an employee working at the store offers to do this for them.

Similarly, during a visit to a multilevel shopping mall, almost everyone chooses to take the escalator instead of the stairs (which tend to be inaccessible). Automobiles, elevators, escalators, telephones, intercoms, remote controls, electric garage door openers—all are modern-day conveniences that minimize the amount of movement and effort required of the human body.

One of the most harmful effects of modern-day technology is an increase in chronic conditions related to a lack of physical activity. These **hypokinetic diseases** include hypertension, heart disease, chronic low back pain, and obesity. (The term "hypo" means low or little, and "kinetic" implies motion.) Lack of adequate physical activity is a fact of modern life that most people can avoid no longer. To enjoy modern-day conveniences and still expect to live life to its fullest, however, one has to make a personalized lifetime exercise program a part of daily living.

Basic Cardiorespiratory Physiology: A Quick Survey

Before we begin to overhaul our bodies with an exercise program, we should understand the mechanisms that we propose to alter and survey the ways by which to measure how well we perform them. CR endurance is a measure of how the pulmonary (lungs), cardiovascular (heart and blood vessels), and muscular systems work together during aerobic activities. As a person breathes, part of the oxygen in the air is taken up by the **alveoli** in the lungs. As blood passes through the alveoli, oxygen is picked up by **hemoglobin** and transported in the blood to the heart. The heart then is responsible for pumping the oxygenated blood through the circulatory system to all organs and tissues of the body.

At the cellular level, oxygen is used to convert food substrates (primarily carbohydrates and fats) through aerobic metabolism into **adenosine triphosphate (ATP)**. This compound provides the energy for physical activity, body functions, and maintenance of a constant internal equilibrium. During physical exertion, more ATP is needed to perform the activity. As a result, the lungs, heart, and blood vessels have to deliver more oxygen to the muscle cells to supply the required energy.

During prolonged exercise, an individual with a high level of CR endurance is able to deliver the required amount of oxygen to the tissues with relative ease. In contrast, the CR system of a person with a low level of endurance has to work much harder, the heart has to work at a higher rate, less oxygen is delivered to the tissues, and consequently, the individual fatigues faster. Hence, a higher capacity to deliver and utilize

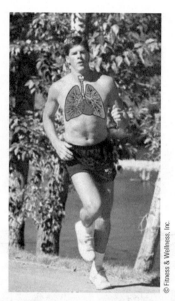

Cardiorespiratory endurance refers to the ability of the lungs, heart, and blood vessels to deliver adequate amounts of oxygen to the cells to meet the demands of prolonged physical activity.

oxygen—called **oxygen uptake**, or VO_2—indicates a more efficient CR system. Measuring oxygen uptake, therefore, is an important way by which to evaluate our CR health.

Aerobic and Anaerobic Exercise

Cardiorespiratory endurance activities often are called **aerobic** exercises. Examples are walking, jogging, swimming, cycling, cross-country skiing, aerobics (including water aerobics), and rope skipping. By contrast, the intensity of **anaerobic** exercise is so high that oxygen cannot be delivered and utilized to produce energy. Because energy production is limited in the absence of oxygen, anaerobic activities can be carried out for only short periods—two to three minutes. The higher the intensity of the activity, the shorter the duration.

Good examples of anaerobic activities are the 100, 200, and 400 meters in track and field, the 100 meters in swimming, gymnastics routines, and strength training. Anaerobic activities do not contribute much to developing the CR system. Only aerobic activities will increase CR endurance. The basic guidelines for CR exercise prescription are set forth later in this chapter.

Critical Thinking

Your friend Joe is not physically active and doesn't exercise. He manages to keep his weight down by dieting and tells you that because he feels and looks good, he doesn't need to exercise. How do you respond to your friend?

Benefits of Aerobic Training

Everyone who participates in a CR or aerobic exercise program can expect a number of beneficial physiological adaptations from training (Figure 6.1). Among them are the following:

1. A higher **maximal oxygen uptake (VO_{2max}).** The amount of oxygen that the body is able to use during exercise increases significantly. This allows the individual to exercise longer and more intensely before becoming fatigued. Depending on the initial fitness level, the increases in VO_{2max} average 15 to 20 percent, although increases greater than 50 percent have been reported in people who have very low initial levels of fitness or who were significantly overweight prior to starting the aerobic exercise program.

2. An increase in the oxygen-carrying capacity of the blood. As a result of training, the red blood cell count goes up. Red blood cells contain hemoglobin, which transports oxygen in the blood.

3. A decrease in **resting heart rate (RHR)** and an increase in cardiac muscle strength. During resting conditions, the heart ejects between 5 and 6 liters of blood per minute (a liter is slightly larger than a quart). This amount of blood, also referred to as **cardiac output**, meets the body's energy demands in the resting state. Like any other muscle, the heart responds to training by increasing in

Key Terms

Hypokinetic diseases "Hypo" denotes "lack of"; therefore, chronic ailments that result from a lack of physical activity.

Alveoli Air sacs in the lungs where oxygen is taken up and carbon dioxide (produced by the body) is released from the blood.

Hemoglobin Iron-containing compound, found in red blood cells, that transports oxygen.

Adenosine triphosphate (ATP) A high-energy chemical compound that the body uses for immediate energy.

Oxygen uptake (VO_2) The amount of oxygen the human body uses.

Aerobic Describes exercise that requires oxygen to produce the necessary energy (ATP) to carry out the activity.

Anaerobic Describes exercise that does not require oxygen to produce the necessary energy (ATP) to carry out the activity.

Maximal oxygen uptake (VO_{2max}) Maximum amount of oxygen the body is able to utilize per minute of physical activity, commonly expressed in milliliters per kilogram per minute (mL/kg/min); the best indicator of cardiorespiratory or aerobic fitness.

Resting heart rate (RHR) Heart rate after a person has been sitting quietly for 15 to 20 minutes.

Cardiac output Amount of blood pumped by the heart in one minute.

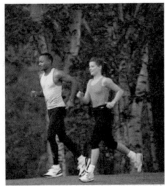
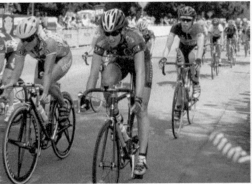
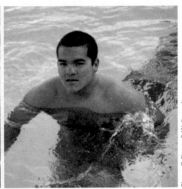

Aerobic activities.

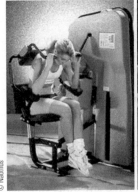
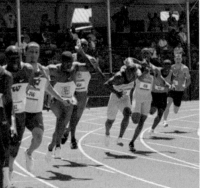
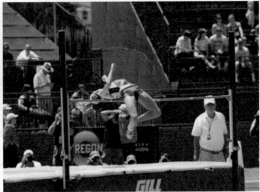

Anaerobic activities.

strength and size. As the heart gets stronger, the muscle can produce a more forceful contraction, which helps the heart to eject more blood with each beat. This **stroke volume** yields a lower heart rate. The lower heart rate also allows the heart to rest longer between beats. Average resting and maximal cardiac outputs, stroke volumes, and heart rates for sedentary, trained, and highly trained (elite) males are shown in Table 6.1. Resting heart rates frequently decrease by 10 to 20 beats per minute (bpm) after only 6 to 8 weeks of training. A reduction of 20 bpm saves the heart about 10,483,200 beats per year. The average heart beats between 70 and 80 bpm. As seen in Table 6.1,

RHRs in highly trained athletes are often around 45 bpm.

4. A lower heart rate at given workloads. When compared with untrained individuals, a trained person has a lower heart rate response to a given task because of greater efficiency of the CR system. Individuals are surprised to find that following several weeks of training, a given **workload** (let's say a 10-minute mile) elicits a much lower heart rate response than their response when they first started training.

5. An increase in the number, size, and capacity of the mitochondria. All energy necessary for cell function is produced in the **mitochondria**. As their size and

Table 6.1	Average Resting and Maximal Cardiac Output, Stroke Volume, and Heart Rate for Sedentary, Trained, and Highly Trained Young Males					
	Resting			Maximal		
	Cardiac Output (L/min)	Stroke Volume (mL)	Heart Rate (bpm)	Cardiac Output (L/min)	Stroke Volume (mL)	Heart Rate (bpm)
Sedentary	5–6	68	74	20	100	200
Trained	5–6	90	56	30	150	200
Highly Trained	5–6	110	45	35	175	200

NOTE: Cardiac output and stroke volume in women are about 25 percent lower than in men.

| Figure 6.1 | Selected benefits of cardiorespiratory (aerobic) fitness. |

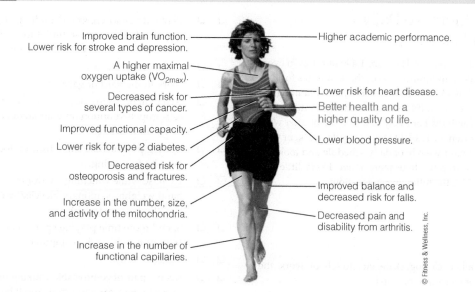

Improved brain function.
Lower risk for stroke and depression.

A higher maximal
oxygen uptake (VO_{2max}).

Decreased risk for
several types of cancer.

Improved functional capacity.

Lower risk for type 2 diabetes.

Decreased risk for
osteoporosis and fractures.

Increase in the number, size,
and activity of the mitochondria.

Increase in the number of
functional capillaries.

Higher academic performance.

Lower risk for heart disease.

Better health and a
higher quality of life.

Lower blood pressure.

Improved balance and
decreased risk for falls.

Decreased pain and
disability from arthritis.

© Fitness & Wellness, Inc.

numbers increase, so does their potential to produce energy for muscular work.

6. An increase in the number of functional capillaries.
Capillaries allow for the exchange of oxygen and
carbon dioxide between the blood and the cells. As
more vessels open up, more gas exchange can take
place, delaying the onset of fatigue during prolonged exercise. This increase in capillaries also
speeds the rate at which waste products of cell
metabolism can be removed. This increased capillar-
ization also occurs in the heart, which enhances the
oxygen delivery capacity to the heart muscle itself.

7. Ability to recover rapidly. Trained individuals have
a faster **recovery time** after exercising. A fit system
is able to more quickly restore any internal equilibrium disrupted during exercise.

8. Lower blood pressure and blood lipids. A regular
aerobic exercise program leads to lower blood pressure (thereby reducing a major risk factor for
stroke) and lower levels of fats (such as cholesterol
and triglycerides), which have been linked to the
formation of atherosclerotic plaque, which ob-
structs the arteries. This decreases the risk for
coronary heart disease (see Chapter 10).

9. An increase in fat-burning enzymes. These enzymes are significant because fat is lost primarily
by burning it in muscle. As the concentration of the
enzymes increases (along with the number and size
of the mitochondria), so does the ability to burn
fat (triglycerides) as opposed to carbohydrates
(glucose/glycogen) during submaximal workloads
(below 85 percent of VO_{2max}).

Physical Fitness Assessment

The assessment of physical fitness serves several
purposes:

- To educate participants regarding their present fitness levels and compare them with health fitness
  and physical fitness standards
- To motivate individuals to participate in exercise
  programs
- To provide a starting point for an individualized
  exercise prescription and to establish realistic
  goals
- To evaluate improvements in fitness achieved
  through exercise programs and adjust exercise
  prescription and fitness goals accordingly
- To monitor changes in fitness throughout the
  years

Key Terms

Stroke volume Amount of blood pumped by the heart in one
beat.

Workload Load (or intensity) placed on the body during physical activity.

Mitochondria Structures within the cells where energy transformations take place.

Capillaries Smallest blood vessels carrying oxygenated blood
to the tissues in the body.

Recovery time Amount of time that the body takes to return
to resting levels after exercise.

Tips to Increase Daily Physical Activity

Adults need recess, too! There are 1,440 minutes in every day. Schedule a minimum of 30 of these minutes for physical activity. With a little creativity and planning, even the person with the busiest schedule can make room for physical activity. For many folks, before or after work or meals is often an available time to cycle, walk, or play. Think about your weekly or daily schedule and look for or make opportunities to be more active. Every little bit helps. Consider the following suggestions:

I PLAN TO
I DID IT

- ❏ ❏ Walk, cycle, jog, skate, etc., to school, work, the store, or place of worship.
- ❏ ❏ Use a pedometer to count your daily steps.
- ❏ ❏ Walk while doing errands.
- ❏ ❏ Get on or off the bus several blocks away.
- ❏ ❏ Park the car farther away from your destination.
- ❏ ❏ At work, walk to nearby offices instead of sending e-mails or using the phone.
- ❏ ❏ Walk or stretch a few minutes every hour that you are at your desk.
- ❏ ❏ Take fitness breaks—walking or doing desk exercises—instead of taking cigarette breaks or coffee breaks.
- ❏ ❏ Incorporate activity into your lunch break (walk to the restaurant).
- ❏ ❏ Take the stairs instead of the elevator or escalator.

- ❏ ❏ Play with children, grandchildren, or pets. Everybody wins. If you find it too difficult to be active after work, try it before work.
- ❏ ❏ Do household tasks.
- ❏ ❏ Work in the yard or garden.
- ❏ ❏ Avoid labor-saving devices. Turn off the self-propelled option on your lawnmower or vacuum cleaner.
- ❏ ❏ Use leg power. Take small trips on foot to get your body moving.
- ❏ ❏ Exercise while watching TV (for example, use hand weights, stationary bicycle/treadmill/stairclimber, or stretch).
- ❏ ❏ Spend more time playing sports than sitting in front of the TV or the computer.
- ❏ ❏ Dance to music.
- ❏ ❏ Keep a pair of comfortable walking or running shoes in your car and office. You'll be ready for activity wherever you go!
- ❏ ❏ Make a Saturday morning walk a group habit.
- ❏ ❏ Learn a new sport or join a sports team.
- ❏ ❏ Avoid carts when golfing.
- ❏ ❏ When out of town, stay in hotels with fitness centers.

Try It Keep a three-day log of all your activities. List the activities performed, time of day, and how long you were engaged in these activities. You may be surprised by your findings.

SOURCE: Adapted from Centers for Disease Control and Prevention, Atlanta, 2005.

Responders versus Nonresponders

Individuals who follow similar training programs show a wide variation in physiological responses. Heredity plays a crucial role in how each person responds to and improves after beginning an exercise program. Several studies have documented that following exercise training, most individuals, called **responders**, readily show improvements, but a few, **nonresponders**, exhibit small or no improvements at all. This concept is referred to as the **principle of individuality**.

After several months of aerobic training, increases in VO$_{2max}$ are between 15 and 20 percent on the average, although individual responses can range from 0 percent (in a few selected cases) to more than 50 percent improvement, even when all participants follow exactly the same training program. Nonfitness and low-fitness participants,

however, should not label themselves as nonresponders based on the previous discussion. Nonresponders constitute less than 5 percent of exercise participants. Although additional research is necessary, lack of improvement in CR endurance among nonresponders might be related to low levels of leg strength. A lower-body strength-training program has been shown to help these individuals improve VO$_{2max}$ through aerobic exercise.[1]

Following your self-assessment of CR fitness, if your fitness level is less than adequate, do not let that discourage you, but do set a priority to be physically active every day. In addition to regular exercise, lifestyle behaviors—walking, taking stairs, cycling to work, parking farther from the office, doing household tasks, gardening, and doing yard work, for example—provide substantial benefits. In this regard, daily **physical activity** and **exercise** habits should be monitored in conjunction with fitness testing to evaluate adherence among nonresponders. After all, it is through increased daily activity that we reap the health benefits that improve our quality of life.

Assessment of Cardiorespiratory Endurance

Cardiorespiratory endurance, CR fitness, or aerobic capacity is determined by the maximal amount of oxygen the human body is able to utilize (the oxygen uptake) per minute of physical activity (VO_{2max}). This value can be expressed in liters per minute (L/min) or milliliters per kilogram per minute (mL/kg/min). The relative value in mL/kg/min is used most often because it considers total body mass (weight) in kilograms. When comparing two individuals with the same absolute value, the one with the lesser body mass will have a higher relative value, indicating that more oxygen is available to each kilogram (2.2 pounds) of body weight. Because all tissues and organs of the body need oxygen to function, higher oxygen consumption indicates a more efficient CR system.

Oxygen uptake expressed in L/min is valuable in determining the caloric expenditure of physical activity. The human body burns about five calories for each liter of oxygen consumed. During aerobic exercise the average person trains between 50 and 85 percent of maximal oxygen uptake.

A person with a maximal oxygen uptake of 3.5 L/min who trains at 60 percent of maximum uses 2.1 (3.5 × .60) liters of oxygen per minute of physical activity. This indicates that 10.5 calories are burned during each minute of exercise (2.1 × 5). If the activity is carried out for 30 minutes, 315 calories (10.5 × 30) have been burned. Because a pound of body fat represents about 3,500 calories, the previous example indicates that this individual would have to exercise for a total of 333 minutes (3,500 ÷ 10.5) to burn the equivalent of a pound of body fat. At 30 minutes per exercise session, approximately 11 sessions would be required to expend the 3,500 calories.

Components of Oxygen Uptake (VO₂)

The amount of oxygen the body actually uses at rest or during submaximal (VO_2) or maximal (VO_{2max}) exercise is determined by the heart rate, the stroke volume, and the amount of oxygen removed from the vascular system (for use by all organs and tissues of the body, including the muscular system).

Heart Rate

Normal heart rate ranges from about 40 bpm during resting conditions in trained athletes to 200 bpm or higher during maximal exercise. The **maximal heart rate**

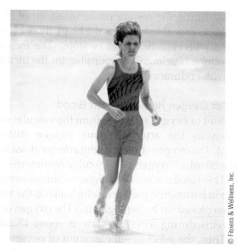

Aerobic fitness leads to better health and a higher quality of life.

© Fitness & Wellness, Inc.

(MHR) that a person can achieve starts to drop by about one beat per year beginning at about 12 years of age. Maximal heart rate in trained endurance athletes is sometimes slightly lower than in untrained individuals. This adaptation to training is thought to allow the heart more time to effectively fill with blood so as to produce a greater stroke volume.

Stroke Volume

Stroke volume ranges from 50 mL per beat (stroke) during resting conditions in untrained individuals to 200 mL at maximum in endurance-trained athletes (see Table 6.1). Following endurance training, stroke volume increases significantly. Some of the increase is the result of a stronger heart muscle, but it also is related to an increase in total blood volume and a greater filling capacity of the

---

Key Terms

Responders Individuals who exhibit improvements in fitness as a result of exercise training.

Nonresponders Individuals who exhibit small or no improvements in fitness as compared to others who undergo the same training program.

Principle of individuality Training concept holding that genetics plays a major role in individual responses to exercise training and these differences must be considered when designing exercise programs for different people.

Physical activity Bodily movement produced by skeletal muscles; requires expenditure of energy and produces progressive health benefits. Examples include walking, taking the stairs, dancing, gardening, yard work, house cleaning, snow shoveling, washing the car, and all forms of structured exercise.

Exercise A type of physical activity that requires planned, structured, and repetitive bodily movement with the intent of improving or maintaining one or more components of physical fitness.

Maximal heart rate (MHR) Highest heart rate for a person, related primarily to age.

ventricles during the resting phase (diastole) of the cardiac cycle. As more blood enters the heart, more blood can be ejected with each heartbeat (systole). The increase in stroke volume is primarily responsible for the increase in VO_{2max} with endurance training.

Amount of Oxygen Removed from Blood

The amount of oxygen removed from the vascular system is known as the **arterial-venous oxygen difference** (a-$\overline{v}O_{2diff}$). The oxygen content in the arteries at sea level is typically 20 mL of oxygen per 100 cubic centimeters (cc) of blood. (This value decreases at higher altitudes because of the drop in barometric pressure, which affects the amount of oxygen picked up by hemoglobin.) The oxygen content in the veins during a resting state is about 15 mL per 100 cc. Thus, the a-$\overline{v}O_{2diff}$—the amount of oxygen in the arteries minus the amount in the veins—at rest is 5 mL per 100 cc. The arterial value remains constant during both resting and exercise conditions. Because of the additional oxygen removed during maximal exercise, the venous oxygen content drops to about 5 mL per 100 cc, yielding an a-$\overline{v}O_{2diff}$ of 15 mL per 100 cc. The latter value may be slightly higher in endurance athletes.

These three factors are used to compute VO_2 using the following equation:

$$VO_2 \text{ in L/min} = (HR \times SV \times \text{a-}\overline{v}O_{2diff}) \div 100,000$$

where

$$HR = \text{heart rate}$$

$$SV = \text{stroke volume}$$

For example, the resting VO_2 (also known as the resting metabolic rate) of an individual with a RHR of 76 bpm and a stroke volume of 79 mL would be

$$VO_2 \text{ in L/min} = (76 \times 79 \times 5) \div 100,000 = 0.3 \text{ L/min}$$

Likewise, the VO_{2max} of a person exercising maximally who achieves a heart rate of 190 bpm and a maximal stroke volume of 120 mL would be

$$VO_{2max} \text{ in L/min} = (190 \times 120 \times 15) \div 100,000$$
$$= 3.42 \text{ L/min}$$

To convert L/min to mL/kg/min, multiply the L/min value by 1,000 and divide by body weight in kilograms. In the above example, if the person weighs 70 kilograms, the VO_{2max} in mL/kg/min would be 48.9 ($3.42 \times 1000 \div 70$).

Critical Thinking

You can improve your relative VO_{2max} without engaging in an aerobic exercise program. • How do you accomplish this? Would you benefit from doing so?

Because the actual measurement of the stroke volume and the a-$\overline{v}O_{2diff}$ is impractical in the fitness setting, VO_2 also is determined through gas (air) analysis. The person being tested breathes into a metabolic cart that measures the difference in oxygen content between the person's exhaled air and the atmosphere. The air we breathe contains 21 percent oxygen; thus, VO_2 can be assessed by establishing the difference between 21 percent and the percent of oxygen left in the air the person exhales, according to the total volume of air taken into the lungs. This type of equipment, however, is expensive. Consequently, several alternative methods of estimating VO_{2max} using limited equipment have been developed. These methods are discussed next.

VO_{2max} is affected by genetics, training, gender, age, and body composition. Although aerobic training can help people attain good or excellent CR fitness, only those with a strong genetic component are able to reach an "elite" level of aerobic capacity (60 to 80 mL/kg/min). Further, VO_{2max} is 15 to 30 percent higher in men. This is related to a greater hemoglobin content, lower body fat (see "Essential and Storage Fat" in Chapter 4, page 122), and larger heart size in men (a larger heart pumps more blood, and thus produces a greater stroke volume). VO_{2max} also decreases by about 1 percent per year starting at age 25. This decrease, however, is only 0.5 percent per year in physically active individuals.

Tests to Estimate VO_{2max}

Even though most CR endurance tests probably are safe to administer to apparently healthy individuals (those with no major coronary risk factors or symptoms), a health history questionnaire (including the PAR-Q), such as found in Activity 1.3 in Chapter 1, should be used as a minimum screening tool prior to exercise testing or participation. The American College of Sports Medicine (ACSM) also recommends that a physician be present for all maximal exercise tests on apparently healthy men 45 or older and women 55 or older.[2] A maximal test is any test that requires the participant's all-out or nearly all-out effort. For submaximal exercise tests, a physician should be present when testing higher-risk/symptomatic individuals or diseased people, regardless of the participants' current age.

Five exercise tests used to assess CR fitness are introduced in this chapter: the 1.5-Mile Run Test, the 1.0-Mile Walk Test, the Step Test, the Astrand-Ryhming Test, and the 12-Minute Swim Test. The procedures for each test are explained in detail in Figures 6.2, 6.3, 6.4, 6.5, and 6.6, respectively.

Several tests are provided in this chapter, so you may choose one depending on time, equipment, and individual physical limitations. For example, people who can't jog or walk can take the Astrand-Ryhming (bicycle) or swim test. You may perform more than one test, but because they are different and they estimate VO_{2max}, they will not necessarily yield the same results. Therefore, to make valid comparisons, you should take the same test when doing pre- and post-assessments. You may record the results of your test(s) in Activity 6.1.

Figure 6.2	Procedure for the 1.5-Mile Run Test.

1. Make sure you qualify for this test. This test is contraindicated for unconditioned beginners, individuals with symptoms of heart disease, and those with known heart disease or risk factors.
2. Select the testing site. Find a school track (each lap is one-fourth of a mile) or a premeasured 1.5-mile course.
3. Have a stopwatch available to determine your time.
4. Conduct a few warm-up exercises prior to the test. Do some stretching exercises, some walking, and slow jogging.
5. Initiate the test and try to cover the distance in the fastest time possible (walking or jogging). Time yourself during the run to see how fast you have covered the distance. If any unusual symptoms arise during the test, do not continue. Stop immediately and retake the test after another 6 weeks of aerobic training.
6. At the end of the test, cool down by walking or jogging slowly for another 3 to 5 minutes. Do not sit or lie down after the test.
7. According to your performance time, look up your estimated maximal oxygen uptake (VO_{2max}) in Table 6.2.

Example: A 20-year-old male runs the 1.5-mile course in 10 minutes and 20 seconds. Table 6.2 shows a VO_{2max} of 49.5 mL/kg/min for a time of 10:20. According to Table 6.8, this VO_{2max} would place him in the "good" cardiorespiratory fitness category.

1.5-Mile Run Test

The 1.5-Mile Run Test is used most frequently to predict VO_{2max} according to the time the person takes to run or walk a 1.5-mile course (see Figure 6.2). VO_{2max} is estimated based on the time the person takes to cover the distance (see Table 6.2).

The only equipment necessary to conduct this test is a stopwatch and a track or premeasured 1.5-mile course. This perhaps is the easiest test to administer, but a note of caution is in order when conducting the test: Given that the objective is to cover the distance in the shortest time, it is considered a maximal exercise test. The 1.5-Mile Run Test should be limited to conditioned individuals who have been cleared for exercise. The test is not recommended for unconditioned beginners, men over age 45 and women over age 55 without proper medical clearance, symptomatic individuals, and those with known disease or risk factors for coronary heart disease. A program of at least 6 weeks of aerobic training is recommended before unconditioned individuals take this test.

1.0-Mile Walk Test

The 1.0-Mile Walk Test can be used by individuals who are unable to run because of low fitness levels or injuries. All that is required is a brisk 1.0-mile walk that will elicit an exercise heart rate of at least 120 bpm at the end of the test.

You will need to know how to take your heart rate by counting your pulse. You can do this by gently placing the middle and index fingers over the radial artery on the inside of the wrist on the side of the thumb or over the carotid artery in the neck just below the jaw

Table 6.2	Estimated Maximal Oxygen Uptake (VO_{2max}) for the 1.5-Mile Run Test

Time	VO_{2max} (mL/kg/min)	Time	VO_{2max} (mL/kg/min)	Time	VO_{2max} (mL/kg/min)
6:10	80.0	10:30	48.6	14:50	34.0
6:20	79.0	10:40	48.0	15:00	33.6
6:30	77.9	10:50	47.4	15:10	33.1
6:40	76.7	11:00	46.6	15:20	32.7
6:50	75.5	11:10	45.8	15:30	32.2
7:00	74.0	11:20	45.1	15:40	31.8
7:10	72.6	11:30	44.4	15:50	31.4
7:20	71.3	11:40	43.7	16:00	30.9
7:30	69.9	11:50	43.2	16:10	30.5
7:40	68.3	12:00	42.3	16:20	30.2
7:50	66.8	12:10	41.7	16:30	29.8
8:00	65.2	12:20	41.0	16:40	29.5
8:10	63.9	12:30	40.4	16:50	29.1
8:20	62.5	12:40	39.8	17:00	28.9
8:30	61.2	12:50	39.2	17:10	28.5
8:40	60.2	13:00	38.6	17:20	28.3
8:50	59.1	13:10	38.1	17:30	28.0
9:00	58.1	13:20	37.8	17:40	27.7
9:10	56.9	13:30	37.2	17:50	27.4
9:20	55.9	13:40	36.8	18:00	27.1
9:30	54.7	13:50	36.3	18:10	26.8
9:40	53.5	14:00	35.9	18:20	26.6
9:50	52.3	14:10	35.5	18:30	26.3
10:00	51.1	14:20	35.1	18:40	26.0
10:10	50.4	14:30	34.7	18:50	25.7
10:20	49.5	14:40	34.3	19:00	25.4

SOURCE: Adapted from K. H. Cooper, "A Means of Assessing Maximal Oxygen Intake," in *Journal of the American Medical Association* 203 (1968): 201–204; M. L. Pollock, J. H. Wilmore, and S. M. Fox III, *Health and Fitness Through Physical Activity* (New York: John Wiley & Sons, 1978); and J. H. Wilmore and D. L. Costill, *Training for Sport and Activity* (Dubuque, IA: Wm. C. Brown Publishers, 1988).

© Cengage Learning 2013

next to the voice box. You should not use the thumb to check the pulse because it has a strong pulse of its own, which can make you miscount. When checking the carotid pulse, do not press too hard, because it may cause a reflex action that slows the heart. For checking the pulse over the carotid artery, some exercise experts recommend that the hand on the same side of the neck (right hand over right carotid artery) be used to avoid excessive pressure on the artery. With minimum experience, however, you can be accurate using either hand as long as you apply only gentle pressure. If available, heart rate monitors can be used to increase the accuracy of heart rate assessment.

VO_{2max} is estimated according to a prediction equation that requires the following data: 1.0-mile walk time, exercise heart rate at the end of the walk, gender, and

Key Terms

Arterial-venous oxygen difference (a-$\bar{v}O_{2diff}$) The amount of oxygen removed from the blood as determined by the difference in oxygen content between arterial and venous blood.

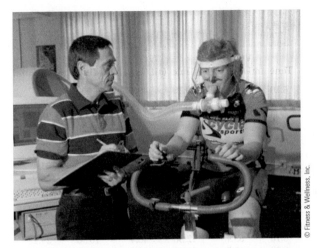

Oxygen uptake (VO₂), as determined through direct gas analysis.

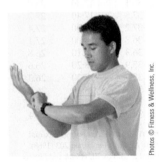

Pulse taken at the radial artery.

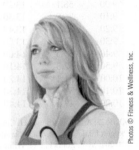

Pulse taken at the carotid artery.

body weight in pounds. The procedure for this test and the equation are given in Figure 6.3.

Step Test

The Step Test requires little time and equipment and can be administered to almost anyone, because a submaximal workload is used to estimate VO_{2max}. Symptomatic and diseased individuals should not take this test. Significantly overweight individuals and those with joint problems in the lower extremities may have difficulty performing the test.

The actual test takes only three minutes. A 15-second recovery heart rate is taken between 5 and 20 seconds following the test (see Figure 6.4 and Table 6.3). The required equipment consists of a bench or gymnasium bleacher 16¼ inches high, a stopwatch, and a metronome.

You also will need to know how to take your heart rate by counting your pulse, as we have just discussed. Once people learn to take their own heart rate, a large group of people can be tested at once, using gymnasium bleachers for the steps.

Astrand-Ryhming Test

Because of its simplicity and practicality, the Astrand-Ryhming Test is one of the most popular tests used to estimate VO_{2max} in the laboratory setting. The test is conducted on a bicycle ergometer and, similar to the Step Test, requires only submaximal workloads and little time to administer.

The cautions given for the Step Test also apply to the Astrand-Ryhming Test. Nevertheless, because the par-

---

| **Figure 6.3** | Procedure for the 1.0-Mile Walk Test. |

1. Select the testing site. Use a 440-yard track (4 laps to a mile) or a premeasured 1.0-mile course.
2. Determine your body weight in pounds prior to the test.
3. Have a stopwatch available to determine total walking time and exercise heart rate.
4. Walk the 1.0-mile course at a brisk pace (the exercise heart rate at the end of the test should be above 120 beats per minute).
5. At the end of the 1.0-mile walk, check your walking time and immediately count your pulse for 10 seconds. Multiply the 10-second pulse count by 6 to obtain the exercise heart rate in beats per minute.
6. Convert the walking time from minutes and seconds to minute units. Because each minute has 60 seconds, divide the seconds by 60 to obtain the fraction of a minute. For instance, a walking time of 12 minutes and 15 seconds would equal 12 + (15 ÷ 60), or 12.25 minutes.
7. To obtain the estimated maximal oxygen uptake (VO_{2max}) in mL/kg/min, plug your values in the following equation:
$VO_{2max} = 88.768 - (0.0957 \times W) + (8.892 \times G) - (1.4537 \times T) - (0.1194 \times HR)$

Where:
W = Weight in pounds
G = Gender (use 0 for women and 1 for men)
T = Total time for the one-mile walk in minutes (see item 6)
HR = Exercise heart rate in beats per minute at the end of the 1.0-mile walk

Example: A 19-year-old female who weighs 140 pounds completed the 1.0-mile walk in 14 minutes 39 seconds with an exercise heart rate of 148 beats per minute. Her estimated VO_{2max} would be:

W = 140 lbs
G = 0 (female gender = 0)
T = 14:39 = 14 + (39 ÷ 60) = 14.65 min
HR = 148 bpm
$VO_{2max} = 88.768 - (0.0957 \times 140) + (8.892 \times 0) - (1.4537 \times 14.65) - (0.1194 \times 148)$
$VO_{2max} = 36.4$ mL/kg/min

SOURCE: Dolgener, F.A., et al. "Validation of the Rockport Fitness Walking Test in College Males and Females," *Research Quarterly for Exercise and Sport* 65 (1994): 152–158.

| **Figure 6.4** | Procedure for the Step Test. |

1. Conduct the test with a bench or gymnasium bleacher 16¼ inches high.
2. Perform the stepping cycle to a four-step cadence (up-up-down-down). Men should perform 24 complete step-ups per minute, regulated with a metronome set at 96 beats per minute. Women perform 22 step-ups per minute, or 88 beats per minute on the metronome.
3. Allow a brief practice period of 5 to 10 seconds to familiarize yourself with the stepping cadence.
4. Begin the test and perform the step-ups for exactly 3 minutes.
5. Upon completing the 3 minutes, remain standing and take your heart rate for a 15-second interval from 5 to 20 seconds into recovery. Convert recovery heart rate to beats per minute (multiply 15-second heart rate by 4).
6. Maximal oxygen uptake (VO_{2max}) in mL/kg/min is estimated

according to the following equations:
Men:
$VO_{2max} = 111.33 - (0.42 \times$ recovery heart rate in bpm)
Women:
$VO_{2max} = 65.81 - (0.1847 \times$ recovery heart rate in bpm)

Example: The recovery 15-second heart rate for a male following the 3-minute step test is found to be 39 beats. His VO_{2max} is estimated as follows:

15-second heart rate = 39 beats
Minute heart rate = 39 × 4 = 156 bpm
$VO_{2max} = 111.33 - (0.42 \times 156) = 45.81$ mL/kg/min
VO_{2max} also can be obtained according to recovery heart rates in Table 6.3.

SOURCE: McArdle, W.D., et al. *Exercise Physiology: Energy, Nutrition, and Human Performance* (Philadelphia: Lea & Febiger, 1986).

ticipant does not have to support his or her own body weight while riding the bicycle, overweight individuals and those with limited joint problems in the lower extremities can take this test.

The bicycle ergometer to be used for this test should allow for the regulation of workloads (see the test procedure in Figure 6.5). Besides the bicycle ergometer, a stop-watch and an additional technician to monitor the heart rate are needed to conduct the test.

The heart rate is taken every minute for six minutes. At the end of the test, the heart rate should be in the range given for each workload in Table 6.5 (generally between 120 and 170 bpm).

When administering the test to older people, good judgment is essential. Low workloads should be used, because if the higher heart rates (around 150 to 170 bpm) are reached, these individuals could be working near or at their maximal capacity, making this an unsafe test without adequate medical supervision. When testing older people, choose workloads so that the final exercise heart rates do not exceed 130 to 140 bpm.

Table 6.3	Predicted Maximal Oxygen Uptake for the Step Test		
15-Sec HR	**HR-bpm**	**Men (mL/kg/min)**	**Women (mL/kg/min)**
30	120	60.9	43.6
31	124	59.3	42.9
32	128	57.6	42.2
33	132	55.9	41.4
34	136	54.2	40.7
35	140	52.5	40.0
36	144	50.9	39.2
37	148	49.2	38.5
38	152	47.5	37.7
39	156	45.8	37.0
40	160	44.1	36.3
41	164	42.5	35.5
42	168	40.8	34.8
43	172	39.1	34.0
44	176	37.4	33.3
45	180	35.7	32.6
46	184	34.1	31.8
47	188	32.4	31.1
48	192	30.7	30.3
49	196	29.0	29.6
50	200	27.3	28.9

© Cengage Learning 2013

12-Minute Swim Test

Similar to the 1.5-Mile Run Test, the 12-Minute Swim Test is considered a maximal exercise test, and the same precautions apply. The objective is to swim as far as possible during the 12-Minute Swim Test (see Figure 6.6).

Unlike land-based tests, predicting VO_{2max} through a swimming test is difficult. A swimming test is practical only for those who are planning to take part in a swimming program or who cannot perform any of the other tests. Differences in skill level, swimming conditioning, and body composition greatly affect the energy requirements (oxygen uptake) of swimming.

Unskilled and unconditioned swimmers can expect lower CR fitness ratings than can be obtained with a land-based test. A skilled swimmer is able to swim more efficiently and expend much less energy than an unskilled swimmer. Improper breathing patterns cause premature fatigue. Overweight individuals are more buoyant in the water, and the larger surface area (body

Figure 6.5	Procedure for the Astrand-Rhyming Test.

1. Adjust the bike seat so the knees are almost completely extended as the foot goes through the bottom of the pedaling cycle.
2. During the test, keep the speed constant at 50 revolutions per minute. Test duration is 6 minutes.
3. Select the appropriate workload for the bike based on gender, age, weight, health, and estimated fitness level. For unconditioned individuals: women, use 300 kpm (kilopounds per meter) or 450 kpm; men, 300 kpm or 600 kpm. Conditioned adults: women, 450 kpm or 600 kpm; men, 600 kpm or 900 kpm.*
4. Ride the bike for 6 minutes and check the heart rate every minute, during the last 15 seconds of each minute. Determine heart rate by recording the time it takes to count 30 pulse beats and then converting to beats per minute using Table 6.4.
5. Average the final two heart rates (5th and 6th minutes). If these two heart rates are not within 5 beats per minute of each other, continue the test for another few minutes until this is accomplished. If the heart rate continues to climb significantly after the 6th minute, stop the test and rest for 15 to 20 minutes. You may then retest, preferably at a lower workload. The final average

heart rate should also fall between the ranges given for each workload in Table 6.5 (men: 300 kpm = 120 to 140 beats per minute; 600 kpm = 120 to 170 beats per minute).

6. Based on the average heart rate of the final 2 minutes and your workload, look up the maximal oxygen uptake (VO_{2max}) in Table 6.5 (for example: men: 600 kpm and average heart rate = 145, VO_{2max} = 2.4 L/min).
7. Correct VO_{2max} using the correction factors found in Table 6.6 (if VO_{2max} = 2.4 and age 35, correction factor = .870. Multiply 2.4 × .870 and final corrected VO_{2max} = 2.09 L/min).
8. To obtain VO_{2max} in mL/kg/min, multiply the VO_{2max} by 1,000 (to convert liters to milliliters) and divide by body weight in kilograms (to obtain kilograms, divide your body weight in pounds by 2.2046).

Example: Corrected VO_{2max} = 2.09 L/min
Body weight = 132 pounds ÷ 2.2046 = 60 kilograms

$$VO_{2max} \text{ in mL/kg/min} = \frac{2.09 \times 1,000}{60} = 34.8 \text{ mL/kg/min}$$

*On the Monark bicycle ergometer, at a speed of 50 revolutions per minute, a load of 1 kp = 300 kpm, 1.5 kp = 450 kpm, 2 kp = 600 kpm, and so forth, with increases of 150 kpm to each half kp.

© Cengage Learning 2013

---

size) produces more friction against movement in the water medium.

Lack of conditioning affects swimming test results as well. An unconditioned skilled swimmer who is in good CR shape because of a regular jogging program will not perform as effectively in a swimming test. Swimming conditioning is important for adequate performance on this test.

Because of these limitations, VO_{2max} cannot be estimated for a swimming test, and the fitness categories given in Table 6.7 are only estimated ratings.

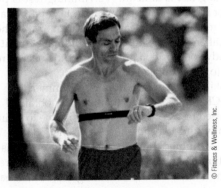

Heart rate monitors increase the accuracy of heart rate assessment.

© Fitness & Wellness, Inc.

Interpreting the Results of Your Maximal Oxygen Uptake

After obtaining your VO_{2max}, you can determine your current level of CR fitness by consulting Table 6.8. Locate the VO_{2max} in your age category, and on the top row you will find your present level of CR fitness. For example, a 19-year-old male with a VO_{2max} of 35 mL/kg/min would be classified in the "average" CR fitness category. After you initiate your personal CR exercise program (see Activity 6.4), you may wish to retest yourself periodically to evaluate your progress.

Principles of CR Exercise Prescription

Before proceeding with the principles of exercise prescription, you should ask yourself if you are willing to give exercise a try. A low percentage of the U.S. population is truly committed to exercise. The first six weeks of the program are most critical. Adherence to exercise is greatly enhanced if you are able to make it through four to six weeks of training. Keep in mind, that all of the benefits of exercise cannot help unless you commit and participate in a lifetime program of physical activity.

Readiness for Exercise

The first step is to ask yourself: Am I ready to start an exercise program? The information provided in Activity 6.2 can help you answer this question. You are evaluated

| Table 6.4 | | Conversion of the Time for 30 Pulse Beats to Pulse Rate per Minute. | | | |

Sec.	bpm	Sec.	bpm	Sec.	bpm
22.0	82	17.3	104	12.6	143
21.9	82	17.2	105	12.5	144
21.8	83	17.1	105	12.4	145
21.7	83	17.0	106	12.3	146
21.6	83	16.9	107	12.2	148
21.5	84	16.8	107	12.1	149
21.4	84	16.7	108	12.0	150
21.3	85	16.6	108	11.9	151
21.2	85	16.5	109	11.8	153
21.1	85	16.4	110	11.7	154
21.0	86	16.3	110	11.6	155
20.9	86	16.2	111	11.5	157
20.8	87	16.1	112	11.4	158
20.7	87	16.0	113	11.3	159
20.6	87	15.9	113	11.2	161
20.5	88	15.8	114	11.1	162
20.4	88	15.7	115	11.0	164
20.3	89	15.6	115	10.9	165
20.2	89	15.5	116	10.8	167
20.1	90	15.4	117	10.7	168
20.0	90	15.3	118	10.6	170
19.9	90	15.2	118	10.5	171
19.8	91	15.1	119	10.4	173
19.7	91	15.0	120	10.3	175
19.6	92	14.9	121	10.2	176
19.5	92	14.8	122	10.1	178
19.4	93	14.7	122	10.0	180
19.3	93	14.6	123	9.9	182
19.2	94	14.5	124	9.8	184
19.1	94	14.4	125	9.7	186
19.0	95	14.3	126	9.6	188
18.9	95	14.2	127	9.5	189
18.8	96	14.1	128	9.4	191
18.7	96	14.0	129	9.3	194
18.6	97	13.9	129	9.2	196
18.5	97	13.8	130	9.1	198
18.4	98	13.7	131	9.0	200
18.3	98	13.6	132	8.9	202
18.2	99	13.5	133	8.8	205
18.1	99	13.4	134	8.7	207
18.0	100	13.3	135	8.6	209
17.9	101	13.2	136	8.5	212
17.8	101	13.1	137	8.4	214
17.7	102	13.0	138	8.3	217
17.6	102	12.9	140	8.2	220
17.5	103	12.8	141	8.1	222
17.4	103	12.7	142	8.0	225

© Cengage Learning 2013

| Table 6.5 | | | | | Maximal Oxygen Uptake (VO_{2max}) Estimates for the Astrand-Ryhming Test | | | | | |

| | Men | | | | | Women | | | | |
| | Workload | | | | | Workload | | | | |
Heart Rate	300	600	900	1200	1500	300	450	600	750	900
120	2.2	3.4	4.8			2.6	3.4	4.1	4.8	
121	2.2	3.4	4.7			2.5	3.3	4.0	4.8	
122	2.2	3.4	4.6			2.5	3.2	3.9	4.7	
123	2.1	3.4	4.6			2.4	3.1	3.9	4.6	
124	2.1	3.3	4.5	6.0		2.4	3.1	3.8	4.5	
125	2.0	3.2	4.4	5.9		2.3	3.0	3.7	4.4	
126	2.0	3.2	4.4	5.8		2.3	3.0	3.6	4.3	
127	2.0	3.1	4.3	5.7		2.2	2.9	3.5	4.2	
128	2.0	3.1	4.2	5.6		2.2	2.8	3.5	4.2	4.8
129	1.9	3.0	4.2	5.6		2.2	2.8	3.4	4.1	4.8
130	1.9	3.0	4.1	5.5		2.1	2.7	3.4	4.0	4.7
131	1.9	2.9	4.0	5.4		2.1	2.7	3.4	4.0	4.6
132	1.8	2.9	4.0	5.3		2.0	2.7	3.3	3.9	4.5
133	1.8	2.8	3.9	5.3		2.0	2.6	3.2	3.8	4.4
134	1.8	2.8	3.9	5.2		2.0	2.6	3.2	3.8	4.4
135	1.7	2.8	3.8	5.1		2.0	2.6	3.1	3.7	4.3
136	1.7	2.7	3.8	5.0		1.9	2.5	3.1	3.6	4.2
137	1.7	2.7	3.7	5.0		1.9	2.5	3.0	3.6	4.2
138	1.6	2.7	3.7	4.9		1.8	2.4	3.0	3.5	4.1
139	1.6	2.6	3.6	4.8		1.8	2.4	2.9	3.5	4.0
140	1.6	2.6	3.6	4.8	6.0	1.8	2.4	2.8	3.4	4.0
141		2.6	3.5	4.7	5.9	1.8	2.3	2.8	3.4	3.9
142		2.5	3.5	4.6	5.8	1.7	2.3	2.8	3.3	3.9
143		2.5	3.4	4.6	5.7	1.7	2.2	2.7	3.3	3.8
144		2.5	3.4	4.5	5.7	1.7	2.2	2.7	3.2	3.8
145		2.4	3.4	4.5	5.6	1.6	2.2	2.7	3.2	3.7
146		2.4	3.3	4.4	5.6	1.6	2.2	2.6	3.2	3.7
147		2.4	3.3	4.4	5.5	1.6	2.1	2.6	3.1	3.6
148		2.4	3.2	4.3	5.4	1.6	2.1	2.6	3.1	3.6
149		2.3	3.2	4.3	5.4		2.1	2.6	3.0	3.5
150		2.3	3.2	4.2	5.3		2.0	2.5	3.0	3.5
151		2.3	3.1	4.2	5.2		2.0	2.5	3.0	3.4
152		2.3	3.1	4.1	5.2		2.0	2.5	2.9	3.4
153		2.2	3.0	4.1	5.1		2.0	2.4	2.9	3.3
154		2.2	3.0	4.0	5.1		2.0	2.4	2.8	3.3
155		2.2	3.0	4.0	5.0		1.9	2.4	2.8	3.2
156		2.2	2.9	4.0	5.0		1.9	2.3	2.8	3.2
157		2.1	2.9	3.9	4.9		1.9	2.3	2.7	3.2
158		2.1	2.9	3.9	4.9		1.8	2.3	2.7	3.1
159		2.1	2.8	3.8	4.8		1.8	2.2	2.7	3.1
160		2.1	2.8	3.8	4.8		1.8	2.2	2.6	3.0
161		2.0	2.8	3.7	4.7		1.8	2.2	2.6	3.0
162		2.0	2.8	3.7	4.6		1.8	2.2	2.6	3.0
163		2.0	2.8	3.7	4.6		1.7	2.2	2.6	2.9
164		2.0	2.7	3.6	4.5		1.7	2.1	2.5	2.9
165		2.0	2.7	3.6	4.5		1.7	2.1	2.5	2.9
166		1.9	2.7	3.6	4.5		1.7	2.1	2.5	2.8
167		1.9	2.6	3.5	4.4		1.6	2.1	2.4	2.8
168		1.9	2.6	3.5	4.4		1.6	2.0	2.4	2.8
169		1.9	2.6	3.5	4.3		1.6	2.0	2.4	2.8
170		1.8	2.6	3.4	4.3		1.6	2.0	2.4	2.7

From I. Astrand, *Acta Physiologica Scandinavica* 49 (1960). Supplementum 169: 45–60.

Table 6.6		Age-Based Correction Factors for Maximal Oxygen Uptake			
Age	Correction Factor	Age	Correction Factor	Age	Correction Factor
14	1.11	32	.909	50	.750
15	1.10	33	.896	51	.742
16	1.09	34	.883	52	.734
17	1.08	35	.870	53	.726
18	1.07	36	.862	54	.718
19	1.06	37	.854	55	.710
20	1.05	38	.846	56	.704
21	1.04	39	.838	57	.698
22	1.03	40	.830	58	.692
23	1.02	41	.820	59	.686
24	1.01	42	.810	60	.680
25	1.00	43	.800	61	.674
26	.987	44	.790	62	.668
27	.974	45	.780	63	.662
28	.961	46	.774	64	.656
29	.948	47	.768	65	.650
30	.935	48	.762		
31	.922	49	.756		

Adapted from I. Astrand, *Acta Physiologica Scandinavica* 49 (1960). Supplementum 169: 45–60.

Table 6.7	12-Minute Swim Test Fitness Categories
Distance (yards)	Fitness Category
≥700	Excellent
500–700	Good
400–500	Average
200–400	Fair
≤200	Poor

Adapted from K. H. Cooper, *The Aerobics Program for Total Well-Being* (New York: Bantam Books, 1982).

Figure 6.6 Procedure for the 12-Minute Swim Test.

1. Enlist a friend to time the test. The only other requisites are a stopwatch and a swimming pool. Do not attempt to do this test in an unsupervised pool.
2. Warm up by swimming slowly and doing a few stretching exercises before taking the test.
3. Start the test and swim as many laps as possible in 12 minutes. Pace yourself throughout the test and do not swim to the point of complete exhaustion.
4. After completing the test, cool down by swimming another 2 or 3 minutes at a slower pace.
5. Determine the total distance you swam during the test and look up your fitness category in Table 6.7.

© Cengage Learning 2013

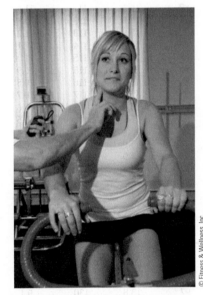

Monitoring heart rate on the carotid artery during the Astrand-Rhyming Test.

© Fitness & Wellness, Inc.

Table 6.8		Cardiorespiratory Fitness Classification According to Maximal Oxygen Uptake (VO₂max)					
			Fitness Category (based on VO_{2max} in mL/kg/min)				
Gender	Age	Poor	Fair	Average	Good	Excellent
Men	<29	<24.9	25–33.9	34–43.9	44–52.9	>53
	30–39	<22.9	23–30.9	31–41.9	42–49.9	>50
	40–49	<19.9	20–26.9	27–38.9	39–44.9	>45
	50–59	<17.9	18–24.9	25–37.9	38–42.9	>43
	60–69	<15.9	16–22.9	23–35.9	36–40.9	>41
	≥70	≤12.9	13–20.9	21–32.9	33–37.9	≥38
Women	<29	<23.9	24–30.9	31–38.9	39–48.9	>49
	30–39	<19.9	20–27.9	28–36.9	37–44.9	>45
	40–49	<16.9	17–24.9	25–34.9	35–41.9	>42
	50–59	<14.9	15–21.9	22–33.9	34–39.9	>40
	60–69	<12.9	13–20.9	21–32.9	33–36.9	>37
	≥70	≤11.9	12–19.9	20–30.9	31–34.9	≥35

■ High physical fitness standard   ■ Health fitness standard
NOTE: See the Chapter 1 discussion on health fitness versus physical fitness.

© Cengage Learning 2013

Cardiorespiratory Endurance Test Results

Name: _____ Date: _____

Course: _____ Section: _____ Gender: _____ Age: _____

Necessary Lab Equipment

1.5-Mile Run: School track or premeasured course and a stopwatch.

1.0-Mile Walk Test: School track or premeasured course and a stopwatch.

Step Test: A bench or gymnasium bleachers 16 ¼ inches high, a metronome, and a stopwatch.

Astrand-Rhyming Test: A bicycle ergometer that allows for regulation of workloads in kilopounds per meter (or watts) and a stopwatch.

12-Minute Swim Test: Swimming pool and a stopwatch.

Objective

To estimate maximal oxygen uptake (VO_{2max}) and cardiorespiratory endurance classification.

Lab Preparation

Wear appropriate exercise clothing including jogging shoes and a swimsuit if required. Be prepared to take the 1.0-Mile Walk Test, the Step Test, the Astrand-Rhyming Test, the 1.5-Mile Run Test, and/or the 12-Minute Swim Test. If more than one test will be conducted, perform them in the order just listed and allow at least 15 minutes between tests. Avoid vigorous physical activity 24 hours prior to this lab.

I. 1.5-Mile Run Test

1.5-Mile Run Time: _____ min and _____ sec VO_{2max} (see Table 6.2, page 195): _____ mL/kg/min

Cardiorespiratory Fitness Category (Table 6.8, page 200): _____

II. 1.0-Mile Walk Test

Weight (W) = _____ lbs   Gender (G) = _____ (female = 0, male = 1)   Time = _____ min and _____ sec

Heart Rate (HR) = _____ bpm

Time in minutes (T) = min + (sec ÷ 60) or T = _____ + (_____ ÷ 60) = _____ min

VO_{2max} = 88.768 − (0.0957 × W) + (8.892 × G) − (1.4537 × T) − (0.1194 × HR)

VO_{2max} = 88.768 − (0.0957 × _____) + (8.892 × _____) − (1.4537 × _____) − (0.1194 × _____)

VO_{2max} = 88.768 − (_____) + (_____) − (_____) − (_____) = _____ mL/kg/min

Cardiorespiratory Fitness Category (Table 6.8, page 200): _____

III. Step Test

15-second recovery heart rate: _____ beats VO_{2max} (Table 6.3, page 197): _____ mL/kg/min

Cardiorespiratory Fitness Category (Table 6.8, page 200): _____

Cardiorespiratory Endurance Test Results (continued)

IV. Astrand-Rhyming Test

Weight (W) = _____ lbs   Weight (BW) in kilograms = (W ÷ 2.2046) = _____ kg   Workload = _____ kpm

Exercise Heart Rates	Time to count 30 beats	Heart Rate (bpm) (from Table 6.4, page 199)		Time to count 30 beats	Heart Rate (bpm) (from Table 6.4, page 199)
First minute:	☐	☐	Fourth minute:	☐	☐
Second minute:	☐	☐	Fifth minute:	☐	☐
Third minute:	☐	☐	Sixth minute:	☐	☐

Average heart rate for the fifth and sixth minutes = _____ bpm

VO_{2max} in L/min (Table 6.5, page 199) = _____ L min   Correction factor (from Table 6.6, page 200) = _____

Corrected VO_{2max} = VO_{2max} in L/min × correction factor = _____ × _____ = _____ L/min

VO_{2max} in mL/kg/min = corrected VO_{2max} in L/min × 1000 ÷ BW in kg = ____ × 1000 ÷ ____ = ____ mL/kg/min

Cardiorespiratory Fitness Category (Table 6.8, page 200): _____

V. 12-Minute Swim Test

Distance swum in 12 minutes: _____ yards

Cardiorespiratory Fitness Category (Table 6.7, page 200): _____

VI. What I Learned and Where I Go From Here:

1. Interpret the results of your cardiorespiratory endurance test(s). Indicate the cardiorespiratory fitness classification you would like to achieve by the end of the term and explain how you are planning to achieve this goal.

_____

_____

_____

_____

_____

_____

_____

2. Briefly discuss the advantages and disadvantages of the cardiorespiratory endurance tests used in this lab.

_____

_____

_____

_____

_____

_____

_____

_____

Exercise Readiness Questionnaire

Name: _____ Date: _____

Course: _____ Section: _____ Gender: _____ Age: _____

Carefully read each statement and circle the number that best describes your feelings in each statement. Please be completely honest with your answers.

	Strongly Agree	Mildly Agree	Mildly Disagree	Strongly Disagree
1. I can walk, ride a bike (or use a wheelchair), swim, or walk in a shallow pool.	4	3	2	1
2. I enjoy exercise.	4	3	2	1
3. I believe exercise can lower the risk for disease and premature mortality.	4	3	2	1
4. I believe exercise contributes to better health.	4	3	2	1
5. I have participated previously in an exercise program.	4	3	2	1
6. I have experienced the feeling of being physically fit.	4	3	2	1
7. I can envision myself exercising.	4	3	2	1
8. I am contemplating an exercise program.	4	3	2	1
9. I am willing to stop contemplating and give exercise a try for a few weeks.	4	3	2	1
10. I am willing to set aside time at least three times a week for exercise.	4	3	2	1
11. I can find a place to exercise (the streets, a park, a YMCA, a health club).	4	3	2	1
12. I can find other people who would like to exercise with me.	4	3	2	1
13. I will exercise when I am moody, fatigued, and even when the weather is bad.	4	3	2	1
14. I am willing to spend a small amount of money for adequate exercise clothing (shoes, shorts, leotards, or swimsuit).	4	3	2	1
15. If I have any doubts about my present state of health, I will see a physician before beginning an exercise program.	4	3	2	1
16. Exercise will make me feel better and improve my quality of life.	4	3	2	1

Scoring Your Test:

This questionnaire allows you to examine your readiness for exercise. You have been evaluated in four categories: mastery (self-control), attitude, health, and commitment. Mastery indicates that you can be in control of your exercise program. Attitude examines your mental disposition toward exercise. Health measures the strength of your convictions about the wellness benefits of exercise. Commitment shows dedication and resolution to carry out the exercise program. Write the number you circled after each statement in the corresponding spaces below. Add the scores on each line to get your totals. Scores can vary from 4 to 16. A score of 12 and above is a strong indicator that that factor is important to you, and 8 and below is low. If you score 12 or more points in each category, your chances of initiating and adhering to an exercise program are good. If you fail to score at least 12 points in three categories, your chances of succeeding at exercise may be slim. You need to be better informed about the benefits of exercise, and a retraining process may be required.

Mastery: 1. [____] + 5. [____] + 6. [____] + 9. [____] = [____]

Attitude: 2. [____] + 7. [____] + 8. [____] + 13. [____] = [____]

Health: 3. [____] + 4. [____] + 15. [____] + 16. [____] = [____]

Commitment: 10. [____] + 11. [____] + 12. [____] + 14. [____] = [____]

Behavior Modification Plan for Cardiorespiratory Endurance

Name: _____ Date: _____

Course: _____ Section: _____ Gender: _____ Age: _____

I. Advantages and disadvantages of starting an exercise program

Advantages: _____

_____

_____

_____

_____

Disadvantages: _____

_____

_____

_____

_____

II. Stage of change for cardiorespiratory exercise

Use Figure 2.5 (page 61) and Table 2.3 (page 60) to identify your current stage of change in regard to participation in a cardiorespiratory

endurance exercise program: [   ]

III. Processes and techniques for change

Identify the processes of change (Table 2.1, page 54) that may help you implement a cardiorespiratory endurance exercise program and list a minimum of three techniques (Table 2.2, page 60) that you will use with each process of change.

Advantages: _____

_____

_____

_____

_____

Disadvantages: _____

_____

_____

_____

_____

in four categories: mastery (self-control), attitude, health, and commitment. The higher you score in any category—mastery, for example—the more important that reason is for you to exercise.

Scores can vary from 4 to 16. A score of 12 or above is a strong indicator that the factor is important to you, whereas 8 or below is low. If you score 12 or more points in each category, your chances of initiating and sticking to an exercise program are good. If you do not score at least 12 points in each of any three categories, your chances of succeeding at exercise may be slim. You need to be better informed about the benefits of exercise, and a retraining process might be helpful to change core values regarding exercise. More tips on how you can become committed to exercise are provided in "Getting Started and Adhering to a Lifetime Exercise Program" (page 216).

Next you will have to decide positively that you will try. Using Activity 6.3, you can list the advantages and disadvantages of incorporating exercise into your lifestyle. Your list might include advantages such as:

- It will make me feel better.
- I will lose weight.
- I will have more energy.
- It will lower my risk for chronic diseases.

Your list of disadvantages might include the following:

- I don't want to take the time.
- I'm too out of shape.
- There's no good place to exercise.
- I don't have the willpower to do it.

When your reasons for exercising outweigh your reasons for not exercising, you will find it easier to try. In Activity 6.3 you will also determine your stage of change for aerobic exercise. Using the information learned in Chapter 2, you can outline specific processes and techniques for change (also see the example in Chapter 9, pages 323–324).

Guidelines for CR Exercise Prescription

In spite of the release of the U.S. Surgeon General's statement on physical activity and health in 1996 indicating that regular moderate physical activity provides substantial health benefits,[3] and the overwhelming evidence validating the benefits of exercise on health and longevity, only about 19 percent of adults in the United States meet minimum recommendations of the ACSM for the improvement and maintenance of CR fitness.[4]

Most people are not familiar with the basic principles of CR exercise prescription. Thus, although they exercise regularly, they do not reap significant improvements in CR endurance.

To develop the CR system, the heart muscle has to be overloaded like any other muscle in the human body. Just as the biceps muscle in the upper arm is developed through strength-training exercises, the heart muscle has to be exercised to increase in size, strength, and efficiency. To better understand how the CR system can be developed, you have to be familiar with the four variables that govern exercise prescription: intensity, mode, duration, and frequency.[5] The acronym **FITT** is sometimes used to describe these variables: *f*requency, *i*ntensity, *t*ype (mode), and *t*ime (quantity and duration). Exercise progression rate is also an important component of the exercise prescription.

First, however, you should be aware that the ACSM recommends that apparently healthy men over age 45 and women over age 55 with one or more risk factor for cardiovascular disease (family history, cigarette smoker, sedentary lifestyle, obesity, high blood pressure, high LDL cholesterol, low HDL cholesterol [see Chapter 10], or prediabetes) get a medical exam and diagnostic graded exercise stress test prior to **vigorous exercise**.[6] The ACSM has defined vigorous exercise as an exercise intensity above 60 percent of maximal capacity. For individuals initiating an exercise program, this intensity is the equivalent of exercise that "substantially increases heart rate and breathing." Symptomatic individuals, or those with known cardiac, pulmonary, or metabolic disease should undergo a medical examination and the exercise test prior to **moderate exercise** (one that "noticeably increases heart rate and breathing").

Intensity of Exercise

When trying to develop the CR system, many people ignore **intensity** of exercise. For muscles to develop, they have to be overloaded to a given point. The training stimulus to develop the biceps muscle, for example, can be accomplished with arm curl exercises with increasing weights. Likewise, the CR system is stimulated by making the heart pump faster for a specified period.

Health and CR fitness benefits result when the person is working between 30 and 85 percent of **heart rate reserve (HRR)** combined with an appropriate duration and frequency of training (see how to calculate intensity, on the next page).[7] Health benefits are achieved when

---

Key Terms

FITT An acronym used to describe the four cardiorespiratory exercise prescription variables: *f*requency, *i*ntensity, *t*ype (mode), and *t*ime (duration).

Vigorous exercise CR exercise that requires an intensity level of approximately 70 percent of capacity.

Intensity In cardiorespiratory exercise, how hard a person has to exercise to improve or maintain fitness.

Heart rate reserve (HRR) The difference between maximal heart rate and resting heart rate.

training at a lower exercise intensity, that is, between 30 and 60 percent of the person's HRR. Even greater health and cardioprotective benefits, and higher and faster improvements in CR fitness (VO_{2max}), however, are achieved primarily through vigorous-intensity programs (at an intensity above 60 percent).[8]

Most people who initiate exercise programs have a difficult time adhering to vigorous-intensity exercise. Thus, unconditioned individuals (those in the "poor" CR fitness category) and older adults should start at a 30 to 40 percent training intensity (TI). For persons in "fair" fitness, training is recommended between 40 and 50 percent TI. For those in the "average" category, a 50 to 60 percent TI is recommended. Active and fit people in the "good" category should exercise between 60 and 70 percent TI, while active persons in the "excellent" fitness category can exercise at the higher TIs between 70 and 85 percent.

Following four to eight weeks of progressive training (depending on your starting TI) at light to moderate (30 to 60 percent) intensities, exercise can be performed between 60 and 85 percent TI. Increases in VO_{2max} are accelerated when the heart is working closer to 85 percent of HRR. Exercise training above 85 percent is recommended only for healthy, performance-oriented individuals and competitive athletes. For most people, training above 85 percent is discouraged to avoid potential cardiovascular problems associated with very-hard-intensity exercise. As intensity increases, exercise adherence decreases and the risk of orthopedic injuries increases.

Intensity of exercise can be calculated easily, and training can be monitored by checking your pulse. To determine the intensity of exercise or **cardiorespiratory training zone** according to heart rate reserve, follow these steps (also refer to Activity 6.4):

1. Estimate your maximal heart rate (MHR)* according to the following formula[9]:

$$MHR = 207 - (.7 \times age)$$

2. Check your resting heart rate (RHR) for a full minute in the evening, after you have been sitting quietly for about 30 minutes reading or watching a relaxing TV show. As explained on pages 195–196, you can check your pulse on the wrist by placing two or three fingers over the radial artery or in the neck, using the carotid artery.

3. Determine the heart rate reserve (HRR) by subtracting the resting heart rate from the maximal heart rate:

$$HRR = MHR - RHR$$

*Recent research indicates that the traditional equation of 220 − age overpredicts MHR in people 40 years and younger and underpredicts MHR in older individuals.

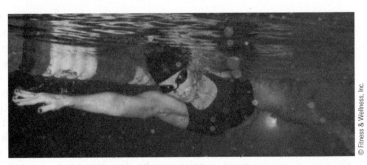

Only those with swimming skill and proper conditioning should take the 12-Minute Swimming Test.

4. Calculate the TIs at 30, 40, 50, 60, 70, and 85 percent. Multiply the heart rate reserve by the respective .30, .40, .50, .60, and .85, and then add the resting heart rate to all four of these figures (e.g., 60% TI = HRR $\times$ .60 + RHR).

Example. The 30, 40, 50, 60, 70, and 85 percent TIs for a 20-year-old with a resting heart rate of 68 bpm would be as follows:

$$MHR: 207 - (.70 \times 20) = 193 \text{ bpm}$$

$$RHR: = 68 \text{ bpm}$$

$$HRR: 193 - 68 = 125 \text{ beats}$$

$$30\% \text{ TI} = (125 \times .30) + 68 = 106 \text{ bpm}$$

$$40\% \text{ TI} = (125 \times .40) + 68 = 118 \text{ bpm}$$

$$50\% \text{ TI} = (125 \times .50) + 68 = 131 \text{ bpm}$$

$$60\% \text{ TI} = (125 \times .60) + 68 = 143 \text{ bpm}$$

$$70\% \text{ TI} = (125 \times .70) + 68 = 155 \text{ bpm}$$

$$85\% \text{ TI} = (125 \times .85) + 68 = 174 \text{ bpm}$$

Light-intensity CR training zone: 106 to 118 bpm
Moderate-intensity CR training zone: 118 to 143 bpm
Vigorous-intensity CR training zone: 143 to 174 bpm

Once you reach the vigorous-intensity CR training zone, continue to exercise between the 60 and 85 TIs to further improve or maintain your CR fitness (see Figure 6.7).

Following a few weeks of training, you may have a considerably lower resting heart rate (10 to 20 beats fewer in 8 to 12 weeks). Therefore, you should recompute your target zone periodically. You can compute your own CR training zone using Activity 6.4. Once you have reached an ideal level of CR endurance, frequent training in the 60 to 85 percent range will allow you to maintain your fitness level.

Moderate- versus Vigorous-Intensity Exercise

As fitness programs became popular in the 1970s, vigorous-intensity exercise (about 70 percent TI) was routinely prescribed for all fitness participants. Follow-

Personalized Cardiorespiratory Exercise Prescription (continued)

III. Cardiorespiratory Exercise Program

The following is your weekly program for development of cardiorespiratory endurance. If you are in the poor or fair cardiorespiratory fitness category, start with week 1. If you are in the average category, you may start at week 5. If you are already active and in the good or excellent category, you may start at week 9 (otherwise start at week 5). After completing the goal for week 12, you can maintain fitness by training between a 70 and 85 percent TI for about 20 to 30 minutes, a minimum of three times per week, on nonconsecutive days. You should also recompute your TIs periodically because you will experience a significant reduction in resting heart rate with aerobic training (approximately 10 to 20 beats in 8 to 12 weeks).

Week	Duration (min)	Frequency	Training Intensity	Heart Rate (bpm)		Physical Activity Perceived Exertion*	
1	15	3	Between 30% and 40%	☐	to ☐	☐	to
2	15	4	Between 30% and 40%			☐	
3	20	4	Between 30% and 40%				
4	20	5	Between 30% and 40%				
5	20	4	Between 40% and 60%	☐	to ☐	☐	to
6	20	5	Between 40% and 60%			☐	
7	30	4	Between 40% and 60%				
8	30	5	Between 40% and 60%				
9	30	4	Between 60% and 85%	☐	to ☐	☐	to
10	30	5	Between 60% and 85%			☐	
11	30–40	5	Between 60% and 85%				
12	30–40	5	Between 60% and 85%				

*See Figure 6.9, page 210.

Maintenance cardiorespiratory training zone (60% to 85% TI): ☐ to ☐ bpm

IV. Briefly state your experience and feelings regarding aerobic exercise.

_____

_____

_____

_____

_____

_____

_____

_____

_____

_____

_____

V. Monitoring Daily Activity

Average total number of daily steps (use 7-day average): ☐

Do you accumulate 10,000 steps on most days of the week (at least five days)?   ☐ Yes ☐ No

risk of cardiovascular disease; whereas the individuals with the highest level of aerobic fitness (also see 100th percentile rank in Figure 6.8) reduce their risk by 64 percent, more than twice the level of risk reduction in the most active group.

Another review of several clinical studies substantiated that vigorous intensity, compared with moderate-intensity exercise, leads to better improvements in coronary heart disease risk factors, including aerobic endurance, blood pressure, and blood glucose control.[13] As a result, the pendulum is again swinging toward vigorous intensity because of the added aerobic benefits, greater protection against disease, and larger energy expenditure that helps with weight management.

Monitoring Exercise Heart Rate

During the first few weeks of an exercise program, you should monitor your exercise heart rate regularly to make sure you are training in the proper zone. Wait until you are about five minutes into the aerobic phase of your exercise session before taking your first reading. When you check your heart rate, count your pulse for 10 seconds, then multiply by six to get the per minute pulse rate. The exercise heart rate will remain at the same level for about 15 seconds following aerobic exercise, then drops rapidly. Do not hesitate to stop during your exercise bout to check your pulse. If the rate is too low, increase the intensity of exercise. If the rate is too high, slow down.

When determining the TI for your own program, you need to consider your personal fitness goals and possible cardiovascular risk factors. Individuals who exercise at around the 50 percent TI still reap significant health benefits—in particular, improvements in the metabolic profile (see "Health Fitness Standards" in Chapter 1, page 21). Training at this lower percentage, however, may place you in only the "average" (moderate fitness) category (see Table 6.8). Exercising at this lower intensity will not allow you to achieve a "good" or "excellent" CR endurance fitness rating (the physical fitness standard). The latter ratings, and even greater health benefits, are obtained by exercising closer to the 85 percent threshold.

Rate of Perceived Exertion

Because many people do not check their heart rate during exercise, an alternative method of prescribing intensity of exercise has been devised using the **physical activity perceived exertion (H-PAPE) scale** (Figure 6.9). This new scale uses phrases based on common terminology used in physical activity and exercise prescription guidelines. Using the scale, a person subjectively rates the perceived exertion or difficulty of exercise when training at different intensity levels. The exercise heart rate then is associated with the corresponding perceived exertion phrase provided.

Figure 6.9   Physical activity perceived exertion scale.

The H-PAPE (Hoeger-Physical Activity Perceived Exertion) Scale provides a subjective rating of the perceived exertion or difficulty of physical activity and exercise when training at a given intensity level. The intensity level is associated with the corresponding perceived exertion phrase provided. These phrases are based on common terminology used in physical activity and exercise prescription guidelines.

Perceived exertion	Training intensity
Light	40%
Moderate	50%
Somewhat hard	60%
Vigorous	70%
Hard	80%
Very hard	90%
All-out effort	100%

SOURCE: Adapted from Hoeger, Werner W. K. "Training for a Walkathon," *Diabetes Self-Management* 24, 4 (2007): 56–68.

For example, if training between 143 (60% TI) and 155 (70% TI) bpm, the person may associate this with training between "somewhat hard" and "vigorous." Some individuals perceive less exertion than others when training at a certain intensity level. Therefore, you have to associate your own inner perception of the task with the phrases given on the scale. You then may proceed to exercise at that rate of perceived exertion.

You must be sure to cross-check your target zone with your perceived exertion during the first weeks of your exercise program. To help you develop this association, you should regularly keep a record of your activities, using the form provided in Activity 6.5. After several weeks of training, you should be able to predict your exercise heart rate just by your own perceived exertion of the intensity of exercise.

Whether you monitor the intensity of exercise by checking your pulse or through the H-PAPE rate, you should be aware that changes in normal exercise conditions will affect the TI. For example, exercising on a hot, humid day or at high altitude increases the heart rate response to a given task, requiring adjustments in the intensity of your exercise.

Mode of Exercise

The **mode**, or type, of exercise that develops the CR system has to be aerobic in nature. Once you have established your CR training zone, any activity or combination of activities that will get your heart rate up to that zone and keep it there for as long as you exercise will give you adequate development. Examples of these activities are walking, jogging, elliptical activity, aerobics, water aerobics, road cycling, spinning, stair climbing, and stationary jogging or cycling. The latter activities require little skill to perform and can be enjoyed by most adults to improve health and fitness. Other aerobic activities such as swimming, cross-country skiing, mountain cycling, rope skipping, racquetball, basketball, and soccer can also be used and are recommended for individuals who already possess the skills to perform these activities or have adequate fitness to learn the necessary skills to safely perform the activity.

Aerobic exercise has to involve the major muscle groups of the body, and it has to be rhythmic and continuous. As the amount of muscle mass involved during exercise increases, so do the demands on the CR system. The activity you choose should be based on your personal preferences, what you most enjoy doing, and your physical limitations. Low-impact activities greatly reduce the risk for injuries. Most injuries to beginners result from high-impact activities. Also, general strength conditioning (see Chapter 7) is recommended prior to initiating an aerobic exercise program for individuals who have been inactive. Strength conditioning can significantly reduce the incidence of injuries.

The amount of strength or flexibility you develop through various activities differs. In terms of CR development, though, the heart doesn't know whether you are walking, swimming, or cycling. All the heart knows is that it has to pump at a certain rate, and as long as that rate is in the desired range, your CR fitness will improve. From a health fitness point of view, training in the lower end of the CR zone will yield substantial health benefits. The closer the heart rate is to the higher end of the CR training zone, however, the greater will be the health benefits and improvements in VO_{2max} (high physical fitness).

Because of the specificity of training, to ascertain changes in fitness, it is recommended that you use the same mode of exercise for training and testing. If your primary mode of training is cycling, it is recommended that you assess VO_{2max} using a bicycle test. For joggers, a field or treadmill running test is best. Swimmers should use a swim test.

Duration of Exercise

The general recommendation is that a person exercise between 20 and 60 minutes per session. For people who have been successful at losing a large amount of weight, however, up to 90 minutes of moderate-intensity activity daily may be required to prevent weight regain.

The duration of exercise is based on how intensely a person trains. The variables are inversely related. If the training is done at around 85 percent, a session of 20 to 30 minutes is sufficient. At about 50 percent intensity, the person should train close to 60 minutes. As mentioned under "Intensity of Exercise," unconditioned people and older adults should train at lower percentages and,

therefore, the activity should be carried out over a longer time.

Although the recommended guideline is 20 to 60 minutes of aerobic exercise per session, in the early stages of conditioning and for individuals who are pressed for time, accumulating 30 minutes or more of moderate-intensity physical activity throughout the day does provide health benefits. Three 10-minute exercise sessions per day (separated by at least 4 hours), at approximately 70 percent of maximal heart rate, have been shown to produce training benefits.[14] Although the increases in VO_{2max} with the latter program were not as large (57 percent) as those found in a group performing a continuous 30-minute bout of exercise per day, the researchers concluded that the accumulation of 30 minutes of moderate-intensity physical activity, conducted for *at least 10 minutes* three times per day, benefits the CR system significantly. Activity bouts of less than 10 minutes in duration do not count toward the 30-minute daily guideline.

Results of this and other similar studies are meaningful because people often mention lack of time as the reason they do not take part in an exercise program. Many think they have to exercise at least 20 continuous minutes to get any benefits at all. Even though a duration of 20 to 30 minutes of continuous vigorous-intensity activity is ideal, short, intermittent physical activity bouts, of at least 10 minutes long each, are beneficial to the CR system.

The 2008 Federal Guidelines for Physical Activity measure duration of exercise in terms of the total quantity of physical activity performed on a weekly basis. Two hours and 30 minutes of moderate-intensity aerobic activity or 1 hour and 15 minutes of vigorous-intensity aerobic activity per week, or an equivalent combination of the two are recommended (30 minutes of moderate-intensity twice per week combined with 20 minutes of vigorous-intensity another two times per week).

Two hours and 30 minutes per week represents the accumulation of 30 minutes of moderate-intensity aerobic activity (done in bouts of at least 10 minutes each) per session/day performed five days per week, whereas 1 hour and 15 minutes is approximately 25 minutes of vigorous-intensity aerobic activity done three times per week. The federal guidelines also indicate that 5 hours of moderate-intensity activity, or 2 hours and 30 minutes of vigorous-intensity activity per week provide additional benefits. Thus, when possible, people are encouraged to go beyond the minimum recommendation.

From a weight management point of view, the recommendation to prevent weight gain is for people to accu-

---

Key Terms

Physical activity perceived exertion (H-PAPE) A perception scale to monitor or interpret the intensity of aerobic exercise.

Mode Form or type of exercise.

mulate 60 minutes of moderate-intensity physical activity most days of the week,[15] whereas 60 to 90 minutes of daily moderate-intensity activity is necessary to prevent weight regain.[16] These recommendations are based on evidence that people who maintain healthy weight typically accumulate between 1 and 1½ hours of physical activity at least five times per week. The duration of exercise should be increased gradually to avoid undue fatigue and exercise-related injuries.

If lack of time is a concern, you should exercise at a vigorous intensity for about 30 minutes, which can burn as many calories as 60 minutes of moderate intensity (also see "The Role of Exercise Intensity and Duration in Weight Management," Chapter 5, page 161), but only 19 percent of adults in the United States typically exercise at a vigorous-intensity level. Novice and overweight exercisers also need proper conditioning prior to vigorous-intensity exercise to avoid injuries or cardiovascular-related problems.

Exercise sessions always should be preceded by a 5 to 10-minute **warm-up** and be followed by a 10-minute **cool-down** period (see Figure 6.7). The purpose of the warm-up is to aid in the transition from rest to exercise. A good warm-up increases extensibility of the muscles and connective tissue, extends joint range of motion, and enhances muscular activity. A warm-up consists of general calisthenics, mild stretching exercises, and walking/jogging/cycling for a few minutes at a lower intensity than the actual target zone. The concluding phase of the warm-up is a gradual increase in exercise intensity to the lower end of the target training zone.

In the cool-down, the intensity of exercise is decreased gradually to help the body return to near resting levels, followed by stretching and relaxation activities. Stopping abruptly causes blood to pool in the exercised body parts, diminishing the return of blood to the heart. Less blood return can cause a sudden drop in blood pressure, dizziness, and faintness, or it can bring on cardiac abnormalities. The cool-down phase also helps dissipate body heat and aid in removing the lactic acid produced during high-intensity exercise.

Frequency of Exercise

The recommended exercise **frequency** for aerobic exercise is three to five days per week. When exercising at 60 to 85 percent of HRR, three 20- to 30-minute exercise sessions per week, on nonconsecutive days, are sufficient to improve (in the early stages) or maintain VO_{2max}. When exercising at a moderate intensity, 30 to 60 minutes five days per week are required.

Research indicates that when vigorous training is conducted more than five days a week, further improvements in VO_{2max} are minimal. Although endurance athletes often train six or seven days per week (often twice per day), their training programs are designed to increase training

---

Behavior Modification Planning

Tips for People Who Have Been Physically Inactive

I PLAN TO **I DID IT**

❑ ❑ Take the sensible approach by starting slowly.

❑ ❑ Begin by choosing moderate-intensity activities you enjoy the most. By choosing activities you enjoy, you'll be more likely to stick with them.

❑ ❑ Gradually build up the time spent exercising by adding a few minutes every few days or so until you can comfortably perform a minimum recommended amount of exercise (20 minutes per day).

❑ ❑ As the minimum amount becomes easier, gradually increase either the length of time exercising or increase the intensity of the activity, or both.

❑ ❑ Vary your activities, both for interest and to broaden the range of benefits.

❑ ❑ Explore new physical activities.

❑ ❑ Reward and acknowledge your efforts.

Try It Fill out the cardiorespiratory exercise prescription in Lab 6D either in your text or online. In your Online Journal or class notebook, describe how well you implement the above suggestions.

SOURCE: Adapted from: Centers for Disease Control and Prevention, Atlanta, 2008.

---

mileage to endure long-distance races (6 to 100 miles) at a high percentage of VO_{2max}, frequently at or above the **anaerobic threshold**.

Although three exercise sessions per week will maintain CR fitness, the importance of regular physical activity in preventing disease and enhancing quality of life has been pointed out clearly by the ACSM, the U.S. Centers for Disease Control and Prevention, and by the President's Council on Physical Fitness and Sports.[17] These organizations along with the U.S. Surgeon General advocate at least 30 minutes of moderate-intensity physical activity on most (defined as five days per week) or preferably all days of the week. This routine has been promoted as an effective way to improve health and quality of life. Further, the Surgeon General states that no one, including older adults, is too old to enjoy the benefits of regular physical activity. Also, be aware that most of the benefits of exercise and activity diminish within two weeks of substantially decreased physical activity and the benefits are completely lost within a few months of inactivity.

Excessive Sitting: A Deadly Proposition

If you meet the guideline and exercise five times per week, but spend most of your day sitting, your lifestyle may be cancelling out the health benefits of the 30-minute exercise session. The human body was created for movement and physical activity. Our society, however, is primarily a sedentary society that lulls us into physical inactivity. Most Americans spend more than half their waking hours sitting: driving to and from work, working at a desk, sitting at the computer, and watching television. Research studies indicate that people who spend most of their day sitting have as much as a 50-percent greater risk of dying prematurely from all causes and an 80-percent greater risk of dying from cardiovascular disease.[18] The data further indicate that death rates are still high for people who spend most of their day sitting, even though they meet the current minimum moderate-physical activity recommendations (30 minutes, at least five times per week).[19] Among many other conditions, excessive sitting leads to weaker muscles, a sluggish central nervous system, increased fatigue, decreased insulin sensitivity, higher blood pressure, decreased activity of lipoprotein lipase (an enzyme that breaks down fats in the blood), and increased cholesterol, LDL cholesterol, and triglycerides. Thus, even if you are meeting the exercise guidelines of physical activity on most days of the week, you should not spend most of the remainder of your day being sedentary.

To minimize inactivity, look to enhance daily **nonexercise activity thermogenesis (NEAT)** or the energy expended doing daily activities not related to exercise. Examples of such activities include:

1. Stand as much as possible while working at home. Place your computer on an elevated stand or shelf and stand while doing work, writing emails, or surfing the Internet. Always stand while answering the phone. Standing triples the energy requirement of doing a similar activity sitting.
2. Use a standing or a treadmill desk. Perform much of your work standing. If at all possible, walk at a light-intensity level while working at your desk. You may find that such practice enhances concentration and work productivity.
3. Use a stability ball for a chair or even a stability ball chair at the office. Such use will enhance body stability, balance, and abdominal, low back, and leg strength.
4. Whenever feasible, hold "walking" instead of conference room meetings.
5. Walk to coworkers' offices to discuss matters with them instead of using the phone or email.
6. Take intermittent breaks. A 10-minute break every hour that you are at the computer to stretch, walk around, or talk to coworkers is quite beneficial.
7. Park farther away or get off the subway, train, or bus several blocks away from the office. When feasible, take the stairs instead of elevators and escalators.

Rate of Progression

How quickly an individual progresses through an exercise program depends on the person's health status, exercise tolerance, and exercise program goals.[20] Initially, only three weekly training sessions of 15 to 20 minutes are recommended to avoid musculo-skeletal injuries. You may then increase the duration by 5 to 10 minutes per week and the frequency so that by the fourth or fifth week you are exercising five times per week (see Activity 6.4). Thereafter, progressively increase frequency, duration, and intensity of exercise until you reach your fitness maintenance goal.

To sum up: Ideally, a person should engage in physical activity six or seven times per week. Based on the previous discussion, to reap both the high-fitness and health-fitness benefits of exercise, a person should do vigorous exercise three times per week for high fitness maintenance, and two to four additional times per week in moderate-intensity activities (see Figure 6.10) to maintain good health. Depending on the intensity of the activity and the health/fitness goals, all exercise sessions should last between 20 and 60 minutes. For adequate weight-management purposes, additional daily physical activity, up to 90 minutes, may be necessary. A summary of the CR exercise prescription guidelines according to the ACSM is provided in Figure 6.11.

Key Terms

Warm-up Starting a workout slowly.

Cool-down Tapering off an exercise session slowly.

Frequency Number of times per week a person engages in exercise.

Anaerobic threshold The highest percentage of the VO_{2max} at which an individual can exercise (maximal steady state) for an extended time without accumulating significant amounts of lactic acid (accumulation of lactic acid forces an individual to slow down the exercise intensity or stop altogether).

Nonexercise activity thermogenesis (NEAT) Energy expended doing everyday activities not related to exercise.

Figure 6.10   The physical activity pyramid.

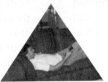
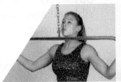

Minimize inactivity

Strength and flexibility: 2–3 days/week

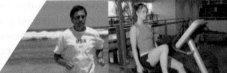
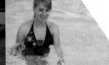

Cardiorespiratory endurance: Exercise 20–60 minutes 3–5 days/week

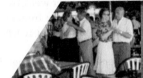
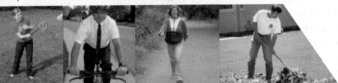

© Cengage Learning 2013

Physical activity: Accumulate 60 to 90 minutes of moderate-intensity activity nearly every day.

Figure 6.11   Cardiorespiratory exercise prescription guidelines.

Mode: Moderate- or vigorous-intensity aerobic activity (examples: walking, jogging, stair climbing, elliptical activity, aerobics, water aerobics, cycling, stair climbing, swimming, cross-country skiing, racquetball, basketball, and soccer)

Intensity: 30% to 85% of heart rate reserve (the training intensity is based on age, health status, initial fitness level, exercise tolerance, and exercise program goals)

Duration: Be active 20 to 90 minutes. At least 20 minutes of continuous vigorous-intensity or 30 minutes of moderate-intensity aerobic activity (the latter may be accumulated in segments of at least 10 minutes in duration each over the course of the day)

Frequency: 3 to 5 days per week for vigorous-intensity aerobic activity to accumulate at least 75 minutes per week, or 5 days per week of moderate-intensity aerobic activity for a minimum total of 150 minutes weekly

Rate of progression:
- Start with three training sessions per week of 15 to 20 minutes
- Increase the duration by 5 to 10 minutes per week and the frequency so that by the fourth or fifth week you are exercising five times per week
- Progressively increase frequency, duration, and intensity of exercise until you reach your fitness goal prior to exercise maintenance

SOURCE: Adapted from American College of Sports Medicine, *ACSM's Guidelines for Exercise Testing and Prescription* (Philadelphia: Wolters Kluwer/Lippincott Williams & Wilkins, 2010).

Fitness Benefits of Aerobic Activities

The contributions of different aerobic activities to the health-related components of fitness vary. Although an accurate assessment of the contributions to each fitness component is difficult to establish, a summary of likely benefits of several activities is provided in Table 6.9. Instead of a single rating or number, ranges are given for some of the categories. The benefits derived are based on the person's effort while participating in the activity.

The nature of the activity often dictates the potential aerobic development. For example, jogging is much more strenuous than walking. The effort during exercise also affects the amount of physiological development. For example, during a low-impact aerobics routine, accentuating all movements (instead of just going through the motions) increases training benefits by orders of magnitude.

Table 6.9 indicates a starting fitness level for each aerobic activity. Attempting to participate in vigorous-intensity activities without proper conditioning often leads to injuries, not to mention discouragement. Beginners should start with light-intensity activities that carry a minimum risk for injuries.

Table 6.9	Ratings for Selected Aerobic Activities

Activity	Recommended Starting Fitness Level[1]	Injury Risk[2]	Potential Cardiorespiratory Endurance Development (VO_{2max})[3,5]	Upper Body Strength Development[3]	Lower Body Strength Development[3]	Upper Body Flexibility Development[3]	Lower Body Flexibility Development[3]	Weight Control[3]	MET Level[4-6]	Caloric Expenditure (cal/hour)[5,6]
Aerobics										
High-Impact Aerobics	A	H	3–4	2	4	3	2	4	6–12	450–900
Moderate-Impact Aerobics	I	M	2–4	2	3	3	2	3	6–12	450–900
Low-Impact Aerobics	B	L	2–4	2	3	3	2	3	5–10	375–750
Step Aerobics	I	M	2–4	2	3–4	3	2	3–4	5–12	375–900
Cross-Country Skiing	B	M	4–5	4	4	2	2	4–5	10–16	750–1,200
Cross-Training	I	M	3–5	2–3	3–4	2–3	1–2	3–5	6–15	450–1,125
Cycling										
Road	I	M	2–5	1	4	1	1	3	6–12	450–900
Stationary	B	L	2–4	1	4	1	1	3	6–10	450–750
Hiking	B	L	2–4	1	3	1	1	3	6–10	450–750
In-Line Skating	I	M	2–4	2	4	2	2	3	6–10	450–750
Jogging	I	M	3–5	1	3	1	1	5	6–15	450–1,125
Jogging, Deep Water	A	L	3–5	2	2	1	1	5	8–15	600–1,125
Racquet Sports	I	M	2–4	3	3	3	2	3	6–10	450–750
Rope Skipping	I	H	3–5	2	4	1	2	3–5	8–15	600–1,125
Rowing	B	L	3–5	4	2	3	1	4	8–14	600–1,050
Spinning	I	L	4–5	1	4	1	1	4	8–15	600–1,125
Stair Climbing	B	L	3–5	1	4	1	1	4–5	8–15	600–1,125
Swimming (front crawl)	B	L	3–5	4	2	3	1	3	6–12	450–900
Walking	B	L	1–2	1	2	1	1	3	4–6	300–450
Walking, Water, Chest-Deep	I	L	2–4	2	3	1	1	3	6–10	450–750
Water Aerobics	B	L	2–4	3	3	3	2	3	6–12	450–900

[1]B = Beginner, I = Intermediate, A = Advanced
[2]L = Low, M = Moderate, H = High
[3]1 = Low, 2 = Fair, 3 = Average, 4 = Good, 5 = Excellent
[4]One MET represents the rate of energy expenditure at rest (3.5 mL/kg/min). Each additional MET is a multiple of the resting value. For example, 5 METs represents an energy expenditure equivalent to five times the resting value, or about 17.5 mL/kg/min.
[5]Varies according to the person's effort (intensity) during exercise.
[6]Varies according to body weight.

© Cengage Learning 2013

In some cases, such as high-impact aerobics and rope skipping, the risk for orthopedic injuries remains high even if the participants are adequately conditioned. These activities should be supplemental only and are not recommended as the sole mode of exercise. Most exercise-related injuries occur as a result of high-impact activities, not high intensity of exercise.

Physicians who work with cardiac patients frequently use metabolic equivalents **(METs)** as an alternative method of prescribing exercise intensity. One MET represents the rate of energy expenditure at rest, that is, 3.5 mL/kg/min. METs are used to measure the intensity of physical activity and exercise in multiples of the resting metabolic rate. At an intensity level of 10 METs, the activity requires a 10-fold increase in the resting energy requirement (or approxi-

> **Key Terms**
>
> **MET** Short for metabolic equivalent, the rate of energy expenditure at rest; 1 MET is the equivalent of a VO_2 of 3.5 mL/kg/min.

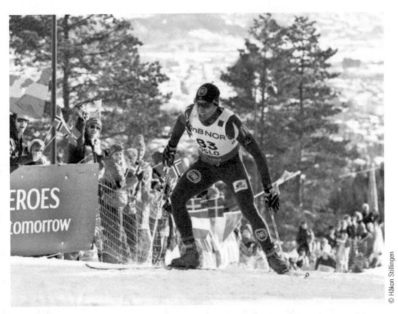

Cross-country skiing requires more oxygen and energy than most other aerobic activities.

mately 35 mL/kg/min). MET levels for a given activity vary according to the effort expended. The MET range for various activities is included in Table 6.9. The harder a person exercises, the higher the MET level.

The effectiveness of various aerobic activities in weight management is charted in Table 6.9. As a general rule, the greater the muscle mass involved in exercise, the better the results. Rhythmic and continuous activities that involve large amounts of muscle mass are most effective in burning calories.

Vigorous-intensity activities increase caloric expenditure as well. Exercising longer, however, compensates for lower intensities. If carried out long enough (45 to 60 minutes five or six times per week), even walking is a good exercise mode for weight management. Additional information on a comprehensive weight management program is given in Chapter 5.

Critical Thinking

Mary started an exercise program last year as a means to lose weight and enhance her body image. She now runs about six miles every day, strength-trains daily, participates in step-aerobics twice per week, and plays tennis or racquetball twice a week. Evaluate her program and make suggestions for improvements.

Getting Started and Adhering to a Lifetime Exercise Program

Following the guidelines provided in Activity 6.4, you may proceed to initiate your own CR endurance program. If you have not been exercising regularly, you might begin by attempting to train five or six times a week for 30 minutes at a time. You might find this discouraging, however, and drop out before getting too far, because you will probably develop some muscle soreness and stiffness and possibly incur minor injuries. Muscle soreness and stiffness and the risk for injuries can be lessened or eliminated by increasing the intensity, duration, and frequency of exercise progressively, as outlined in Activity 6.4.

Once you have determined your exercise prescription, the difficult part begins: starting and sticking to a lifetime exercise program. Although you may be motivated after reading about the benefits to be gained from physical activity, lifelong dedication and perseverance are necessary to reap and maintain good fitness.

The first few weeks probably will be the most difficult for you, but where there's a will, there's a way. Once you begin to see positive changes, it won't be as hard. Soon you will develop a habit of exercising that will be deeply satisfying and will bring about a sense of self-accomplishment. The suggestions provided in the accompanying Behavior Modification Planning box (see page 217) have been used successfully to help change behavior and adhere to a lifetime exercise program.

Tips to Enhance Exercise Compliance

I PLAN TO
I DID IT

❏ ❏ 1. Set aside a regular time for exercise. If you don't plan ahead, it is a lot easier to skip. On a weekly basis, using red ink, schedule your exercise time into your day planner. Next, hold your exercise hour "sacred." Give exercise priority equal to the most important school or business activity of the day. If you are too busy, attempt to accumulate 30 to 60 minutes of daily activity by doing separate 10-minute sessions throughout the day. Try reading the mail while you walk, taking stairs instead of elevators, walking the dog, or riding the stationary bike as you watch the evening news.

❏ ❏ 2. Exercise early in the day, when you will be less tired and the chances of something interfering with your workout are minimal; thus, you will be less likely to skip your exercise session.

❏ ❏ 3. Select aerobic activities you enjoy. Exercise should be as much fun as your favorite hobby. If you pick an activity you don't enjoy, you will be unmotivated and less likely to keep exercising. Don't be afraid to try out a new activity, even if that means learning new skills.

❏ ❏ 4. Combine different activities. You can train by doing two or three different activities the same week. This cross-training may reduce the monotony of repeating the same activity every day. Try lifetime sports. Many endurance sports, such as racquetball, basketball, soccer, badminton, roller skating, cross-country skiing, and body surfing (paddling the board), provide a nice break from regular workouts.

❏ ❏ 5. Use the proper clothing and equipment for exercise. A poor pair of shoes, for example, can make you more prone to injury, discouraging you from the beginning.

❏ ❏ 6. Find a friend or group of friends to exercise with. Social interaction will make exercise more fulfilling. Besides, exercise is harder to skip if someone is waiting to go with you.

❏ ❏ 7. Set goals and share them with others. Quitting is tougher when someone else knows what you are trying to accomplish. When you reach a targeted goal, reward yourself with a new pair of shoes or a jogging suit.

❏ ❏ 8. Purchase a pedometer (step counter) and build up to 10,000 steps per day. These 10,000 steps may include all forms of daily physical activity combined. Pedometers motivate people toward activity because they track daily activity, provide feedback on activity level, and remind the participant to enhance daily activity.

❏ ❏ 9. Don't become a chronic exerciser. Overexercising can lead to chronic fatigue and injuries. Exercise should be enjoyable, and in the process you should stop and smell the roses.

❏ ❏ 10. Exercise in different places and facilities. This will add variety to your workouts.

❏ ❏ 11. Exercise to music. People who listen to fast-tempo music tend to exercise more vigorously and longer. Using headphones when exercising outdoors, however, can be dangerous. Even indoors, it is preferable not to use headphones so you still can be aware of your surroundings.

❏ ❏ 12. Keep a regular record of your activities. Keeping a record allows you to monitor your progress and compare it against previous months and years (see Figure 6.11, page 214).

❏ ❏ 13. Conduct periodic assessments. Improving to a higher fitness category is often a reward in itself, and creating your own rewards is even more motivating.

❏ ❏ 14. Listen to your body. If you experience pain or unusual discomfort, stop exercising. Pain and aches are an indication of potential injury. If you do suffer an injury, don't return to your regular workouts until you are fully recovered. You may cross-train using activities that don't aggravate your injury (for instance, swimming instead of jogging).

❏ ❏ 15. If a health problem arises, see a physician. When in doubt, it's better to be safe than sorry.

Try It The most difficult challenge about exercise is to keep going once you start. The above behavioral change tips will enhance your chances for exercise adherence. In your Online Journal or class notebook, describe which suggestions were most useful.

Cardiorespiratory Exercise Record Form

Name: _____ Course: _____ Section: _____ Gender: _____ Age: _____

Date: _____

Month: _____

Date	Body Weight	Exercise HR	Type of Activity	Dist. in Miles	Time in Min.	H-PAPE*	Daily Steps
1							
2							
3							
4							
5							
6							
7							
8							
9							
10							
11							
12							
13							
14							
15							
16							
17							
18							
19							
20							
21							
22							
23							
24							
25							
26							
27							
28							
29							
30							
31							
Total							

*Physical activity perceived exertion.

Month: _____

Date	Body Weight	Exercise HR	Type of Activity	Dist. in Miles	Time in Min.	H-PAPE*	Daily Steps
1							
2							
3							
4							
5							
6							
7							
8							
9							
10							
11							
12							
13							
14							
15							
16							
17							
18							
19							
20							
21							
22							
23							
24							
25							
26							
27							
28							
29							
30							
31							
Total							

*Physical activity perceived exertion.

Cardiorespiratory Exercise Record Form (continued)

Name: _____ Date: _____ Course: _____ Section: _____ Gender: _____ Age: _____

Month: _____

Date	Body Weight	Exercise HR	Type of Activity	Dist. in Miles	Time in Min.	H-PAPE*	Daily Steps
1							
2							
3							
4							
5							
6							
7							
8							
9							
10							
11							
12							
13							
14							
15							
16							
17							
18							
19							
20							
21							
22							
23							
24							
25							
26							
27							
28							
29							
30							
31							
						Total	

*Physical activity perceived exertion.

Month: _____

Date	Body Weight	Exercise HR	Type of Activity	Dist. in Miles	Time in Min.	H-PAPE*	Daily Steps
1							
2							
3							
4							
5							
6							
7							
8							
9							
10							
11							
12							
13							
14							
15							
16							
17							
18							
19							
20							
21							
22							
23							
24							
25							
26							
27							
28							
29							
30							
31							
						Total	

*Physical activity perceived exertion.

A Lifetime Commitment to Fitness

The benefits of fitness can be maintained only through a regular lifetime program. Exercise is not like putting money in the bank. It doesn't help much to exercise four or five hours on Saturday and not do anything else the rest of the week. If anything, exercising only once a week is not safe for unconditioned adults.

The time involved in losing the benefits of exercise varies among the different components of physical fitness and also depends on the person's condition before the interruption. In regard to CR endurance, it has been estimated that 4 weeks of aerobic training are completely reversed in two consecutive weeks of physical inactivity. But if you have been exercising regularly for months or years, two weeks of inactivity won't hurt you as much as it will someone who has exercised only a few weeks. As a rule, after 48 to 72 hours of aerobic inactivity, the CR system starts to lose some of its capacity.

To maintain fitness, you should keep up a regular exercise program, even during vacations. If you have to interrupt your program for reasons beyond your control, you should not attempt to resume training at the same level you left off but, rather, build up gradually again.

Even the greatest athletes on earth, if they were to stop exercising, would be, after just a few years, at about the same risk for disease as someone who has never done any physical activity. Staying with a physical fitness program long enough brings about positive physiological and psychological changes. Once you are there, you will not want to have it any other way.

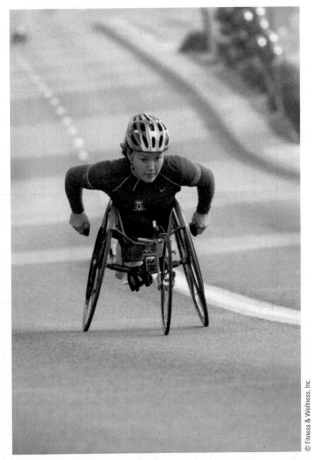

© Fitness & Wellness, Inc.

Physically challenged people can participate and derive health and fitness benefits through a vigorous-intensity exercise program.

Assess Your Behavior

1. Do you consciously attempt to incorporate as much physical activity as possible in your daily living (walk, take stairs, cycle, participate in sports and recreational activities)?

2. Are you accumulating at least 30 minutes of moderate-intensity physical activity over a minimum of five days per week?

3. Is aerobic exercise in the appropriate target zone a priority in your life a minimum of three times per week for at least 20 minutes per exercise session?

4. Do you own a pedometer and do you accumulate 10,000 or more steps on most days of the week?

5. Have you evaluated your aerobic fitness and do you meet at least the health fitness category?

Assess Your Knowledge

Evaluate how well you understand the concepts presented in this chapter using the chapter-specific quizzing available in the online materials at www.cengagebrain.com.

1. CR endurance is determined by
   a. the amount of oxygen the body is able to utilize per minute of physical activity.
   b. the length of time it takes the heart rate to return to 120 bpm following the 1.5-Mile Run Test.
   c. the difference between the maximal heart rate and the resting heart rate.
   d. the product of the heart rate and blood pressure at rest versus exercise.
   e. the time it takes a person to reach a heart rate between 120 and 170 bpm during the Astrand-Ryhming test.

2. Which of the following is not a benefit of aerobic training?
   a. higher VO_{2max}
   b. increase in red blood cell count
   c. decrease in resting heart rate
   d. increase in heart rate at a given workload
   e. increase in functional capillaries

3. The oxygen uptake for a person with an exercise heart rate of 130, a stroke volume of 100, and an a-$\overline{v}O_{2diff}$ of 10 is
   a. 130,000 mL/kg/min.
   b. 1,300 L/min.
   c. 1.3 L/min.
   d. 130 mL/kg/min.
   e. 13 mL/kg/min.

4. The oxygen uptake, in mL/kg/min, for a person with a VO_2 of 2.0 L/min who weighs 60 kilograms is
   a. 120.
   b. 26.5.
   c. 33.3.
   d. 30.
   e. 120,000.

5. The Step Test estimates VO_{2max} according to
   a. how long a person is able to sustain the proper Step Test cadence.
   b. the lowest heart rate achieved during the test.
   c. the recovery heart rate following the test.

d. the difference between the maximal heart rate achieved and the resting heart rate.
   e. the exercise heart rate and the total stepping time.

6. An "excellent" CR fitness rating, in mL/kg/min, for young male adults is about
   a. 10.
   b. 20.
   c. 30.
   d. 40.
   e. 50.

7. How many minutes would a person training at 2.0 L/min have to exercise to burn the equivalent of one pound of fat?
   a. 700
   b. 350
   c. 120
   d. 60
   e. 20

8. The vigorous-intensity CR training zone for a 22-year-old individual with a resting heart rate of 68 bpm is
   a. 120 to 148.
   b. 132 to 156.
   c. 138 to 164.
   d. 146 to 179.
   e. 154 to 188.

9. Which of the following activities does not contribute to the development of CR endurance?
   a. light-impact aerobics
   b. jogging
   c. 400-yard dash
   d. racquetball
   e. All of these activities contribute to its development.

10. The recommended duration for each cardiorespiratory training session is
    a. 10 to 20 minutes.
    b. 15 to 30 minutes.
    c. 20 to 60 minutes.
    d. 45 to 70 minutes.
    e. 60 to 120 minutes.

Correct answers can be found at the back of the book.

Muscular Strength and Endurance

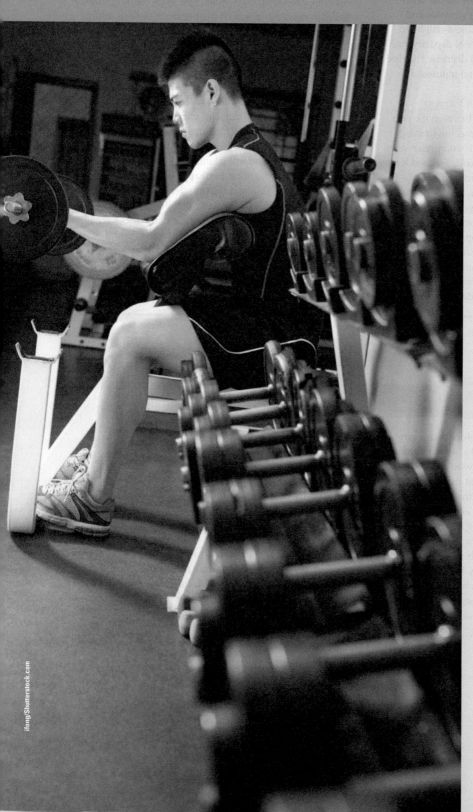

ifong/Shutterstock.com

"Progressive resistance strength training provides significant improvements in functional capacity, fitness, health, and overall well-being."

Objectives

- ▸ **Explain** the importance of adequate muscular strength levels in maintaining good health and well-being.
- ▸ **Clarify** misconceptions about strength fitness.
- ▸ **Define** muscular strength and muscular endurance.
- ▸ **Be able to assess** muscular strength and endurance and learn to interpret test results according to health fitness and physical fitness standards.
- ▸ **Identify** the factors that affect strength.
- ▸ **Understand** the principles of overload and specificity of training for strength development.
- ▸ **Learn** dietary guidelines for optimum strength development.
- ▸ **Become** familiar with core strength training and realize its importance for overall quality of life.
- ▸ **Become acquainted** with two distinct strength-training programs—with weights and without weights.

CENGAGE brain.com

Chart your achievements for strength tests.

Visit www.cengagebrain.com to access course materials and companion resources for this text including quiz questions designed to check your understanding of the chapter contents. See the preface on page xv for more information.

Which is more important for good health: aerobic fitness or muscular strength? They are both important. During the initial fitness boom in the 1970s and 1980s, the emphasis was almost exclusively on aerobic fitness. We now know that both aerobic fitness and muscular strength contribute to health, fitness, work capacity, and overall quality of life. Among many health benefits, aerobic fitness is important in the prevention of cardiovascular diseases and some types of cancer; whereas muscular fitness will build strong muscles and bones, increase functional capacity, prevent osteoporosis and type 2 diabetes, and decrease the risk for low back pain and other musculoskeletal injuries.

Should I do aerobic exercise or strength training first? Ideally, allow some recovery hours between the two types of training. If you can't afford the time, the training order should be based on your fitness goals and preferences. Unless extremely exhausting, aerobics provides a good lead into strength training. Excessive fatigue can lead to bad form while lifting and may result in injury. If your primary goal is strength development, lift first, as you'll be less fatigued and will end up with a more productive workout. On the other hand, if you are trying to develop the cardiorespiratory system or enhance caloric expenditure for weight-loss purposes, heavy lower body lifting will make it very difficult to sustain a good cardio workout thereafter. Thus, evaluate your goals, and select the training order accordingly.

Do big muscles turn into fat when the person stops training? Muscle and fat tissue are two completely different types of tissue. Just as an apple will not turn into an orange, muscle tissue cannot turn into fat or vice versa. Muscle cells increase and decrease in size according to your training program. If you train quite hard, muscle cells increase in size. This increase is limited in women due to hormonal differences compared with men. When one stops training, muscle cells again decrease in size. If the person maintains a high caloric intake without physical training, however, fat cells will increase in size as weight (fat) is gained.

What strength-training exercises are best to get an abdominal "six-pack"? Most men tend to store body fat around the waist, while women do so around the hips. There are, however, no "miracle" exercises to spot-reduce. Multiple sets of abdominal curl-ups, crunches, reverse crunches, or sit-ups performed three to five times per week will strengthen the abdominal musculature but will not be sufficient to allow the muscles to appear through the layer of fat between the skin and the muscles. The total energy (caloric) expenditure of a few sets of abdominal exercises will not be sufficient to lose a significant amount of weight (fat). If you want to get a "washboard stomach" (or, for women, achieve shapely hips), you need to engage in a moderate to vigorous aerobic and strength-training program combined with a moderate reduction in daily caloric intake (diet).

Real Life Story Jason's Experience

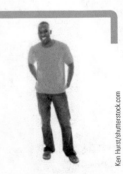

Ken Hurst/shutterstock.com

When I lifted weights with my friends before taking my fitness class, I would show off by trying to lift more than they could. I was really competitive and would do whatever it took to lift as much or more weight than my friends. I was even using really bad form to beat them. When I would do a biceps curl, I would lift my elbows and arch my back and use the momentum to swing the weight up. On the bench press, I would arch my back and bounce the weight off my chest to lift it up. And with squats, I would cheat by doing a shallow squat, not really bending my legs that much. When we covered strength training in class, we talked about proper form and going through the full range of motion. In the weight room, my instructor helped me use correct form. I finally realized that the mistakes I was making were actually keeping me from getting stronger. I made the corrections that my instructor showed me. I didn't like that I had to decrease the amount of weight I was using at first, but eventually I improved and increased my strength. Now I am able to lift more than I did before, this time using correct form!

Personal Understanding of Muscular Fitness Concepts

I. Good muscular strength is not a critical component for adequate health fitness. _____ Yes _____ No

II. Even though body weight may not drop or even increase as a result of a progressive resistance strength-training program, circumference measurements (inches) and percent body fat may decrease. _____ True _____ False

III. Performing at least one set within the RM zone for each exercise produces substantial strength development. _____ Yes _____ No

IV. A periodized strength-training program is frequently used to maximize muscular strength and endurance gains. _____ Yes _____ No

V. Single-joint exercises are more effective than multiple-joint exercises for strength development. _____ Yes _____ No

The benefits of **strength training** or **resistance training** on health and well-being are well documented. The need for strength fitness is not confined to highly trained athletes, fitness enthusiasts, and individuals who have jobs that require heavy muscular work.

Benefits of Strength Training

A well-planned strength-training program leads to increased muscle strength and endurance, power, muscle tone, and tendon and ligament strength—all of which help to improve and maintain everyday functional physical capacity. Strength is a basic health-related fitness component and is an important wellness component for optimal performance in daily activities such as sitting, walking, running, lifting and carrying objects, doing housework, and enjoying recreational activities. Strength also is of great value in improving posture, personal appearance, and self-image; in developing sports skills; in promoting stability of joints; and in meeting certain emergencies in life.

From a health standpoint, increasing strength helps to increase or maintain muscle and a higher resting metabolic rate; encourages weight loss and maintenance, preventing obesity; lessens the risk for injury; reduces chronic low back pain; alleviates arthritic pain; aids in childbearing; improves bone density, preventing osteoporosis; improves cholesterol levels, decreases triglyceride levels, and reduces high blood pressure, thus reducing the risk for cardiovascular disease; and promotes psychological well-being.

Regular strength training also helps control blood sugar. Much of the blood glucose from food consumption goes to the muscles, where it is stored as glycogen. When muscles are not used, muscle cells may become insulin resistant, and glucose cannot enter the cells,

thereby increasing the risk for type 2 diabetes. Following 16 weeks of strength training, a group of diabetic men and women improved their blood sugar control, gained strength, increased lean body mass, lost body fat, and lowered blood pressure.[1]

Furthermore, with time, the heart rate and blood pressure response to lifting a heavy resistance (a weight) decreases. This adaptation reduces the demands on the cardiovascular system when you perform activities such as carrying a child, the groceries, or a suitcase.

Muscular Strength and Aging

In the older adult population, muscular strength may be the most important health-related component of physical fitness. Although proper cardiorespiratory endurance is necessary to help maintain a healthy heart, good strength contributes more to independent living than any other fitness component. Older adults with good strength levels can successfully perform most **activities of daily living**.

A common occurrence as people age is **sarcopenia**, the loss of lean body mass, strength, and function.

Strength training A program designed to improve muscular strength and/or endurance through a series of progressive resistance (weight) training exercises that overload the muscle system and cause physiological development.

Resistance training See Strength training.

Activities of daily living Everyday behaviors that people normally do to function in life (cross the street, carry groceries, lift objects, do laundry, sweep floors).

Sarcopenia Age-related loss of lean body mass, strength, and function.

How much of this loss is related to the aging process itself or to actual physical inactivity and faulty nutrition is unknown. And whereas thinning of the bones from osteoporosis renders them prone to fractures, the gradual loss of muscle mass and ensuing frailty are what lead to falls and subsequent loss of function in older adults. Strength training helps to slow the age-related loss of muscle function. Protein deficiency, seen in some older adults, also contributes to loss of lean tissue.

More than anything else, older adults want to enjoy good health and to function independently. Many of them, however, are confined to nursing homes because they lack sufficient strength to move about. They cannot walk very far, and many have to be helped in and out of beds, chairs, and tubs.

A strength-training program can enhance quality of life tremendously, and nearly everyone can benefit from it. Only people with advanced heart disease are advised to refrain from strength training. Inactive adults between the ages of 56 and 86 who participated in a 12-week strength-training program increased their lean body mass by about 3 pounds, lost about 4 pounds of fat, and increased their resting metabolic rate by almost 7 percent.[2] In other research, leg strength improved by as much as 200 percent in previously inactive adults over age 90.[3] As strength improves, so does the ability to move about, the capacity for independent living, and enjoyment of life during the "golden years." More specifically, good strength enhances quality of life in that it

- improves balance and restores mobility,
- makes lifting and reaching easier,
- decreases the risk for injuries and falls, and
- stresses the bones and preserves bone mineral density, thereby decreasing the risk for osteoporosis.

Another benefit of maintaining a good strength level is its relationship to human **metabolism**. A primary outcome of a strength-training program is an increase in muscle mass or size (lean body mass), known as muscle **hypertrophy**.

Muscle tissue uses more energy than does fatty tissue. That is, your body expends more calories to maintain muscle than to maintain fat. All other factors being equal, if two individuals both weigh 150 pounds but have different amounts of muscle mass, the one with more muscle mass will have a higher **resting metabolism**. Even small increases in muscle mass have a long-term positive effect on metabolism.

Loss of lean tissue also is thought to be a primary reason for the decrease in metabolism as people grow older. Contrary to some beliefs, metabolism does not have to slow down significantly with aging. It is not so much that metabolism slows down, it's that we slow down. Lean body mass decreases with sedentary living, which in turn slows down the resting metabolic rate. Thus, if people continue eating at the same rate as they age, body fat increases.

Daily energy requirements decrease an average of 360 calories between age 26 and age 60.[4] Participating in a strength-training program can offset much of the decline and prevent and reduce excess body fat. One research study found an increase in resting metabolic rate of 35 calories per pound of muscle mass in older adults who participated in a strength-training program.[5]

Gender Differences

A common misconception about physical fitness concerns women in strength training. Because of the increase in muscle mass typically seen in men, some women think that a strength-training program will result in their developing large musculature.

Even though the quality of muscle in men and women is the same, endocrinological differences do not allow women to achieve the same amount of muscle hypertrophy (size) as men. Men also have more muscle fibers, and because of the sex-specific male hormones, each individual fiber has more potential for hypertrophy. On the average, following 6 months of training, women can achieve up to a 50-percent increase in strength but only a 10-percent increase in muscle size.

The idea that strength training allows women to develop muscle hypertrophy to the same extent as men is as false as the notion that playing basketball will turn women into giants. Masculinity and femininity are established by genetic inheritance, not by the amount of physical activity. Variations in the extent of masculinity and femininity are determined by individual differences in hormonal secretions of androgen, testosterone, estrogen, and progesterone. Women with a bigger-than-average build often are inclined to participate in sports because of their natural physical advantage. As a result, many people have associated women's participation in sports and strength training with large muscle size.

As the number of females who participate in sports has increased steadily, the myth of strength training in women leading to large increases in muscle size has abated somewhat. For example, per pound of body weight, female gymnasts are among the strongest athletes in the world. These athletes engage regularly in vigorous strength-training programs. Yet, female gymnasts have some of the most well-toned and graceful figures of all women.

Improved body appearance has become the rule rather than the exception for women who participate in strength-training programs. Some of the most attractive female movie stars also train with weights to further improve their personal image.

Nonetheless, you may ask, "If weight training does not masculinize women, why do so many women body

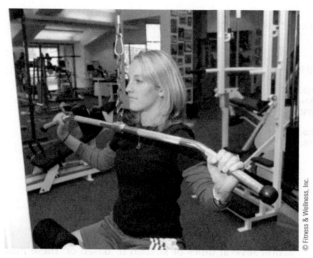

© Fitness & Wellness, Inc.

Improved body appearance has become the rule rather than the exception for women who participate in strength-training exercises.

builders develop such heavy musculature?" In the sport of body building, the athletes follow intense training routines consisting of two or more hours of constant weight lifting with short rest intervals between sets. Many body-building training routines call for back-to-back exercises using the same muscle groups. The objective of this type of training is to pump extra blood into the muscles. This additional fluid makes the muscles appear much bigger than they do in a resting condition. Based on the intensity and the length of the training session, the muscles can remain filled with blood, appearing measurably larger for an hour or longer after completing the training session. Performing such routines is a common practice before competitions. Therefore, in real life, these women are not as muscular as they seem when they are participating in a contest.

In the sport of body building (among others), a big point of controversy is the use of **anabolic steroids** and human growth hormones. These hormones produce detrimental and undesirable side effects, even more so in women (such as hypertension, fluid retention, decreased breast size, deepening of the voice, and whiskers and other atypical body hair growth), which some women deem tolerable. Anabolic steroid use in general—except for medical reasons and when carefully monitored by a physician—can lead to serious health consequences.

Critical Thinking

What role should strength training have in a fitness program? • Should people be motivated for the health fitness benefits, or should they participate to enhance their body image? • What are your feelings about individuals (male or female) with large body musculature?

Selected Detrimental Effects From Using Anabolic Steroids

- Liver tumors
- Hepatitis
- Hypertension
- Reduction of high-density lipoprotein (HDL) cholesterol
- Elevation of low-density lipoprotein (LDL) cholesterol
- Hyperinsulinism
- Impaired pituitary function
- Impaired thyroid function
- Mood swings
- Aggressive behavior
- Increased irritability
- Acne
- Fluid retention
- Decreased libido
- HIV infection (via injectable steroids)
- Prostate problems (men)
- Testicular atrophy (men)
- Reduced sperm count (men)
- Clitoral enlargement (women)
- Decreased breast size (women)
- Increased body and facial hair (irreversible in women)
- Deepening of the voice (irreversible in women)

Use of anabolic steroids by female body builders and female track-and-field athletes is not uncommon. Athletes use anabolic steroids to remain competitive at the highest level. During the 2004 Olympic Games in Athens, Greece, two women shot putters, including the gold medal winner (later stripped of the medal), were expelled from the games for using steroids. Women who take steroids undoubtedly will build heavy musculature, and if they take them long enough, the steroids will produce masculinizing effects.

Key Terms

Metabolism All energy and material transformations that occur within living cells; necessary to sustain life.

Hypertrophy An increase in the size of the cell, as in muscle hypertrophy.

Resting metabolism Amount of energy (expressed in milliliters of oxygen per minute or total calories per day) an individual requires during resting conditions to sustain proper body function.

Anabolic steroids Synthetic versions of the male sex hormone testosterone, which promotes muscle development and hypertrophy.

| **Figure 7.1** | Changes in body composition as a result of a combined aerobic and strength-training program. |

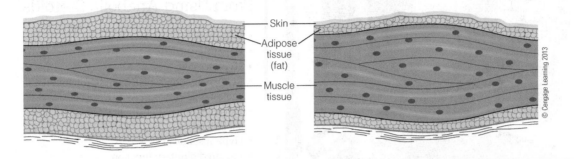

To prevent steroid use, the International Federation of Body Building instituted a mandatory steroid-testing program for women participating in the Miss Olympia contest. When drugs are not used to promote development, improved body image is the rule rather than the exception among women who participate in body building, strength training, and sports in general.

Changes in Body Composition

A benefit of strength training, accentuated even more when combined with aerobic exercise, is a decrease in adipose or fatty tissue around muscle fibers themselves. This decrease is often greater than the amount of muscle hypertrophy (see Figure 7.1). Therefore, losing inches but not body weight is common.

Because muscle tissue is more dense than fatty tissue (and despite the fact that inches are lost during a combined strength-training and aerobic program), people, especially women, often become discouraged because they cannot see the results readily on the scale. They can offset this discouragement by determining body composition regularly to monitor their changes in percent body fat rather than simply measuring changes in total body weight (see Chapter 4).

Assessment of Muscular Strength and Endurance

Although muscular strength and endurance are interrelated, they do differ. **Muscular strength** is the ability to exert maximum force against resistance. **Muscular endurance** is the ability of a muscle to exert submaximal force repeatedly over time.

Muscular endurance (also referred to as "localized muscular endurance") depends to a large extent on muscular strength. Weak muscles cannot repeat an action several times or sustain it. Based on these principles, strength tests and training programs have been designed to measure and develop absolute muscular strength, muscular endurance, or a combination of the two.

Muscular strength is usually determined by the maximal amount of resistance (weight)—**one repetition maximum** or **1 RM**—that an individual is able to lift in a single effort. Although this assessment yields a good measure of absolute strength, it does require considerable time, because the 1 RM is determined through trial and error. For example, strength of the chest muscles is frequently measured through the bench press exercise. If an individual has not trained with weights, he may try 100 pounds and lift this resistance easily. After adding 50 pounds, he fails to lift the resistance. Then he decreases resistance by 20 or 30 pounds. Finally, after several trials, the 1 RM is established.

Using this method, a true 1 RM might be difficult to obtain the first time an individual is tested, because fa-

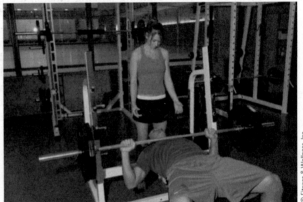

The maximal amount of resistance that an individual is able to lift in one single effort (1 repetition maximum or 1RM) is a measure of absolute strength.

tigue becomes a factor. By the time the 1 RM is established, the person already has made several maximal or near-maximal attempts.

In contrast, muscular endurance typically is established by the number of repetitions an individual can perform against a submaximal resistance or by the length of time a given contraction can be sustained. For example: How many push-ups can an individual do? Or how many times can a 30-pound resistance be lifted? Or how long can a person hold a chin-up?

If time is a factor and only one test item can be done, the Hand Grip Strength Test, described in Figure 7.2, is commonly used to assess strength. This test, though, provides only a weak correlation with overall body strength. Two additional strength tests are provided in Figures 7.3 and 7.4. Activity 7.1 also offers you the opportunity to assess your own level of muscular strength or endurance with all three tests. You may take one or more of these tests, according to your time and the facilities available.

In strength testing, several body sites should be assessed, because muscular strength and muscular endurance are both highly specific. A high degree of strength

---

Figure 7.2 Procedure for the Hand Grip Strength Test.

1. Adjust the width of the dynamometer* so the middle bones of your fingers rest on the distant end of the dynamometer grip.
2. Use your dominant hand for this test. Place your elbow at a 90° angle and about 2 inches away from the body.
3. Now grip as hard as you can for a few seconds. Do not move any other body part as you perform the test (do not flex or extend the elbow, do not move the elbow away or toward the body, and do not lean forward or backward during the test).
4. Record the dynamometer reading in pounds (if reading is in kilograms, multiply by 2.2046).
5. Three trials are allowed for this test. Use the highest reading for your final test score. Look up your percentile rank for this test in Table 7.1.
6. Based on your percentile rank, obtain the hand grip strength fitness category according to the following guidelines:

Percentile Rank	Fitness Category
≥90	Excellent
70–80	Good
50–60	Average
30–40	Fair
≤20	Poor

*A Lafayette model 78010 dynamometer is recommended for this test (Lafayette Instruments Co., Sagamore and North 9th Street, Lafayette, IN 47903).

© Cengage Learning 2013

---

or endurance in one body part does not necessarily indicate similarity in other parts, so no single strength test provides a good assessment of overall body strength. Accordingly, exercises for the strength tests were selected to include the upper body, lower body, and abdominal regions.

Before strength testing, you should become familiar with the procedures for the respective tests. For safety reasons, always take at least one friend with you whenever you train with weights or undertake any type of strength assessment. Also, these are different tests, so to make valid comparisons, you should use the same test for pre- and post-assessments. The following are your options.

Muscular Strength: Hand Grip Strength Test

As indicated previously, when time is a factor, the Hand Grip Test can be used to provide a rough estimate of strength. Unlike the next two tests, this one is isometric (involving static contraction, discussed later in the chapter). If the proper grip is used, no finger motion or body movement is visible during the test. The test procedure is given in Figure 7.2, and percentile ranks based on your results are provided in Table 7.1. You can record the results of this test in Activity 7.1.

Changes in strength are more difficult to evaluate with the Hand Grip Strength Test. Most strength-training programs are dynamic in nature (body segments are moved through a range of motion), whereas this test provides an isometric assessment. Further, grip-strength exercises seldom are used in strength training, and increases in strength are specific to the body parts exercised. This test, however, can be used to supplement the following strength tests.

Muscular Endurance Test

Three exercises were selected to assess the endurance of the upper body, lower body, and midbody muscle groups (see Figure 7.3). The advantage of the Muscular Endurance Test is that it does not require strength-training equipment—only a stopwatch, a metronome, a bench or gymnasium bleacher 16¼ inches high, a cardboard strip 3½ inches wide by 30 inches long, and a

---

Key Terms

Muscular strength The ability of a muscle to exert maximum force against resistance (e.g., 1 repetition maximum [or 1 RM] on the bench press exercise).

Muscular endurance The ability of a muscle to exert submaximal force repeatedly over time.

One repetition maximum (1 RM) The maximum amount of resistance an individual is able to lift in a single effort.

Table 7.1	Scoring Table for Hand Grip Strength Test	
Percentile Rank	Men	Women
99	153	101
95	145	94
90	141	91
80	139	86
70	132	80
60	124	78
50	122	74
40	114	71
30	110	66
20	100	64
10	91	60
5	76	58

◻ High physical fitness standard

◻ Health fitness standard

© Cengage Learning 2013

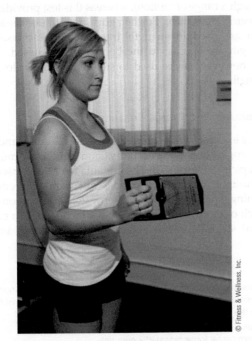

© Fitness & Wellness, Inc.

The hand grip tests strength.

partner. A percentile rank is given for each exercise according to the number of repetitions performed (see Table 7.2). An overall endurance rating can be obtained by totaling the number of points obtained on each exercise. Record the results of this test in Activity 7.1 and Appendix A.

Muscular Strength and Endurance Test

In the Muscular Strength and Endurance Test, you will lift a submaximal resistance as many times as possible using the six strength-training exercises listed in Figure 7.4. The resistance for each lift is determined according to selected percentages of body weight shown in Figure 7.4 and Activity 7.1.

With this test, if an individual does only a few repetitions, primarily absolute strength will be measured. For those who are able to do a lot of repetitions, the test will be an indicator of muscular endurance. If you are not familiar with the different lifts, see the illustrations provided at the end of this chapter.

A strength/endurance rating is determined according to the maximum number of repetitions you are able to perform on each exercise. Fixed-resistance strength units are necessary to administer all but the abdominal exercises in this test (see "Dynamic Training" on pages 238–239 for an explanation of fixed-resistance equipment).

A percentile rank for each exercise is given based on the number of repetitions performed (see Table 7.3). As with the Muscular Endurance Test, an overall muscular strength/endurance rating is obtained by totaling the number of points obtained on each exercise.

If no fixed-resistance equipment is available, you can still perform the test using different equipment. In that case, though, the percentile rankings and strength fitness categories may not be completely accurate because a certain resistance (e.g., 50 pounds) is seldom the same on two different strength-training machines (e.g., Universal Gym versus Nautilus). The industry has no standard calibration procedure for strength equipment. Consequently, if you lift a certain resistance for a specific exercise (e.g., bench press) on one machine, you may or may not be able to lift the same amount for this exercise on a different machine.

Even though the percentile ranks may not be valid across different equipment, test results can be used to evaluate changes in fitness. For example, you may be able to do 7 repetitions during the initial test, but if you can perform 14 repetitions after 12 weeks of training, that's a measure of improvement. Results of the Muscular Strength and Endurance Test can be recorded in Activity 7.1.

Figure 7.3 Muscular Endurance Test.

Three exercises are conducted on this test: bench jumps, modified dips (men) or modified push-ups (women), and bent-leg curl-ups or abdominal crunches. All exercises should be conducted with the aid of a partner. The correct procedure for performing each exercise is as follows:

Bench jump. Using a bench or gymnasium bleacher 16¼" high, attempt to jump up onto and down off of the bench as many times as possible in 1 minute. If you cannot jump the full minute, you may step up and down. A repetition is counted each time both feet return to the floor.

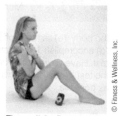

Figure 7.3a Bench jump

Modified dip. Men only: Using a bench or gymnasium bleacher, place the hands on the bench with the fingers pointing forward. Have a partner hold your feet in front of you. Bend the hips at approximately 90° (you also may use three sturdy chairs: Put your hands on two chairs placed by the sides of your body and place your feet on the third chair in front of you). Lower your body by flexing the elbows until they reach a 90° angle, then return to the starting position (also see Exercise 6 at the end of this chapter). Perform the repetitions to a two-step cadence (down-up) regulated with a metronome set at 56 beats per minute. Perform as many continuous repetitions as possible. Do not count any more repetitions if you fail to follow the metronome cadence.

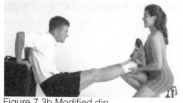

Figure 7.3b Modified dip

Modified push-up. Women only: Lie down on the floor (face down), bend the knees (feet up in the air), and place the hands on the floor by the shoulders with the fingers pointing forward. The lower body will be supported at the knees (as opposed to the feet) throughout the test (see Figure 7.3c). The chest must touch the floor on each repetition. As with the modified dip exercise (above), perform the repetitions to a two-step cadence (up-down) regulated with a metronome set at 56 beats per minute. Perform as many continuous repetitions as possible. Do not count any more repetitions if you fail to follow the metronome cadence.

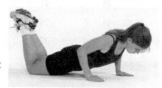

Figure 7.3c Modified push-up

Bent-leg curl-up. Lie down on the floor (face up) and bend both legs at the knees at approximately 100°. The feet should be on the floor, and you must hold them in place yourself throughout the test. Cross the arms in front of the chest, each hand on the opposite shoulder. Now raise the head off the floor, placing the chin against the chest. This is the starting and finishing position for each curl-up (see Figure 7.3d). **The back of the head may not come in contact with the floor, the hands cannot be removed from the shoulders, nor may the feet or hips be raised off the floor at any time during the test. The test is terminated if any of these four conditions occur.**

When you curl up, the upper body must come to an upright position before going back down (see Figure 7.3e). The repetitions are performed to a two-step cadence (up-down)

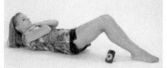

Figure 7.3d Bent-leg curl-up

regulated with the metronome set at 40 beats per minute. For this exercise, you should allow a brief practice period of 5 to 10 seconds to familiarize yourself with the cadence (the *up* movement is initiated with the first beat, then you must wait for the next beat to initiate the *down* movement; one repetition is accomplished every two beats of the metronome). Count as many repetitions as you are able to perform following the proper cadence. The test is also terminated if you fail to maintain the appropriate cadence or if you accomplish 100 repetitions. Have your partner check the angle at the knees throughout the test to make sure to maintain the 100° angle as close as possible.

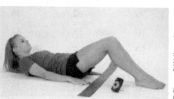

Figure 7.3e Bent-leg curl-up

Abdominal crunch. This test is recommended only for individuals who are unable to perform the bent-leg curl-up test because of susceptibility to low back injury. Exercise form must be carefully monitored during the test. Several authors and researchers have indicated that proper form during this test is extremely difficult to control. Subjects often slide their bodies, bend their elbows, or shrug their shoulders during the test. Such actions facilitate the performance of the test and misrepresent the actual test results. Biomechanical factors also limit the ability to perform this test. Further, lack of spinal flexibility keeps some individuals from being able to move the full 3½" range of motion. Others are unable to keep their heels on the floor during the test. The validity of this test as an effective measure of abdominal strength or abdominal endurance has also been questioned through research.

Tape a 3½" × 30" strip of cardboard onto the floor. Lie down on the floor in a supine position (face up) with the knees bent at approximately 100°. The feet should be on the floor, and you must hold them in place yourself throughout the test. Straighten out your arms and place them on the floor alongside the trunk with the palms down and the fingers fully extended. The fingertips of both hands should barely touch the closest edge of the cardboard (see Figure 7.3f). Bring the head off the floor until the chin is 1" to 2" away from your chest. Keep the head in this position during the entire test (do not move the head by flexing or extending the neck). You are now ready to begin the test.

Perform the repetitions to a two-step cadence (up-down) regulated with a metronome set at 60 beats per minute. As you curl up, slide the fingers over the cardboard until the fingertips reach the far edge (3½") of the board (see Figure 7.3g), then return to the starting position.

Allow a brief practice period of 5 to 10 seconds

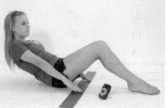

Figure 7.3f Abdominal crunch test

Figure 7.3g Abdominal crunch test

to familiarize yourself with the cadence. Initiate the *up* movement with the first beat and the *down* movement with the next beat. Accomplish one repetition every two beats of the metronome. Count as many repetitions as you are able to perform following the proper cadence. You may not count a repetition if the fingertips fail to reach the distant edge of the cardboard.

Terminate the test if you (a) fail to maintain the appropriate cadence, (b) bend the elbows, (c) shrug the shoulders, (d) slide

(continued)

Figure 7.3	Muscular Endurance Test. (continued)

the body, (e) lift heels off the floor, (f) raise the chin off the chest, (g) accomplish 100 repetitions, or (h) no longer can perform the test. Have your partner check the angle at the knees throughout the test to make sure that the 100° angle is maintained as closely as possible.

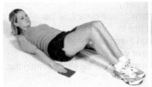 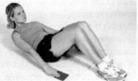

Figure 7.3h   Figure 7.3i
Abdominal crunch test performed with a Crunch-Ster Curl-Up Tester.

For this test you may also use a Crunch-Ster Curl-Up Tester, available from Novel Products.* An illustration of the test performed with this equipment is provided in Figures 7.3h and 7.3i.

According to the results, look up your percentile rank for each exercise in the far left column of Table 7.2 and determine your

muscular endurance fitness category according to the following classification:

Average Score	Fitness Category	Points
≥90	Excellent	5
70–80	Good	4
50–60	Average	3
30–40	Fair	2
≤20	Poor	1

Look up the number of points assigned for each fitness category above. Total the number of points and determine your overall strength endurance fitness category according to the following ratings:

Total Points	Strength Endurance Category
≥13	Excellent
10–12	Good
7–9	Average
4–6	Fair
≤3	Poor

*Novel Products, Inc. Figure Finder Collection, P.O. Box 408, Rockton, IL 61072-0408. 1-800-323-5143, Fax 815-624-4866.

Table 7.2	Muscular Endurance Scoring Table

Percentile Rank	Men				Women			
	Bench Jumps	Modified Dips	Bent-Leg Curl-Ups	Abdominal Crunches	Bench Jumps	Modified Push-Ups	Bent-Leg Curl-Ups	Abdominal Crunches
99	66	54	100	100	58	95	100	100
95	63	50	81	100	54	70	100	100
90	62	38	65	100	52	50	97	69
80	58	32	51	66	48	41	77	49
70	57	30	44	45	44	38	57	37
60	56	27	31	38	42	33	45	34
50	54	26	28	33	39	30	37	31
40	51	23	25	29	38	28	28	27
30	48	20	22	26	36	25	22	24
20	47	17	17	22	32	21	17	21
10	40	11	10	18	28	18	9	15
5	34	7	3	16	26	15	4	0

▭ High physical fitness standard   ▭ Health fitness standard

© Cengage Learning 2013

Figure 7.4	Muscular Strength and Endurance Test.

1. Familiarize yourself with the six lifts used for this test: lat pull-down, leg extension, bench press, bent-leg curl-up or abdominal crunch,* leg curl, and arm curl. Graphic illustrations for each lift are given at the end of this chapter. For the leg curl exercise, the knees should be flexed to 90°. A description and illustration of the bent-leg curl-up and the abdominal crunch exercises are provided in Figure 7.3. On the leg extension lift, maintain the trunk in an upright position.
2. Determine your body weight in pounds.
3. Determine the amount of resistance to be used on each lift. To obtain this number, multiply your body weight by the percent given below for each lift.

Lift	Percent of Body Weight	
	Men	**Women**
Lat Pull-Down	.70	.45
Leg Extension	.65	.50
Bench Press	.75	.45
Bent-Leg Curl-Up or Abdominal Crunch*	NA**	NA**
Leg Curl	.32	.25
Arm Curl	.35	.18

*The abdominal crunch exercise should be used only by individuals who suffer or are susceptible to low back pain.
**NA = not applicable—see Figure 7.3.

4. Perform the maximum continuous number of repetitions possible.
5. Based on the number of repetitions performed, look up the percentile rank for each lift in the left column of Table 7.3.
6. The individual strength fitness category is determined according to the following classification:

Percentile Rank	Fitness Category	Points
≥90	Excellent	5
70–80	Good	4
50–60	Average	3
30–40	Fair	2
≤20	Poor	1

7. Look up the number of points assigned for each fitness category under item 6 above. Total the number of points and determine your overall strength fitness category according to the following ratings:

Total Points	Strength Category
≥25	Excellent
19–24	Good
13–18	Average
7–12	Fair
≤6	Poor

8. Record your results in Activity 7.1.

Table 7.3	Muscular Strength and Endurance Scoring Table

	Men							Women						
Percentile Rank	Lat Pull-Down	Leg Extension	Bench Press	Bent-Leg Curl-Up	Abdominal Crunch	Leg Curl	Arm Curl	Lat Pull-Down	Leg Extension	Bench Press	Bent-Leg Curl-Up	Abdominal Crunch	Leg Curl	Arm Curl
99	30	25	26	100	100	24	25	30	25	27	100	100	20	25
95	25	20	21	81	100	20	21	25	20	21	100	100	17	21
90	19	19	19	65	100	19	19	21	18	20	97	69	12	20
80	16	15	16	51	66	15	15	16	13	16	77	49	10	16
70	13	14	13	44	45	13	12	13	11	13	57	37	9	14
60	11	13	11	31	38	11	10	11	10	11	45	34	7	12
50	10	12	10	28	33	10	9	10	9	10	37	31	6	10
40	9	10	7	25	29	8	8	9	8	5	28	27	5	8
30	7	9	5	22	26	6	7	7	7	3	22	24	4	7
20	6	7	3	17	22	4	5	6	5	1	17	21	3	6
10	4	5	1	10	18	3	3	3	3	0	9	15	1	3
5	3	3	0	3	16	1	2	2	1	0	4	0	0	2

☐ High physical fitness standard   ☐ Health fitness standard

Muscular Strength and Endurance Assessment

Name: _____ Date: _____

Course: _____ Section: _____ Gender: _____ Age: _____

I. Hand Grip Strength Test

Instructions are provided in Figure 7.2, page 229. Perform the test according to the instructions and look up your results in Table 7.1, page 230.

Hand used: ☐ Right ☐ Left

Reading: [____] lbs.

Fitness category (see Figure 7.2, page 229): [_____]

II. Muscular Endurance Test

Conduct this test using the guidelines provided in Figure 7.3, pages 231–232, and Table 7.2, page 232. Record your repetitions, fitness category, and points in the spaces provided below.

Exercise	Metronome Cadence	Repetitions	Fitness Category	Points
Bench jumps	none	[ ]	[ ]	[ ]
Modified dips—men only	56 bpm	[ ]	[ ]	[ ]
Modified push-ups—women only	56 bpm	[ ]	[ ]	[ ]
Bent-leg curl-ups	40 bpm	[ ]	[ ]	[ ]
Abdominal crunches	60 bpm	[ ]	[ ]	[ ]

Total Points: [____]

Overall muscular endurance fitness category (see end of Figure 7.3, page 232): [_____]

Muscular Strength and Endurance Assessment (continued)

III. Muscular Strength and Endurance Test

Perform the Muscular Strength and Endurance Test according to the procedure outlined in Figure 7.4, page 233. Record the results, fitness category, and points in the appropriate blanks provided below.

Body weight: [＿＿＿＿] lbs.

Lift	Percent of Body Weight (pounds)		Resistance	Repetitions	Fitness Category	Points
	Men	Women				
Lat pull-down	.70	.45				
Leg extension	.65	.50				
Bench press	.75	.45				
Bent-leg curl-up or abdominal crunch	NA*	NA*				
Leg curl	.32	.25				
Arm curl	.35	.18				

*Not applicable—no resistance required. Use test described in Figure 7.3, pages 231–232.

Overall muscular strength fitness category (see Figure 7.4, page 233): [＿＿＿＿＿＿＿]

IV. Muscular Strength and Endurance Goals

Indicate the muscular strength/endurance category that you would like to achieve by the end of the term: [＿＿＿＿＿]

Behavior Modification

Briefly state your feelings about your current strength level and indicate how you are planning to achieve your strength objective:

_____

_____

_____

_____

_____

_____

_____

_____

_____

_____

_____

Strength-Training Prescription

The capacity of muscle cells to exert force increases and decreases according to the demands placed upon the muscular system. If muscle cells are overloaded beyond their normal use, such as in strength-training programs, the cells increase in size (hypertrophy) and strength. If the demands placed on the muscle cells decrease, such as in sedentary living or required rest because of illness or injury, the cells **atrophy** and lose strength. A good level of muscular strength is important to develop and maintain fitness, health, and total well-being.

Factors That Affect Strength

Several physiological factors combine to create muscle contraction and subsequent strength gains: neural stimulation, type of muscle fiber, overload, specificity of training, training volume, and periodization. Basic knowledge of these concepts is important to understand the principles involved in strength development.

Neural Function

Within the neuromuscular system, single **motor neurons** branch and attach to multiple muscle fibers. The motor neuron and the fibers it innervates (supplies with nerves) form a **motor unit**. The number of fibers that a motor neuron can innervate varies from just a few in muscles that require precise control (e.g., eye muscles) to as many as 1,000 or more in large muscles that do not perform refined or precise movements.

Stimulation of a motor neuron causes the muscle fibers to contract maximally or not at all. Variations in the number of fibers innervated and the frequency of their stimulation determine the strength of the muscle contraction. As the number of fibers innervated and frequency of stimulation increase, so does the strength of the muscular contraction.

Neural adaptations are prominent in the early stages of strength training. In novice participants, significant strength increases seen during the first two to three weeks of training are largely related to enhanced neural function by increasing motor neuron stimulation and muscle fiber recruitment (skill acquisition). Long-term strength development is primarily related to increased physiological adaptation within the muscle(s) and to a lesser extent to continued neural adaptations.

Types of Muscle Fiber

The human body has two basic types of muscle fibers: (a) slow-twitch or red fibers and (b) fast-twitch or white fibers. **Slow-twitch fibers** have a greater capacity for aerobic work. **Fast-twitch fibers** have a greater capacity for anaerobic work and produce more overall force. The latter are important for quick and powerful movements commonly used in strength-training activities.

The proportion of slow- and fast-twitch fibers is determined genetically and consequently varies from one person to another. Nevertheless, training increases the functional capacity of both types of fiber, and more specifically, strength training increases their ability to exert force.

During muscular contraction, slow-twitch fibers always are recruited first. As the force and speed of muscle contraction increase, the relative importance of the fast-twitch fibers increases. To activate the fast-twitch fibers, an activity must be intense and powerful.

Overload

Strength gains are achieved in two ways:

1. Through increased ability of individual muscle fibers to generate a stronger contraction
2. By recruiting a greater proportion of the total available fibers for each contraction

These two factors combine in the **overload principle**. The demands placed on the muscle must be increased systematically and progressively over time, and the resistance must be of a magnitude significant enough to cause physiological adaptation. In simpler terms, just like all other organs and systems of the human body, to increase in physical capacity, muscles have to be taxed repeatedly beyond their accustomed loads. Because of this principle, strength training also is called progressive resistance training.

Several procedures can be used to overload in strength training[6]:

1. Increasing the intensity (resistance of amount of weight used)
2. Increasing the number of repetitions at the current intensity
3. Increasing or decreasing the speed at which the repetitions are performed
4. Decreasing the rest interval for endurance improvements (with lighter resistances) or lengthening the rest interval for strength and power development (with higher resistances)
5. Increasing the volume (sum of the repetitions performed multiplied by the resistance used)
6. Using any combination of the above

Specificity of Training

Training adaptations are specific to the impetus applied. In strength training, the principle of **specificity of training** holds that for a muscle to increase in strength or endurance, the training program must be specific to obtain the desired effects (see also the discussion on resistance on pages 240–241).

The principle of specificity also applies to activity or sport-specific development and is commonly referred to as **specific adaptation to imposed demand (SAID) training**. The SAID principle implies that if an individual is attempting to improve specific sport skills, the strength-training exercises performed should resemble as closely as possible the movement patterns encountered in that particular activity or sport.

For example, a soccer player who wishes to become stronger and faster would emphasize exercises that will develop leg strength and power. In contrast, an individual recovering from a lower-limb fracture initially exercises to increase strength and stability, and subsequently muscle endurance.

Training Volume

Volume is the sum of all the repetitions performed multiplied by the resistances used during a strength-training session. Volume frequently is used to quantify the amount of work performed in a given training session. For example, an individual who does three sets of six repetitions with 150 pounds has performed a training volume of 2,700 ($3 \times 6 \times 150$) for this exercise. The total training volume can be obtained by totaling the volume of all exercises performed.

The volume of training done in a strength-training session can be modified by changing the total number of exercises performed, the number of sets done per exercise, or the number of repetitions performed per set. Athletes typically use high training volumes and low intensities to achieve muscle hypertrophy, and low volumes and high intensities to increase strength and power.

Periodization

The concept of **periodization** (variation) entails systematically altering training variables over time to keep the program challenging and lead to greater strength development. Periodization means cycling one's training objectives (hypertrophy, strength, and endurance), with each phase of the program lasting anywhere from 2 to 12 weeks. Training variables altered include resistance (weight lifted), number of repetitions, number of sets, and/or number of exercises performed.

The periodized training approach is popular among athletes and is frequently used to prevent **overtraining**. Training volume should not increase by more than 5 percent from one phase to the next. Periodization now is popular among fitness participants who wish to achieve maximal strength gains. Over the long run, for intermediate and advanced participants, the periodized approach has been shown to be superior to nonperiodized training (using the same exercises, sets, and repetitions repeatedly).

Three types of periodized training, based on program design and objectives, are commonly used. These are:

- **Classical Periodization.** The classical or linear model is used by individuals seeking maximal strength development. It starts with an initial high volume of training using low resistances. In subsequent cycles, the program gradually switches to a lower volume and higher resistances.
- **Reverse Periodization.** A model used primarily by individuals seeking greater muscular endurance.

Also a linear model, it is opposite to the classical model. The resistances are highest at the beginning of training with a low volume, subsequently followed by progressive decreases in resistances and increases in training volume.

- **Undulating Periodization.** This model uses a combination of volumes and resistances within a cycle by alternating in a nonlinear fashion (randomly or systematically) among the muscular fitness components: strength, hypertrophy, power, and endurance. The undulating model compares favorably, and in some cases, it is even superior to the classical and reverse models.

Understanding all five training concepts that affect strength (neural stimulation, muscle fiber types, overload, specificity, and periodization) discussed thus far is required to design an effective strength-training program.

Principles Involved in Strength Training

Because muscular strength and endurance are important in developing and maintaining overall fitness and well-being, the principles necessary to develop a strength-

Key Terms

Atrophy Decrease in the size of a cell.

Motor neurons Nerves connecting the central nervous system to the muscle.

Motor unit The combination of a motor neuron and the muscle fibers that neuron innervates.

Slow-twitch fibers Muscle fibers with greater aerobic potential and slow speed of contraction.

Fast-twitch fibers Muscle fibers with greater anaerobic potential and fast speed of contraction.

Overload principle Training concept that the demands placed on a system (cardiorespiratory or muscular) must be increased systematically and progressively over time to cause physiological adaptation (development or improvement).

Specificity of training Principle that training must be done with the specific muscle(s) the person is attempting to improve.

Specific adaptation to imposed demand (SAID) training Training principle stating that, for improvements to occur in a specific activity, the exercises performed during a strength-training program should resemble as closely as possible the movement patterns encountered in that particular activity.

Volume (in strength training) The sum of all repetitions performed multiplied by the resistance used during a training session.

Periodization A training approach that divides the season into cycles using a systematic variation in intensity and volume of training to enhance fitness and performance.

Overtraining An emotional, behavioral, and physical condition marked by increased fatigue, decreased performance, persistent muscle soreness, mood disturbances, and feelings of "staleness" or "burnout" as a result of excessive physical training.

training program have to be understood, just as in the prescription for cardiorespiratory endurance. These principles are mode, resistance, sets, frequency, and volume of training. The key factor in successful muscular strength development, however, is the individualization of the program according to these principles and the person's goals, as well as the magnitude of the individual's effort during training itself.[7]

Mode of Training

Two types of training methods are used to improve strength: isometric (static) and dynamic (previously called "isotonic"). In **isometric training**, muscle contractions produce little or no movement, such as pushing or pulling against an immovable object or holding a given position against resistance for a given period of time. In dynamic training, the muscle contractions produce movement, such as extending the knees with resistance on the ankles (leg extension). The specificity of training principle applies here, too. To increase isometric versus dynamic strength, an individual must use static instead of dynamic training to achieve the desired results.

Isometric Training

Isometric training does not require much equipment. Because strength gains with isometric training are specific to the angle of muscle contraction, this type of training is beneficial in a sport such as gymnastics, which requires regular static contractions during routines. As presented in Chapter 8, however, isometric training is a critical component of health conditioning programs for the low back (see "Preventing and Rehabilitating Low Back Pain," pages 284–288) and for spinal-stabilization musculature and healthy posture. Selected exercises, in particular core exercises, are recommended as a part of a comprehensive strength-training program.

Dynamic Training

Dynamic training is the most common mode for strength training. The primary advantage is that strength is gained through the full **range of motion**. Most daily activities are dynamic in nature. We are constantly lifting, pushing, and pulling objects, and strength is needed through a complete range of motions. Another advantage is that improvements are measured easily by the amount lifted.

Dynamic training consists of two action phases when an exercise is performed: (1) **concentric** or **positive resistance** and (2) **eccentric** or **negative resistance**. In the concentric phase, the muscle shortens as it contracts to overcome the resistance. In the eccentric phase, the muscle lengthens to overcome the resistance. For example, during a bench press exercise, when the person lifts the resistance from the chest to full-arm extension, the triceps muscle on the back of the upper arm shortens to extend (straighten) the elbow. During the eccentric phase, the same triceps muscle is used to lower the weight during elbow flexion, but the muscle lengthens slowly to avoid dropping the resistance. Both motions work the same muscle against the same resistance.

Eccentric muscle contractions allow us to lower weights in a smooth, gradual, and controlled manner. Without eccentric contractions, weights would be suddenly dropped on the way down. Because the same muscles work when you lift and lower a resistance, always be sure to execute both actions in a controlled manner. Failure to do so diminishes the benefits of the training program and increases the risk for injuries. Eccentric contractions seem to be more effective in producing muscle hypertrophy but result in greater muscle soreness.[8]

Dynamic training programs can be conducted without weights; using exercise bands; and with **free weights**, **fixed-resistance** machines, **variable-resistance** machines, or isokinetic equipment. When you perform dynamic exercises without weights (e.g., pull-ups and push-ups), with free weights, or with fixed-resistance machines, you

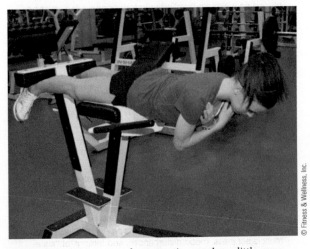

In isometric training, muscle contraction produces little or no movement.

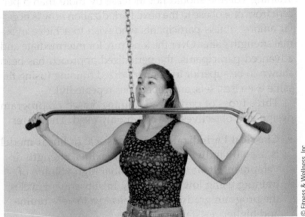

In dynamic training, muscle contraction produces movement in the respective joint.

match the user's force through the range of motion. The mode of training that an individual selects depends mainly on the type of equipment available and the specific objective the training program is attempting to accomplish.

The benefits of isokinetic and variable-resistance training are similar to those of the other dynamic training methods. Theoretically, strength gains should be better because maximum resistance is applied at all angles. Research, however, has not shown this type of training to be more effective than other modes of dynamic training.

Free Weights versus Machines in Dynamic Training

The most popular weight-training devices available during the first half of the 20th century were plate-loaded barbells (free weights). Strength-training machines were developed in the middle of the century but did not become popular until the 1970s. With subsequent technological improvements to these machines, a debate arose over which of the two training modalities was better.

Free weights require that the individual balance the resistance through the entire lifting motion. Thus, one could logically assume that free weights are a better training modality because additional stabilizing muscles are needed to balance the resistance as it is moved through the range of motion. Research, however, has not shown any differences in strength development between the two exercise modalities.[9]

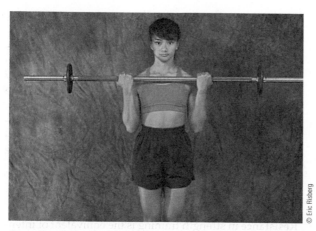
Strength-training can be done using free weights.

move a constant resistance through a joint's full range of motion. The greatest resistance that can be lifted equals the maximum weight that can be moved at the weakest angle of the joint. This is because of changes in length of muscle and angle of pull as the joint moves through its range of motion. This type of training is also referred to as **dynamic constant external resistance** or DCER.

As strength training became more popular, new strength-training machines were developed. This technology brought about **isokinetic training** and variable-resistance training programs, which require special machines equipped with mechanical devices that provide differing amounts of resistance, with the intent of overloading the muscle group maximally through the entire range of motion. A distinction of isokinetic training is that the speed of the muscle contraction is kept constant because the machine provides resistance to

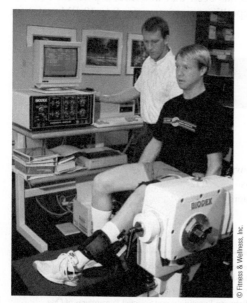
In isokinetic training, the speed of muscle contraction is constant.

Key Terms

Isometric training Strength-training method referring to a muscle contraction that produces little or no movement, such as pushing or pulling against an immovable object.

Range of motion Entire arc of movement of a given joint.

Dynamic training Strength-training method referring to a muscle contraction with movement.

Concentric Describes shortening of a muscle during muscle contraction.

Positive resistance The lifting, pushing, or concentric phase of a repetition during a strength-training exercise.

Eccentric Describes lengthening of a muscle during muscle contraction.

Negative resistance The lowering or eccentric phase of a repetition during a strength-training exercise.

Free weights Barbells and dumbbells.

Fixed resistance Type of exercise in which a constant resistance is moved through a joint's full range of motion (dumbbells, barbells, machines using a constant resistance).

Variable resistance Training using special machines equipped with mechanical devices that provide differing amounts of resistance through the range of motion.

Dynamic constant external resistance (DCER) See Fixed resistance.

Isokinetic training Strength-training method in which the speed of the muscle contraction is kept constant because the equipment (machine) provides an accommodating resistance to match the user's force (maximal) through the range of motion.

Advantages of Free Weights

Following are the advantages of using free weights instead of machines in a strength-training program:

- Cost: Free weights are much less expensive than most exercise machines. On a limited budget, free weights are a better option.
- Variety: A bar and a few plates can be used to perform many exercises to strengthen most muscles in the body.
- Portability: Free weights can be easily moved from one area or station to another.
- Coordination: Free weights require greater muscular coordination that mimic movement requirements of specific tasks.
- Balance: Free weights require that a person balance the weight through the entire range of motion. This feature involves additional stabilizing muscles to keep the weight moving properly.
- One size fits all: People of almost all ages can use free weights. A drawback of machines is that individuals who are at the extremes in terms of height or limb length often do not fit into the machines. In particular, small women and adolescents are at a disadvantage.

Advantages of Machines

Strength-training machines have the following advantages over free weights:

- Safety: Machines are safer because spotters are rarely needed to monitor exercises.
- Selection: A few exercises—such as hip flexion, hip abduction, leg curls, lat pull-downs, and neck exercises—can be performed only with machines.
- Variable resistance: Most machines provide variable resistance. Free weights provide only fixed resistance.
- Isolation: Individual muscles are better isolated with machines because stabilizing muscles are not used to balance the weight during the exercise.
- Time: Exercising with machines requires less time because you can set the resistance quickly by using a selector pin instead of having to manually change dumbbells or weight plates on both sides of a barbell.
- Flexibility: Most machines can provide resistance over a greater range of movement during the exercise, thereby contributing to more flexibility in the joints. For example, a barbell pullover exercise provides resistance over a range of 100 degrees, whereas a weight machine may allow for as much as 260 degrees.
- Rehabilitation: Machines are more useful during injury rehabilitation. A knee injury, for instance, is practically impossible to rehab using free weights, whereas with a weight machine, small loads can be easily selected through a limited range of motion.
- Skill acquisition: Learning a new exercise movement—and performing it correctly—is faster because the machine controls the direction of the movement.

Although each modality has pros and cons, muscles do not know whether the source of a resistance is a barbell, a dumbbell, a Universal Gym machine, a Nautilus machine, or a simple cinder block. What determines the extent of a person's strength development is the quality of the program and the individual's effort during the training program itself—not the type of equipment used. Currently, the general recommendation is that both machines and free weights be used by beginners and intermediate participants, whereas advanced participants are encouraged to use primarily free weights.

Resistance

Resistance in strength training is the equivalent of intensity in cardiorespiratory exercise prescription. To stimulate strength development, the general recommendation has been to use a resistance of approximately 80 percent of the maximum capacity (1 RM). For example, a person with a 1 RM of 150 pounds should work with about 120 pounds (150 × .80).

The number of repetitions that one can perform at 80 percent of the 1 RM varies among exercises (i.e., bench press, lat pull-down, leg curl; see Table 7.4). Data indicate that the total number of repetitions performed at a certain percentage of the 1 RM depends on the amount of muscle mass involved (bench press versus triceps extension) and whether it is a single- or multi-joint exercise (leg press versus leg curl). In trained and untrained subjects alike, the number of repetitions is greater with larger muscle mass involvement and multi-joint exercises.[10]

Because of the time factor involved in constantly determining the 1 RM on each lift to ensure that the person is indeed working around 80 percent, the accepted rule for many years has been that individuals perform between 8 and 12 repetitions maximum (or 8 to 12 RM zone) for

Table 7.4	Number of Repetitions Performed at 80 Percent of the One Repetition Maximum (1 RM)			
	Trained		**Untrained**	
Exercise	**Men**	**Women**	**Men**	**Women**
Leg press	19	22	15	12
Lat pull-down	12	10	10	10
Bench press	12	14	10	10
Leg extension	12	10	9	8
Sit-up*	12	12	8	7
Arm curl	11	7	8	6
Leg curl	7	5	6	6

*Sit-up exercise performed with weighted plates on the chest and feet held in place with an ankle strap.

SOURCE: W. W. K. Hoeger, D. R. Hopkins, S. L. Barette, and D. F. Hale, "Relationship Between Repetitions and Selected Percentages of One Repetition Maximum: A Comparison Between Untrained and Trained Males and Females," *Journal of Applied Sport Science Research* 4, no. 2 (1990): 47–51.

adequate strength gains.[11] For instance, if a person is training with a resistance of 120 pounds and cannot lift it more than 12 times—that is, the person reaches volitional fatigue at or before 12 repetitions—the training stimulus (weight used) is adequate for strength development. Once the person can lift the resistance more than 12 times, the resistance is increased by 5 to 10 pounds and the person again should build up to 12 repetitions. This is referred to as **progressive resistance training**.

Strength development, however, also can occur when working with less than 80 percent of the 1 RM (60 percent to 80 percent). Although the 8 to 12 RM zone is the most commonly prescribed resistance training zone, benefits do accrue when working below 8 RM or above 12 RM. If the main objective of the training program is muscular endurance, 15 to 25 repetitions per set are recommended. Older adults and individuals susceptible to musculoskeletal injuries are encouraged to work with 10 to 15 repetitions using moderate resistances (about 50 percent to 60 percent of the 1 RM).

In both young and older individuals, all repetitions should be performed at a moderate velocity (about 1 second concentric and 1 second eccentric), as such yields the greatest strength gains. For advanced training, varying training velocity between sets, from very slow to fast, are recommended.

Elite strength and power athletes typically work between 1 and 6 RM, but they often shuffle training (periodized training) with a different number of repetitions and sets for selected periods (weeks) of time. Body builders tend to work with moderate resistance levels (60 to 85 percent of the 1 RM) and perform 8 to 20 repetitions to near fatigue. A foremost objective of body building is to increase muscle size. Moderate resistance promotes blood flow to the muscles, "pumping up the muscles" (also known as "the pump"), which makes them look much larger than they do in a resting state.

From a general fitness point of view, a moderate resistance of only about 50 percent should be used initially while learning proper form and lifting technique. Following the first two weeks of training, working near a 10-repetition threshold seems to improve overall performance most effectively. We live in a dynamic world in which muscular strength and endurance are both required to lead an enjoyable life. Working around 10 RM produces good results in terms of strength, endurance, and hypertrophy. To maximize training development, advanced participants are encouraged to cycle between 1 and 12 RM.

Sets

In strength training, a **set** is the number of repetitions performed for a given exercise. For example, a person lifting 120 pounds eight times has performed one set of eight repetitions ($1 \times 8 \times 120$). For general fitness, the recommendation is two to four sets per exercise (ad-

vanced participants often train with up to six sets per exercise).

When performing multiple sets using the RM zone with the same resistance, if the person truly performs 12 RM to muscle fatigue (or close to it), in subsequent sets fewer RM will be performed (perhaps 10, 9, and 7 RM). Because of the characteristics of muscle fiber, the number of sets the exerciser can do is limited. As the number of sets increases, so does the amount of muscle fatigue and subsequent recovery time.

When time is a factor, and although multiple-set training is most beneficial, single-set programs are still effective, as long as the single set is performed within the RM zone to muscular fatigue. You may also choose to do two sets for multi-joint exercises (bench press, leg press, lat pull-down) and a single RM-zone set for single-joint exercises (arm curl, triceps extension, knee extension).

A recommended program for beginners in their first year of training is one or two light warm-up sets per exercise, using about 50 percent of the 1 RM (no warm-up sets are necessary for subsequent exercises that use the same muscle group), followed by one to four sets to near fatigue per exercise. Maintaining a resistance and effort that will temporarily fatigue the muscle (volitional exhaustion) from the number of repetitions selected in at least one of the sets is crucial to achieve optimal progress. Because of the lower resistances used in body building, four to eight sets can be done for each exercise.

To avoid muscle soreness and stiffness, new participants ought to build up gradually to the three to four sets of maximal repetitions. They can do this by performing only one set of each exercise with a lighter resistance on the first day of training, two sets of each exercise on the second day—the first light and the second with the required resistance to volitional exhaustion. If you choose to do so, you can increase to three sets on the third day—one light and two heavy. After that, a person should be able to perform anywhere from two to four sets as planned.

The time necessary to recover between sets depends mainly on the resistance used during each set. In strength training, the energy to lift heavy weights is derived primarily from the system involving adenosine triphosphate (ATP) and creatine phosphate (CP) or phosphagen (see Chapter 3, "Energy (ATP) Production," pages 107–108). Ten seconds of maximal exercise nearly depletes the CP stores in the exercised muscle(s). These stores are replenished in about 3 to 5 minutes of recovery.

***

Key Terms

Resistance Amount of weight lifted.

Progressive resistance training A gradual increase of resistance over a period of time.

Set A fixed number of repetitions; one set of bench press might be 10 repetitions.

Based on this principle, rest intervals between sets vary in length depending on the program goals and are dictated by the amount of resistance used in training. Short rest intervals of less than 2 minutes are commonly used when one is trying to develop local muscular endurance. Moderate rest intervals of 2 to 4 minutes are used for strength development. Long intervals of more than 4 minutes are used when one is training for power development.[12] Using these guidelines, individuals training for health fitness purposes might allow 2 minutes of rest between sets. Body builders, who use lower resistances, should rest no more than 1 minute to maximize the "pumping" effect.

For individuals who are trying to maximize strength gains, the exercise program will be more time-effective if two or three exercises are alternated that require different muscle groups, called **circuit training**. In this way, an individual will not have to wait 2 to 3 minutes before proceeding to a new set on a different exercise. For example, the bench press, leg extension, and abdominal curl-up exercises may be combined so that the person can go almost directly from one exercise set to the next.

Men and women alike should observe the guidelines given previously. Many women do not follow them. They erroneously believe that training with low resistances and many repetitions is best to enhance body composition and maximize energy expenditure. Unless a person is seeking to increase muscular endurance for a specific sport-related activity, the use of low resistances and high repetitions is not recommended to achieve optimal strength-fitness goals and maximize long-term energy expenditure.

Frequency

In the early stages of training, strength training should be done through a total body workout two to three times a week. Training can be performed more frequently if using a split-body routine, that is, upper body one day and lower body the next. After a maximum strength workout, the trained muscles should be rested at least 2 days (about 48 hours) to allow adequate recovery. If not completely recovered in 2 to 3 days, the person most likely is overtraining and therefore not reaping the full benefits of the program. In that case, the person should do fewer sets of exercises than in the previous workout. A summary of strength-training guidelines for health fitness purposes is provided in Figure 7.5.

To achieve significant strength gains, a minimum of 8 weeks of consecutive training is necessary. After an individual has achieved a recommended strength level, from a health fitness standpoint, one to two training session per week will be sufficient to maintain it. Highly trained athletes have to train twice a week to maintain their strength levels.

Frequency of strength training for body builders varies from person to person. Because they use moderate resistance, daily or even two-a-day workouts are common.

| Figure 7.5 | Strength-training guidelines. |

Mode: Select 8 to 10 dynamic strength-training exercises that involve the body's major muscle groups and include opposing muscle groups (chest and upper back, abdomen and lower back, front and back of the legs).

Resistance: Sufficient resistance to perform 8 to 12 repetitions maximum for muscular strength and 15 to 25 repetitions to near fatigue for muscular edurance. Older adults and injury prone individuals should use 10 to 15 repetitions with moderate resistance (50% to 60% of their 1 RM).

Sets: 2 to 4 sets per exercise with 2 to 3 minutes recovery between sets for optimal strength development. Less than 2 minutes per set if exercises are alternated that require different muscle groups (chest and upper back) or between muscular endurance sets.

Frequency: 2 to 3 days per week on nonconsecutive days. More frequent training can be done if different muscle groups are exercised on different days. (Allow at least 48 hours between strength-training sessions of the same muscle group.)

SOURCE: Adapted from American College of Sports Medicine, *ACSM's Guidelines for Exercise Testing and Prescription* (Philadelphia: Wolters Kluwer/Lippincott Williams & Wilkins, 2010).

The frequency depends on the amount of resistance, number of sets performed per session, and the person's ability to recover from the previous exercise bout (see Table 7.5). The latter often is dictated by level of conditioning.

Exercise Variations

Multiple-joint and single-joint exercises are used in strength training. Multiple-joint exercises, such as the squat, bench press, and lat pull down, require more skill and complex neural responses. Multiple-joint exercises allow you to lift more weight and develop more strength.

Table 7.5	Guidelines for Various Strength-Training Programs			
Strength-Training Program	Resistance	Sets	Rest Between Sets*	Frequency (workouts per week)**
General fitness	8–12 reps max	2–4	2–3 min	2–3
Muscular endurance	15–25 reps	2–4	1–2 min	2–3
Maximal strength	1–6 reps max	2–5	3 min	2–3
Body building	8–20 reps near max	3–8	up to 1 min	4–12

*Recovery between sets can be decreased by alternating exercises that use different muscle groups.

**Weekly training sessions can be increased by using a split-body routine.

© Cengage Learning 2013

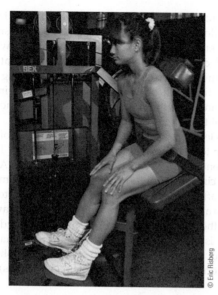

From a health-fitness standpoint, one to two strength-training sessions per week are sufficient to maintain strength.

Single-joint exercises, such as the arm curl or knee extension, are used to target specific muscles for further development. Both are recommended for a comprehensive training program.

Many strength-training exercises can be performed bilaterally and unilaterally. Muscle activation differs between the two modes. Unilateral training can enhance selected sport skills, such as single-leg jumping, high jumping, and single-arm throwing. Unilateral training is also used extensively in rehab programs. For example, bilateral concentric knee extension followed by unilateral eccentric knee flexion is strongly recommended for individuals with weak knees and to prevent potential knee problems (see Exercise 28B). Both modes of training are recommended to maximize strength gains.

Plyometrics

Strength, speed, and explosiveness are all crucial for success in athletics. All three of these factors are enhanced with a progressive resistance-training program, but greater increases in speed and explosiveness are thought to be possible with **plyometric exercise**. The objective is to generate the greatest amount of force in the shortest time. A solid strength base is necessary before attempting plyometric exercises.

Plyometric training is popular in sports that require powerful movements, such as basketball, volleyball, sprinting, jumping, and gymnastics. A typical plyometric exercise involves jumping off and back onto a box, attempting to rebound as quickly as possible on each jump. Box heights are increased progressively from about 12 to 22 inches.

The bounding action attempts to take advantage of the stretch-recoil and stretch reflex characteristics of muscle. The rapid stretch applied to the muscle during contact with the ground is thought to augment muscle contraction, leading to more explosiveness. Plyometrics can be used, too, for strengthening upper body muscles. An example is doing push-ups so the extension of the arms is forceful enough to drive the hands (and body) completely off the floor during each repetition.

A drawback of plyometric training is its higher risk for injuries compared with conventional modes of progressive resistance training. For instance, the potential for injury in rebound exercise escalates with the increase in box height or the number of repetitions.

Strength Gains

A common question by many strength-training participants is: How quickly can strength gains be observed? Strength-training studies have revealed that most of the strength gains are seen in the first 8 weeks of training. The amount of improvement, however, is related to previous training status. Increases of 40 percent are seen in individuals with no previous strength-training experience, 16 percent in previously strength-trained people, and 10 percent in advanced individuals.[13] Adhering to a periodized strength-training program can yield further improvements (see "Periodization," Chapter 9).

Critical Thinking

Your roommate started a strength-training program last year and has seen good results. He is now strength training on a nearly daily basis and taking performance-enhancing supplements hoping to accelerate results. What are your feelings about his program? • What would you say (and not say) to him?

Strength-Training Exercises

The strength-training programs introduced on pages 254–270 provide a complete body workout. The major muscles of the human body referred to in the exercises are pointed out in Figure 7.6 and with the exercises themselves at the end of the chapter.

Key Terms

Circuit training Alternating exercises by performing them in a sequence of three to six or more.

Plyometric exercise Explosive jump training, incorporating speed and strength training to enhance explosiveness.

Only a minimum of equipment is required for the first program, Strength-Training Exercises without Weights (Exercises 1 through 14). You can conduct this program in your own home. Your body weight is used as the primary resistance for most exercises. A few exercises call for a friend's help or some basic implements from around your house to provide greater resistance.

Strength-Training Exercises with Weights (Exercises 15 through 37) require machines as shown in the accompanying photographs. These exercises can be conducted on either fixed-resistance or variable-resistance equipment. Many of these exercises also can be performed with free weights. The first 13 of these exercises (15 to 27) are recommended to get a complete workout. You can do these exercises as circuit training. If time is a factor, as a minimum perform the first nine (15 through 23) exercises. Exercises 28 to 37 are supplemental or can replace some of the basic 13 (e.g., substitute Exercise 29 or 30 for 15; 31 for 16; 33 for 19; 34 for 24; 35 for 26; 32 for 27). Exercises 38 to 46 are stability ball exercises that can be used to complement your workout. Some of these exercises can also take the place of others that you use to strengthen similar muscle groups.

Selecting different exercises for a given muscle group is recommended between training sessions (e.g., chest press for bench press). No evidence indicates that a given exercise is best for a given muscle group. Changing exercises works the specific muscle group through a different range of motion and may change the difficulty of the exercise. Alternating exercises is also beneficial to avoid the monotony of repeating the same training program each training session.

Dietary Guidelines for Strength Development

Individuals who wish to enhance muscle growth and strength during periods of intense strength training should increase protein intake from .8 gram per kilogram of body weight per day to about 1.5 grams per kilogram of body weight per day. An additional 500 daily calories are also recommended to optimize muscle mass gain. If protein intake is already at 1.5 grams per kilogram of body weight, the additional 500 calories should come primarily from complex carbohydrates to provide extra nutrients to the body and glucose for the working muscles.

The time of day when carbohydrates and protein are consumed in relation to the strength-training workout also plays a role in promoting muscle growth. Studies suggest that consuming a pre-exercise snack consisting of a combination of carbohydrates and protein is beneficial to muscle development. The carbohydrates supply energy for training, and the availability of amino acids (the building blocks of protein) in the blood during training enhances muscle building. A peanut butter, turkey, or tuna sandwich, milk or yogurt and fruit, or nuts and fruit consumed 30 to 60 minutes before training are excellent choices for a pre-workout snack.

Consuming a carbohydrate/protein snack immediately following strength training and a second snack an hour thereafter further promotes muscle growth and strength development. Post-exercise carbohydrates help restore muscle glycogen depleted during training and, in combination with protein, induce an increase in blood insulin and growth hormone levels. These hormones are essential to the muscle-building process.

Muscle fibers also absorb a greater amount of amino acids up to 48 hours following strength training. The first hour, nonetheless, seems to be the most critical. A higher level of circulating amino acids in the bloodstream immediately after training is believed to increase protein synthesis to a greater extent than amino acids made available later in the day. A ratio of 4 to 1 grams of carbohydrates to protein is recommended for a post-exercise snack—for example, a snack containing 40 grams of carbohydrates (160 calories) and 10 grams of protein (40 calories).

Core Strength Training

The trunk (spine) and pelvis are referred to as the "core" of the body. Core muscles include the abdominal muscles (rectus, transversus, and internal and external obliques), hip muscles (front and back), and spinal muscles (lower and upper back muscles). These muscle groups are responsible for maintaining the stability of the spine and pelvis.

Many of the major muscle groups of the legs, shoulders, and arms attach to the core. A strong core allows a person to perform activities of daily living with greater ease, improve sports performance through a more effective energy transfer from large to small body parts, and decrease the incidence of low back pain. **Core strength training** also contributes to better posture and balance.

Interest in core strength training programs has increased. A major objective of core training is to exercise the abdominal and lower back muscles in unison. Furthermore, individuals should spend as much time training the back muscles as they do the abdominal muscles. Besides enhancing stability, core training improves dynamic balance, which is often required during physical activity and participation in sports.

Key core training exercises include the abdominal crunch and bent-leg curl-up, reverse crunch, pelvic tilt, lateral bridge, prone bridge, leg press, seated back, lat pull-down, back extension, lateral trunk flexion, supine bridge, and pelvic clock (Exercises 4, 11, 12, 13, 14, 16, 20, 24, 36, and 37 in this chapter and Exercises 26 and 27 in Chapter 8, respectively). Stability ball exercises 38 through 46 are also used to strengthen the core.

When core training is used in athletic conditioning programs, athletes attempt to mimic the dynamic skills they use in their sport. To do so, they use special equipment such as balance boards, stability balls, and foam pads. Using this equipment allows the athletes to train the core while seeking balance and stability in a sport-specific manner.

Figure 7.6 Major muscles of the human body.

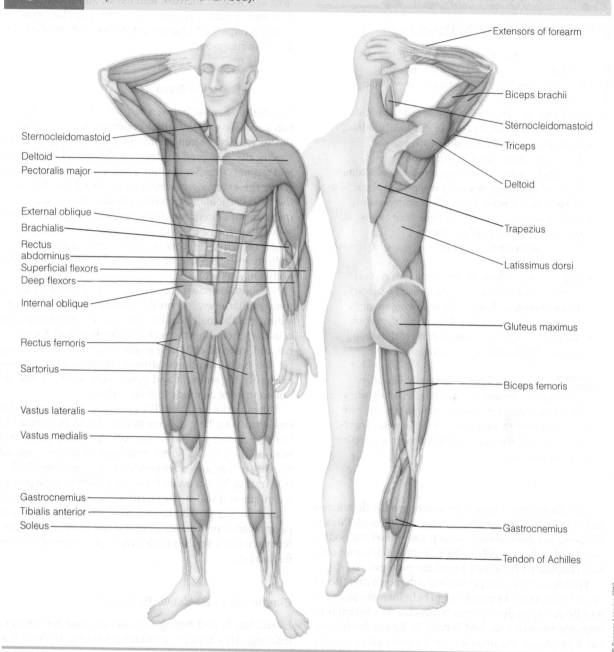

Extensors of forearm

Biceps brachii

Sternocleidomastoid

Triceps

Deltoid

Trapezius

Latissimus dorsi

Gluteus maximus

Biceps femoris

Gastrocnemius

Tendon of Achilles

Sternocleidomastoid

Deltoid

Pectoralis major

External oblique

Brachialis

Rectus abdominus

Superficial flexors

Deep flexors

Internal oblique

Rectus femoris

Sartorius

Vastus lateralis

Vastus medialis

Gastrocnemius

Tibialis anterior

Soleus

© Cengage Learning 2013

Pilates Exercise System

Pilates exercises have become increasingly popular in recent years. Previously, Pilates training was used primarily by dancers, but now this exercise modality is embraced by a large number of fitness participants, rehab patients, models, actors, and even professional athletes. Pilates studios, college courses, and classes at health clubs are available nationwide.

Key Terms

Core strength training A program designed to strengthen the abdominal, hip, and spinal muscles (the core of the body).

Pilates A training program that uses exercises designed to help strengthen the body's core by developing pelvic stability and abdominal control; exercises are coupled with focused breathing patterns.

Behavior Modification Planning

Healthy Strength Training

- Make a progressive resistance strength-training program a priority in your weekly schedule.
- Strength train at least once a week; even better, twice a week.
- Find a facility where you feel comfortable training and where you can get good professional guidance.
- Learn the proper technique for each exercise.
- Train with a friend or group of friends.
- Consume a pre-exercise snack consisting of a combination of carbohydrates and some protein about 30 to 60 minutes before each strength-training session.
- Use a minimum of 8 to 10 exercises that involve all major muscle groups of your body.
- Perform at least one set of each exercise to near muscular fatigue.
- To enhance protein synthesis, consume one post-exercise snack with a 4-to-1 gram ratio of carbohydrates to protein immediately following strength training; and a second snack one hour thereafter.
- Allow at least 48 hours between strength-training sessions that involve the same muscle groups.

Try It   Attend the school's fitness or recreation center and have an instructor or fitness trainer help you design a progressive resistance strength-training program. Train twice a week for the next 4 weeks. Thereafter, evaluate the results and write down your feelings about the program.

The Pilates training system was originally developed in the 1920s by German physical therapist Joseph Pilates. He designed the exercises to help strengthen the body's core by developing pelvic stability and abdominal control, coupled with focused breathing patterns.

Pilates exercises are performed either on a mat (floor) or with specialized equipment to help increase strength and flexibility of deep postural muscles. The intent is to improve muscle tone and length (a limber body), instead of increasing muscle size (hypertrophy). Pilates mat classes focus on body stability and proper body mechanics. The exercises are performed in a slow, controlled, precise manner. When performed properly, these exercises require intense concentration. Initially, Pilates training should be conducted under the supervision of certified instructors with extensive Pilates teaching experience.

Fitness goals of Pilates programs include better flexibility, muscle tone, posture, spinal support, body balance, low back health, sports performance, and mind–body awareness. Individuals with loose or unstable joints benefit from Pilates because the exercises are designed to enhance joint stability. The Pilates program is also used to help lose weight, increase lean tissue, and manage stress. Although Pilates programs are quite popular, more research is required to corroborate the benefits attributed to this training system.

Stability Exercise Balls

A stability exercise ball is a large flexible and inflatable ball used for exercises that combines the principles of Pilates with core strength training. Stability exercises are specifically designed to develop abdominal, hip, chest, and spinal muscles by addressing core stabilization while the exerciser maintains a balanced position over the ball. Particular emphasis is placed on correct movement and maintenance of proper body alignment to involve as much of the core as possible. Although the primary objective is core strength and stability, many stability exercises can be performed to strengthen other body areas as well.

Stability exercises are thought to be more effective than similar exercises on the ground. For instance, just sitting on the ball requires the use of stabilizing core muscles (including the rectus abdominis and the external and internal obliques) to keep the body from falling off the ball. Traditional strength-training exercises are primarily for strength and power development and do not contribute as much to body balance.

When performing stability exercises, choose a ball size based on your height. Your thighs should be parallel to the floor when you sit on the ball. A slightly larger ball may be used if you suffer from back problems. Several stability ball exercises are provided on pages 268–270. For best results, have a trained specialist teach you the proper technique and watch your form while you learn the exercises. Individuals who have a weak muscular system or poor balance or who are over the age of 65 should perform stability exercises under the supervision of a qualified trainer.

Elastic-Band Resistive Exercise

Elastic bands and tubing can also be used for strength training. This type of constant-resistance training has increased in popularity and can be used to supplement traditional strength training as it has shown to help increase strength, mobility, functional ability (particularly in older adults), and to aid in the rehab of many types of injuries. Some of the advantages to using this type of training include low cost, versatility (you can create resistance in almost all angles and directions of the range of motion), use of a large number of exercises to work all joints of the body, and they provide a great way to work out while traveling (exercise bands can be easily packed in a suitcase). This type of resistance training can also add variety to your routine workout.

Figure 7.7   Sample elastic-band resistive exercises.

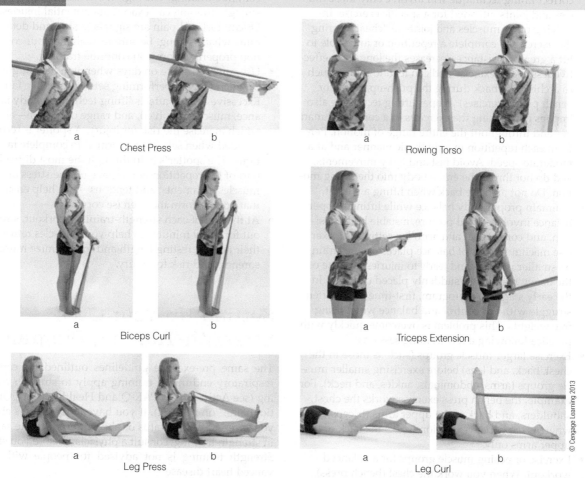

Chest Press

Rowing Torso

Biceps Curl

Triceps Extension

Leg Press

Leg Curl

© Cengage Learning 2013

Elastic-band resistive exercise workouts can be just as challenging as with free weights or machines. Due to the constant resistance provided by the bands or tubing, the training may appear more difficult to some individuals because the resistance is used both during the eccentric and concentric phases of the repetition. Additionally, the bands can be used by beginners and strength-trained individuals. That is because several different tension cords (up to eight bands) are available and all participants can progress through various resistance levels.

At the beginning, it may be a little confusing trying to determine how to use the bands and create the proper loops to grip the bands. The assistance of a training video, an instructor, or a personal trainer is helpful. The bands can be wrapped around a post, a door knob, or you can stand on them as well for some of the exercises. A few sample exercises with elastic-band resistive exercises are provided in Figure 7.7. Instructional booklets are available for purchase with your elastic band or tubing.

Exercise Safety Guidelines

As you prepare to design your strength-training program, keep the following guidelines in mind:

- Select exercises that will involve all major muscle groups: chest, shoulders, back, legs, arms, hip, and trunk.
- Select exercises that will strengthen the core. Use controlled movements and start with light-to-moderate resistances. (Later, athletes may use explosive movements with heavier resistances.)
- Never lift weights alone. Always have someone work out with you in case you need a spotter or help with an injury. When you use free weights, one to two spotters are recommended for certain exercises (e.g., bench press, squats, and overhead press).
- Prior to lifting weights, warm up properly by performing a light- to moderate-intensity aerobic activity (5 to 7 minutes) and some gentle stretches for a few minutes.

- Use proper lifting technique for each exercise. The correct lifting technique will involve only those muscles and joints intended for a specific exercise. Involving other muscles and joints to "cheat" during the exercise to complete a repetition or to be able to lift a greater resistance decreases the long-term effectiveness of the exercise and can lead to injury (such as arching the back during the push-up, squat, or bench press exercises). Proper lifting technique also implies performing the exercises in a controlled manner and throughout the entire range of motion. Perform each repetition in a rhythmic manner and at a moderate speed. Avoid fast and jerky movements, and do not throw the entire body into the lifting motion. Do not arch the back when lifting a weight.
- Maintain proper body balance while lifting. Proper balance involves good posture, a stable body position, and correct seat and arm/leg settings on exercise machines. Loss of balance places undue strain on smaller muscles and leads to injuries because of the heavy resistances suddenly placed on them. In the early stages of a program, first-time lifters often struggle with bar control and balance when using free weights. This problem is overcome quickly with practice following a few training sessions.
- Exercise larger muscle groups (such as those in the chest, back, and legs) before exercising smaller muscle groups (arms, abdominals, ankles, and neck). For example, the bench press exercise works the chest, shoulders, and back of the upper arms (triceps), whereas the triceps extension works the back of the upper arms only.
- Exercise opposing muscle groups for a balanced workout. When you work the chest (bench press), also work the back (rowing torso). If you work the biceps (arm curl), also work the triceps (triceps extension).
- Breathe naturally. Inhale during the eccentric phase (bringing the weight down), and exhale during the concentric phase (lifting or pushing the weight up). Practice proper breathing with lighter weights when you are learning a new exercise.
- Avoid holding your breath while straining to lift a weight. Holding your breath increases the pressure inside the chest and abdominal cavity greatly, making it nearly impossible for the blood in the veins to return to the heart. Although rare, a sudden high intrathoracic pressure may lead to dizziness, blackout, stroke, heart attack, or hernia.
- Based on the program selected, allow adequate recovery time between sets of exercises (see Table 7.5).

- If you experience unusual discomfort or pain, discontinue training. The high tension loads used in strength training can exacerbate potential injuries. Discomfort and pain are signals to stop and determine what's wrong. Be sure to evaluate your condition properly before you continue training.
- Use common sense on days when you feel fatigued or when you are performing sets to complete fatigue. Excessive fatigue affects lifting technique, body balance, muscles involved, and range of motion—all of which increase the risk for injury. A spotter is recommended when sets are performed to complete fatigue. The spotter's help through the most difficult part of the repetition will relieve undue stress on muscles, ligaments, and tendons—and help ensure that you perform the exercise correctly.
- At the end of each strength-training workout, stretch out for a few minutes to help your muscles return to their normal resting length and to minimize muscle soreness and risk for injury.

Setting Up Your Own Strength-Training Program

The same pre-exercise guidelines outlined for cardiorespiratory endurance training apply to strength training (see Activity 1.3, "PAR-Q and Health History Questionnaire," on page 34). If you have any concerns about your present health status or ability to participate safely in strength training, consult a physician before you start. Strength training is not advised for people with advanced heart disease.

Before you proceed to write your strength-training program, you should determine your stage of change for this fitness component in Activity 7.2 at the end of the chapter. Next, if you are prepared to do so, and depending on the facilities available, you can choose one of the training programs outlined in this chapter (use Activity 7.2). Once you begin your strength-training program, you may use the form provided in Activity 7.3 to keep a record of your training sessions.

You should base the resistance, number of repetitions, and sets you use with your program on your current strength-fitness level and the amount of time that you have for your strength workout. If you are training for reasons other than general health fitness, review Table 7.5 for a summary of the guidelines.

Designing Your Strength-Training Program

Name: _____ Date: _____

Course: _____ Section: _____ Gender: _____ Age: _____

I. Stage of Change for Muscular Strength or Endurance

Using Figure 2.5 (page 61) and Table 2.3 (page 60), identify your current stage of change for participation in a muscular strength or muscular endurance program:

II. Instructions

Select one of the two strength-training exercise programs. Perform all of the recommended exercises and, with the exception of the abdominal curl-up exercises, determine the resistance required to do approximately 10 repetitions maximum. For "Strength-Training Exercises without Weights," simply indicate the total number of repetitions performed. For the abdominal crunches or curl-up exercises, perform or build up to about 20 repetitions.

1. Strength-Training Exercises without Weights

Exercise	Repetitions
Step-up	
Rowing torso	
Push-up	
Abdominal crunch or bent-leg curl-up	
Leg curl	
Modified dip	
Pull-up or arm curl	
Heel raise	
Leg abduction and adduction	
Reverse crunch	
Pelvic tilt	
Lateral bridge	
Prone bridge	

Designing Your Strength-Training Program (continued)

2. Strength-Training Exercises with Weights

Exercise	Repetitions	Resistance
Bench press, shoulder press, or chest press (select and circle one)		
Leg press or squat (select one)		
Abdominal crunch or bent-leg curl-up		N/A
Rowing torso		
Arm curl or upright rowing (select one)		
Leg curl or seated leg curl (select one)		
Seated back		
Heel raise		
Lat pull-down or bent-arm pullover (select one)		
Rotary torso		
Triceps extension or dip (select one)		
Leg extension		
Back extension		

III. Your Personalized Strength-Training Program

Once you have performed the strength-training exercises with or without weights (or both), and depending on your personal preference (strength versus endurance), design your strength-training program selecting a minimum of eight exercises. Indicate the number of sets, repetitions, and approximate resistance that you will use. Also state the days of the week, time, and facility that will be used for this program.

Strength-training days: M☐ T☐ W☐ Th☐ F☐ Sa☐ Su☐   Time of day: _____   Facility: _____

	Exercise	Sets / Reps / Resistance		Exercise	Sets / Reps / Resistance
1.			9.		
2.			10.		
3.			11.		
4.			12.		
5.			13.		
6.			14.		
7.			15.		
8.			16.		

Strength-Training Record Form

Name: _____   Date: _____   Course: _____   Section: _____   Gender: _____   Age: _____

Date										
Exercise	St/Reps/Res*	St/Reps/Res*	St/Reps/Res*	St/Reps/Res*	St/Reps/Res*	St/Reps/Res*	St/Reps/Res*	St/Reps/Res*	St/Reps/Res*	St/Reps/Res*

*St/Reps/Res = Sets, Repetitions, and Resistance (e.g., 1/6/125 = 1 set of 6 repetitions with 125 pounds)

Strength-Training Record Form (continued)

Name: _____ Date: _____ Course: _____ Section: _____ Gender: _____ Age: _____

Date											
Exercise	St/Reps/Res*	St/Reps/Res*	St/Reps/Res*	St/Reps/Res*	St/Reps/Res*	St/Reps/Res*	St/Reps/Res*	St/Reps/Res*	St/Reps/Res*	St/Reps/Res*	St/Reps/Res*

*St/Reps/Res = Sets, Repetitions, and Resistance (e.g., 1/6/125 = 1 set of 6 repetitions with 125 pounds)

Assess Your Behavior

1. Are your strength levels sufficient to perform tasks of daily living (climbing stairs, carrying a backpack, opening jars, doing housework, mowing the yard) without requiring additional assistance or feeling unusually fatigued?

2. Do you regularly participate in a strength-training program that includes all major muscle groups of the body, and do you perform at least one set of each exercise to near fatigue?

Assess Your Knowledge

Evaluate how well you understand the concepts presented in this chapter using the chapter-specific quizzing available in the online materials at www.cengagebrain.com.

1. The ability of a muscle to exert submaximal force repeatedly over time is known as
   a. muscular strength.
   b. plyometric training.
   c. muscular endurance.
   d. isokinetic training.
   e. isometric training.

2. In older adults, each additional pound of muscle tissue increases resting metabolism by
   a. 10 calories.
   b. 17 calories.
   c. 23 calories.
   d. 35 calories.
   e. 50 calories.

3. The Hand Grip Strength Test is an example of
   a. an isometric test.
   b. an isotonic test.
   c. a dynamic test.
   d. an isokinetic test.
   e. a plyometric test.

4. A 70th-percentile rank places an individual in the _____ fitness category.
   a. excellent
   b. good
   c. average
   d. fair
   e. poor

5. During an eccentric muscle contraction,
   a. the muscle shortens as it overcomes the resistance.
   b. there is little or no movement during the contraction.
   c. a joint has to move through the entire range of motion.
   d. the muscle lengthens as it contracts.
   e. the speed is kept constant throughout the range of motion.

6. The training concept stating that the demands placed on a system must be increased systematically and progressively over time to cause physiological adaptation is referred to as
   a. the overload principle.
   b. positive-resistance training.
   c. specificity of training.
   d. variable-resistance training.
   e. progressive resistance.

7. A set in strength training refers to
   a. the starting position for an exercise.
   b. the recovery time required between exercises.
   c. a given number of repetitions.
   d. the starting resistance used in an exercise.
   e. the sequence in which exercises are performed.

8. For health fitness, the recommendation of the American College of Sports Medicine is that a person should perform a maximum of between
   a. 1 and 6 reps.
   b. 4 and 10 reps.
   c. 8 and 12 reps.
   d. 10 and 25 reps.
   e. 20 and 30 reps.

9. Plyometric training frequently is used to help with performance in
   a. gymnastics.
   b. basketball.
   c. volleyball.
   d. sprinting.
   e. all of these sports.

10. The posterior deltoid, rhomboids, and trapezius muscles can be developed with the
    a. bench press.
    b. lat pull-down.
    c. rotary torso.
    d. squat.
    e. rowing torso.

Correct answers can be found at the back of the book.

EXERCISE 1 STEP-UP

Action: Step up and down using a box or chair approximately 12 to 15 inches high (a). Conduct one set using the same leg each time you step up, and then conduct a second set using the other leg. You also could alternate legs on each step-up cycle. You may increase the resistance by holding a child or an object in your arms (b). Hold the child or object close to the body to avoid increased strain in the lower back.

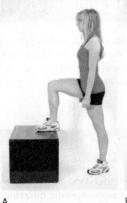
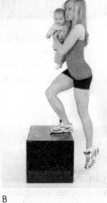

Muscles Developed: Gluteal muscles, quadriceps, gastrocnemius, and soleus

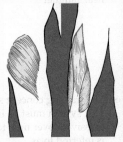
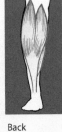

Back   Front   Back

A   B

EXERCISE 2 ROWING TORSO

Action: Raise your arms laterally (abduction) to a horizontal position and bend your elbows to 90°. Have a partner apply enough pressure on your elbows to gradually force your arms forward (horizontal flexion) while you try to resist the pressure. Next, reverse the action, horizontally forcing the arms backward as your partner applies sufficient forward pressure to create resistance.

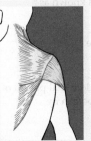
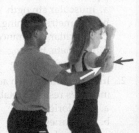

Muscles Developed: Posterior deltoid, rhomboids, and trapezius

Back

EXERCISE 3 PUSH-UP

Action: Maintaining your body as straight as possible (a), flex the elbows, lowering the body until you almost touch the floor (b), then raise yourself back up to the starting position. If you are unable to perform the push-up as indicated, decrease the resistance by supporting the lower body with the knees rather than the feet (c).

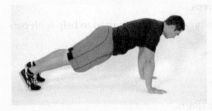
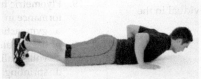
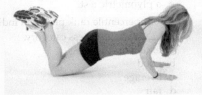

A   B   C

Muscles Developed: Triceps, deltoid, pectoralis major, abdominals, and erector spinae

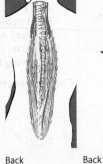
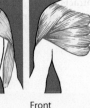
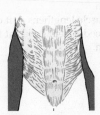

Back   Back   Front   Front

Photos © Fitness & Wellness, Inc.

© Fitness & Wellness, Inc.

Photos © Fitness & Wellness, Inc.

EXERCISE 4 ABDOMINAL CRUNCH AND BENT-LEG CURL-UP

Action: Start with your head and shoulders off the floor, arms crossed on your chest, and knees slightly bent (a). The greater the flexion of the knee, the more difficult the curl-up. Now curl up to about 30° (abdominal crunch—illustration b) or curl up all the way (abdominal curl-up—illustration c), then return to the starting position without letting the head or shoulders touch the floor or allowing the hips to come off the floor. If you allow the hips to raise off the floor and the head and shoulders to touch the floor, you most likely will "swing up" on the next crunch or curl-up, which minimizes the work of the abdominal muscles. If you cannot curl up with the arms on the chest, place the hands by the side of the hips or even help yourself up by holding on to your thighs (d and e). Do not perform the sit-up exercise with your legs completely extended, because this will strain the lower back.

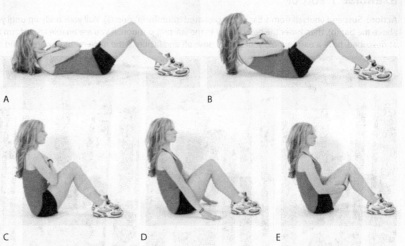

A   B

C   D   E

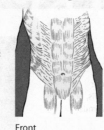

Muscles Developed: Abdominal muscles and hip flexors

Front

Note: The abdominal curl-up exercise should be used only by individuals of at least average fitness without a history of lower back problems. New participants and those with a history of lower back problems should use the abdominal crunch exercise in its place.

EXERCISE 5 LEG CURL

Action: Lie on the floor face down. Cross the right ankle over the left heel (a). Apply resistance with your right foot while you bring the left foot up to 90° at the knee joint (b). Apply enough resistance so the left foot can only be brought up slowly. Repeat the exercise, crossing the left ankle over the right heel.

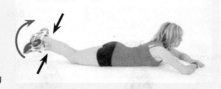

A   B

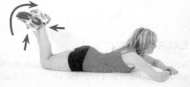

Muscles Developed: Hamstrings (and quadriceps)

Front   Back

EXERCISE 6 MODIFIED DIP

Action: Place your hands on a box or gymnasium bleacher. The feet are supported and held in place by an exercise partner (a). Dip down at least to a 90° angle at the elbow joint (b), and then return to the starting position.

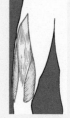

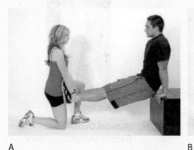

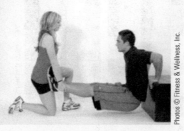

A   B

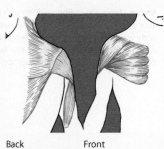

Back   Front

Muscles Developed: Triceps, deltoid, and pectoralis major

Chapter 7 Muscular Strength and Endurance   **255**

EXERCISE 7 PULL UP

Action: Suspend yourself from a bar with a pronated (thumbs-in) grip (a). Pull your body up until your chin is above the bar (b), then lower the body slowly to the starting position. If you are unable to perform the pull-up as described, have a partner hold your feet to push off and facilitate the movement upward (c and d).

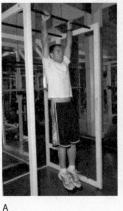 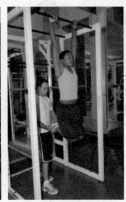 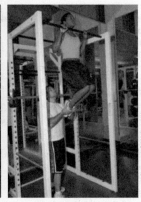

A   B   C   D

Photos © Fitness & Wellness, Inc.

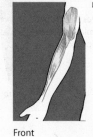 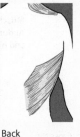

Muscles Developed:
Biceps, brachioradialis, brachialis, trapezius, and latissimus dorsi

Front   Back

EXERCISE 8 ARM CURL

Action: Using a palms-up grip, start with the arm completely extended and, with the aid of a backpack filled with books as needed (a), curl up as far as possible (b), then return to the initial position. Repeat the exercise with the other arm.

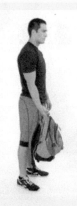 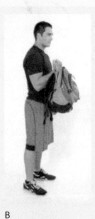

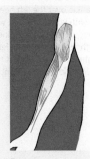

A   B

Photos © Fitness & Wellness, Inc.

Front

Muscles Developed: Biceps, brachioradialis, and brachialis

EXERCISE 9 HEEL RAISE

Action: From a standing position with feet flat on the floor or at the edge of a step (a), raise and lower your body weight by moving at the ankle joint only (b). For added resistance, have someone else hold your shoulders down as you perform the exercise.

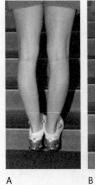 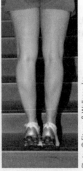

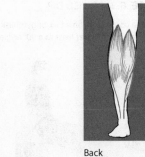

A   B

Photos © Fitness & Wellness, Inc.

Back

Muscles Developed:
Gastrocnemius and soleus

EXERCISE 10 LEG ABDUCTION AND ADDUCTION

Action: Both participants sit on the floor. The person on the left places the feet on the inside of the other person's feet. Simultaneously, the person on the left presses the legs laterally (to the outside—abduction), while the person on the right presses the legs medially (adduction). Hold the contraction for 5 to 10 seconds. Repeat the exercise at all three angles, and then reverse the pressing sequence: The person on the left places the feet on the outside and presses inward while the person on the right presses outward.

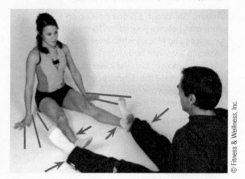

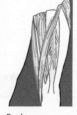

Muscles Developed: Hip abductors (rectus femoris, sartori, gluteus medius and minimus) and adductors (pectineus, gracilis, dductor magnus, adductor longus, and adductor brevis)

Back

EXERCISE 11 REVERSE CRUNCH

Action: Lie on your back with arms to the sides and knees and hips flexed at 90° (a). Now attempt to raise the pelvis off the floor by lifting vertically from the knees and lower legs (b). This is a challenging exercise that may be difficult for beginners to perform.

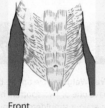

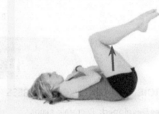

Front   A

B

Muscles Developed: Abdominals

EXERCISE 12 PELVIC TILT

Action: Lie flat on the floor with the knees bent at about a 90° angle (a). Tilt the pelvis by tightening the abdominal muscles, flattening your back against the floor, and raising the lower gluteal area ever so slightly off the floor (b). Hold the final position for several seconds.

Areas Stretched: Low back muscles and ligaments

Areas Strengthened: Abdominal and gluteal muscles

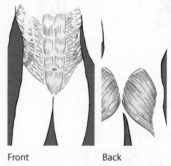

Front   Back

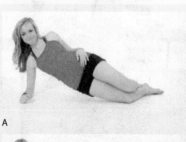

A

B

EXERCISE 13 LATERAL BRIDGE

Action: Lie on your side with legs bent (a: easier version) or straight (b: harder version) and support the upper body with your arm. Straighten your body by raising the hip off the floor and hold the position for several seconds. Repeat the exercise with the other side of the body.

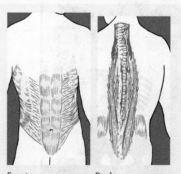

Front   Back

Muscles Developed: Abdominals (obliques and transversus abdominus) and quadratus lumborum (lower back)

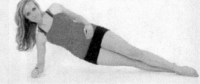

A

B

EXERCISE 14 PRONE BRIDGE

Action: Starting in a prone position on a floor mat, balance yourself on the tips of your toes and elbows while attempting to maintain a straight body from heels to shoulders (do not arch the lower back [a]). You can increase the difficulty of this exercise by placing your hands in front of you and straightening the arms (b).

Muscles Developed: Anterior and posterior muscle groups of the trunk and pelvis

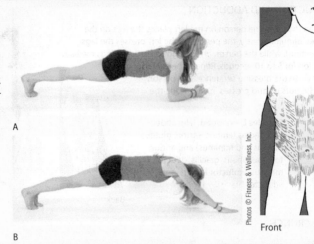

A

B

Front   Back

Photos © Fitness & Wellness, Inc.

Strength-Training Exercises with Weights

EXERCISE 15 BENCH (CHEST) PRESS

Muscles Developed: Pectoralis major, triceps, and deltoid

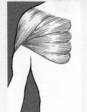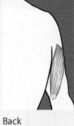

Front   Back

Free Weights: Lie on the bench with arms extended and have one or two spotters help you place the barbell directly over your shoulders (a). Lower the weight to your chest (b) and then push it back up until you achieve full extension of the arms. Do not arch the back during this exercise.

Machine: From a seated position, grasp the bar handles (a) and press forward until the arms are completely extended (b), then return to the original position. Do not arch the back during this exercise.

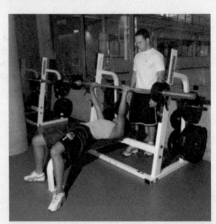

A

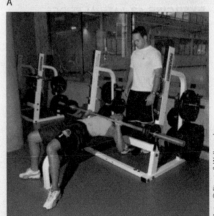

B

Photos © Fitness & Wellness, Inc.

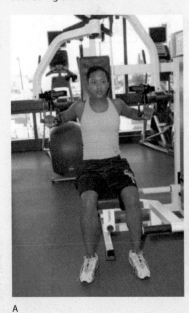

A   B

Photos © Fitness & Wellness, Inc.

EXERCISE 16 LEG PRESS

Action: From a sitting position with the knees flexed at about 100° and both feet on the footrest (a), extend the legs fully (b), then return slowly to the starting position.

Muscles Developed: Quadriceps and gluteal muscles

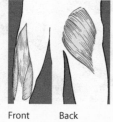

Front   Back

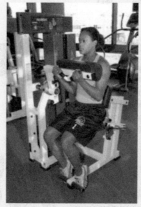

A

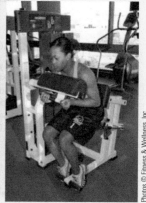

B

EXERCISE 17 ABDOMINAL CRUNCH

Action: Sit in an upright position. Grasp the handles in front of the chest pad and crunch forward. Return slowly to the original position.

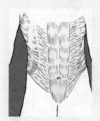

Muscles Developed: Abdominals

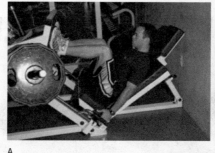

A

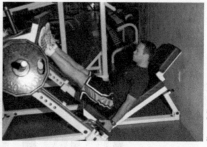

B

EXERCISE 18A ROWING TORSO

Action: Sit in the machine and grasp the handles in front of you (a). Press back as far as possible, drawing the shoulder blades together (b). Return to the original position.

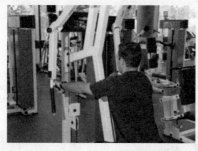

A

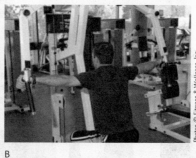

B

Back

Muscles Developed: Posterior deltoid, rhomboids, and trapezius

EXERCISE 18B BENT-OVER LATERAL RAISE

Action: Bend over with your back straight and knees bent at about 5 to 10° (a). Hold one dumbbell in each hand. Raise the dumbbells laterally to about shoulder level (b) and then slowly return them to the starting position.

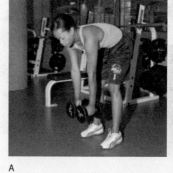

A

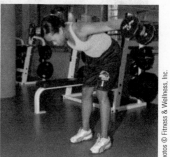

B

Chapter 7 Muscular Strength and Endurance **259**

EXERCISE 19 LEG CURL

Action: Lie with the face down on the bench, legs straight, and place the back of the feet under the padded bar (a). Curl up to at least 90° (b), and return to the original position.

Muscles Developed:
Hamstrings

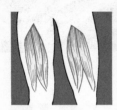

Back

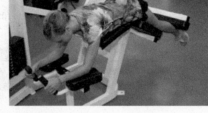

A   A

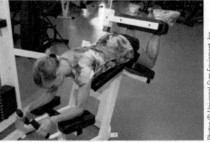

EXERCISE 20 SEATED BACK

Action: Sit in the machine with your trunk flexed and the upper back against the shoulder pad. Place the feet under the padded bar and hold on with your hands to the bars on the sides (a). Start the exercise by pressing backward, simultaneously extending the trunk and hip joints (b). Slowly return to the original position.

Muscles Developed: Erector spinae and gluteus maximus

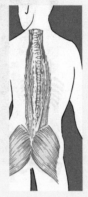

Back

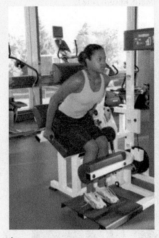

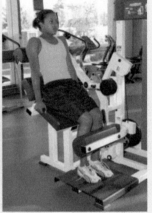

A   B

EXERCISE 21 CALF PRESS

Machine: Start with your feet flat on the plate (a). Now extend the ankles by pressing on the plate with the balls of your feet (b).

Free Weights: In a standing position, place a barbell across the shoulders and upper back. Grip the bar by the shoulders (a). Raise your heels off the floor or step box as far as possible (b) and then slowly return them to the starting position.

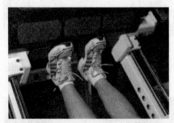

A

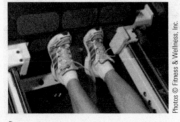

B

Back
Muscles Developed: Gastrocnemius, soleus

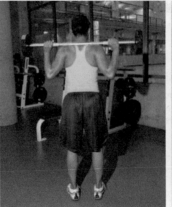

A

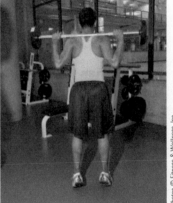

B

EXERCISE 22 LEG (HIP) ADDUCTION

Action: Adjust the pads on the inside of the thighs as far out as the desired range of motion to be accomplished during the exercise (a). Press the legs together until both pads meet at the center (b). Slowly return to the starting position.

Muscles Developed: Hip adductors (pectineus, gracilis, adductor magnus, adductor longus, and adductor brevis)

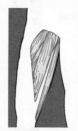

Front

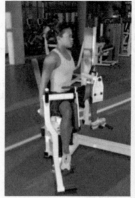

A

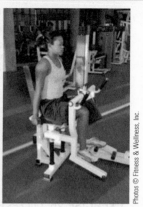

B

EXERCISE 23 LEG (HIP) ABDUCTION

Action: Place your knees together with the pads directly outside the knees (a). Press the legs laterally out as far as possible (b). Slowly return to the starting position.

Muscles Developed: Hip abductors (rectus femoris, sartori, gluteus medius, and minimus)

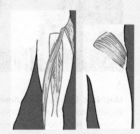

Front   Back

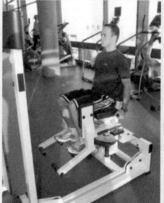

A

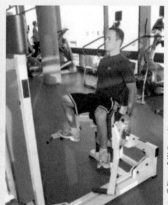

B

EXERCISE 24 LAT PULL-DOWN

Action: Starting from a sitting position, hold the exercise bar with a wide grip (a). Pull the bar down in front of you until it reaches the upper chest (b), then return to the starting position.

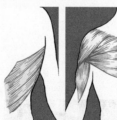

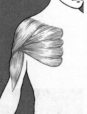

Back   Front

Muscles Developed: Latissimus dorsi, pectoralis major, and biceps

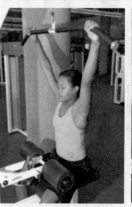

A

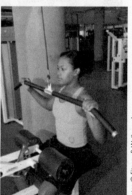

B

Photos © Fitness & Wellness, Inc.

EXERCISE 25 ROTARY TORSO

Action: Stand with your feet slightly apart. Place a barbell across your shoulders and upper back, holding on to the sides of the barbell. Now gently, and in a controlled manner, twist your torso to one side as far as possible and then do so in the opposite direction.

Muscles Developed: Internal and external obliques (abdominal muscles)

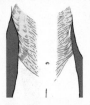

Front

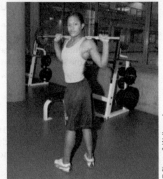

EXERCISE 26 TRICEPS EXTENSION

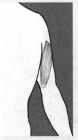

Muscles Developed: Triceps

Back

Machine: Sit in an upright position and grasp the bar behind the shoulders (a). Fully extend the arms (b) and then return to the original position.

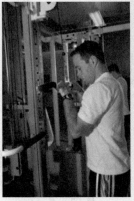

A   B

Machine: Using a palms-down grip, grasp the bar slightly closer than shoulder-width and start with the elbows almost completely bent (a). Extend the arms fully (b), then return to starting position.

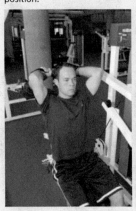

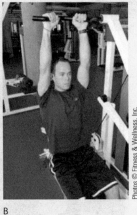

A   B

Free Weights: In a standing position, hold a barbell with both hands overhead and with the arms in full extension (a). Slowly lower the barbell behind your head (b) and then return it to the starting position.

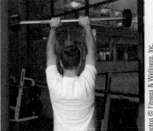

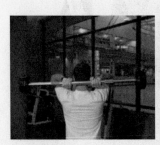

A   B

EXERCISE 27 ARM CURL

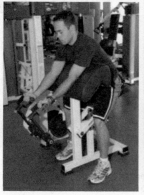

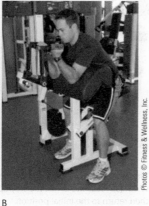

A   B

Machine: Using a supinated (palms-up) grip, start with the arms almost completely extended (a). Curl up as far as possible (b), then return to the starting position.

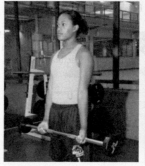

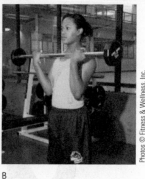

A   B

Free Weights: Standing upright, hold a barbell in front of you at about shoulder width with arms extended and the hands in a thumbs-out position (supinated grip) (a). Raise the barbell to your shoulders (b) and slowly return it to the starting position.

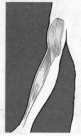

Muscles Developed: Biceps, brachioradialis, and brachialis

Front

EXERCISE 28A LEG EXTENSION

Action: Sit in an upright position with the feet under the padded bar and grasp the handles at the sides (a). Extend the legs until they are completely straight (b), then return to the starting position.

Muscles Developed: Quadriceps

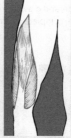

Front

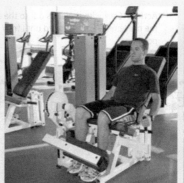

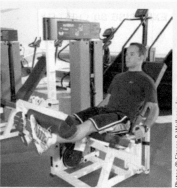

A   B

EXERCISE 28B UNILATERAL ECCENTRIC KNEE FLEXION

Action: Using a moderate resistance, raise the padded bar by extending both knees (a and b). Next, remove the left foot from the padded bar while holding the bar in place with the right leg (c). Now slowly lower the resistance (padded bar) to about 45 degrees (d). Return the left foot to the padded bar and once again press the bar up to full knee extension. Alternate legs by releasing the right foot next and lower the resistance with the left foot. Repeat the exercise about 10 times with each leg. This exercise is quite helpful to strengthen weak knees and prevent potential future knee problems.

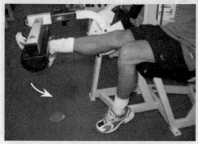

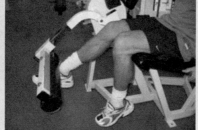

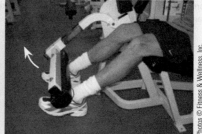

C   D   E

EXERCISE 29 SHOULDER PRESS

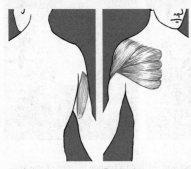

Back   Front

Muscles Developed: Triceps, deltoid, and pectoralis major

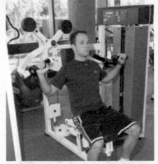 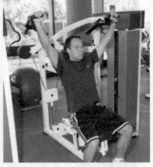

A   B

Photos © Fitness & Wellness, Inc.

Machine: Sit in an upright position and grasp the bar wider than shoulder width (a). Press the bar all the way up until the arms are fully extended (b), then return to the initial position.

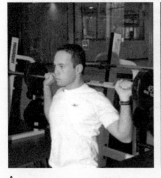

A   B

Photos © Fitness & Wellness, Inc.

Free Weights: Place a barbell on your shoulders (a) and press the weight overhead until complete extension of the arms is achieved (b). Return the weight to the original position. Be sure not to arch the back or lean back during this exercise.

EXERCISE 30 CHEST FLY

Action: Start with the arms out to the side, and grasp the handle bars with the arms straight (a). Press the movement arms forward until they are completely in front of you (b). Slowly return to the starting position.

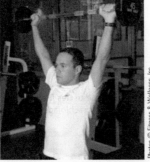

Muscles Developed: Pectoralis major and deltoid

Front

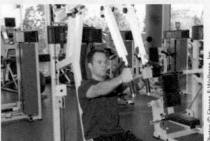

A   B

Photos © Fitness & Wellness, Inc.

BENT-ARM FLY

Action: Lie down on your back on a bench and hold a dumbbell in each hand directly overhead (a). Keeping your elbows slightly bent, lower the weights laterally to a horizontal position (b) and then bring them back up to the starting position.

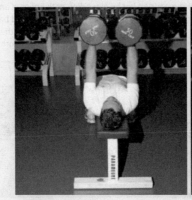 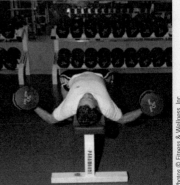

A   B

Photos © Fitness & Wellness, Inc.

EXERCISE 31 SQUAT

Machine: Place the shoulders under the pads and grasp the the handles in front of you (a). Slowly bend the knees to about 120° (b). Return to the starting position.

Muscles Developed: Quadriceps, gluteus maximus, erector spinae

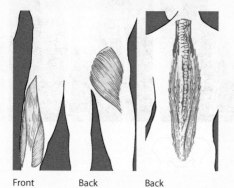

Front   Back   Back

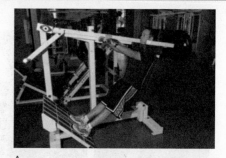

A

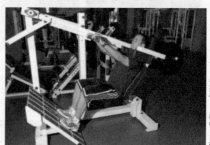

B

Free Weights: From a standing position, and with a spotter to each side, support a barbell over your shoulders and upper back (a). Keeping your head up and back straight, bend at the knees and the hips until you achieve an approximate 120° angle at the knees (b). Return to the starting position. *Do not perform this exercise alone.* If no spotters are available, use a squat rack to ensure that you will not get trapped under a heavy weight.

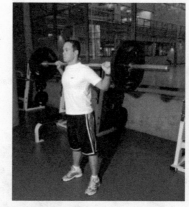

A

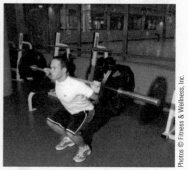

B

EXERCISE 32 UPRIGHT ROWING

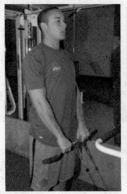

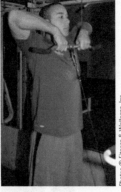

A   B

Photos © Fitness & Wellness, Inc.

Machine: Start with the arms extended and grip the handles with the palms down (a). Pull all the way up to the chin (b), then return to the starting position.

Free Weights: Hold a barbell in front of you, with the arms fully extended and hands in a thumbs-in (pronated) grip less than shoulder-width apart (a). Pull the barbell up until it reaches shoulder level (b) and then slowly return it to the starting position.

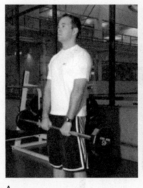

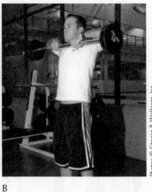

A   B

Photos © Fitness & Wellness, Inc.

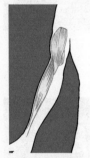

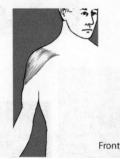

Front   Front   Back

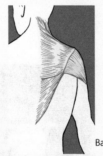

Muscles Developed: Biceps, brachioradialis, brachialis, deltoid, and trapezius

EXERCISE 33 SEATED LEG CURL

Action: Sit in the unit and place the thigh pad over the upper thighs. With legs extended, place the back of the feet over the lower-leg pad (a). Flex the knees until you reach a 90° to 100° angle (b). Slowly return to the starting position.

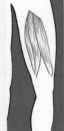

Muscles Developed: Hamstrings

Back

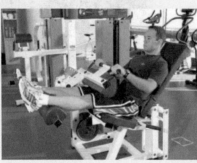

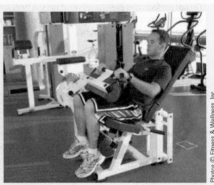

A   B

Photos © Fitness & Wellness, Inc.

EXERCISE 34 BENT-ARM PULLOVER

Action: Lie on your back on an exercise bench with your head over the edge of the bench. Hold a barbell over your chest with the hands less than shoulder-width apart (a). Keeping the elbows shoulder-width apart, lower the weight over your head until your shoulders are completely extended (b). Slowly return the weight to the starting position.

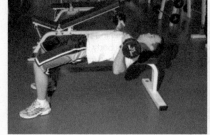

A

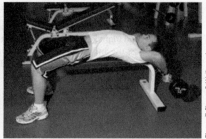

B

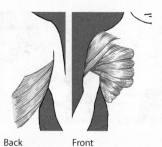

Back   Front

Muscles Developed: Latissimus dorsi, pectoral muscles, deltoid, and serratus anterior

EXERCISE 35 DIP

Action: Start with the elbows flexed (a), then extend the arms fully (b), and return slowly to the initial position.

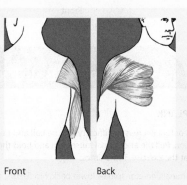

Front   Back

Muscles Developed: Triceps, deltoid, and pectoralis major

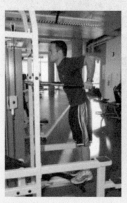

A   B

EXERCISE 36 BACK EXTENSION

Action: Place your feet under the ankle pad and the hips over the padded seat. Start with the trunk in a flexed position and the arms crossed over the chest (a). Slowly extend the trunk to a horizontal position (b), hold the extension for 2 to 5 seconds, then slowly flex (lower) the trunk to the original position.

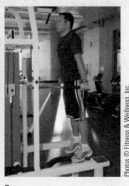

A   B

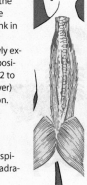

Back

Muscles Developed: Erector spinae, gluteus maximus, and quadratus lumborum (lower back)

EXERCISE 37 LATERAL TRUNK FLEXION

Action: Lie sideways on the padded seat with the right foot under the left side of the padded ankle pad (right knee slightly bent) and the left foot stabilized behind the vertical bar. Cross the arms over the abdomen or chest and start with the body in a straight line. Raise (flex) your upper body about 30 to 40° and then slowly return to the starting position.

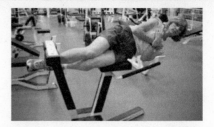

A

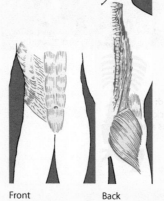

Front   Back

Muscles Developed: Erector spinae, rectus abdominus, internal and external abdominal obliques, quadratus lumborum, gluteal muscles

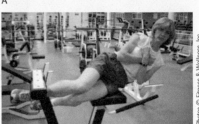

B

Photos © Fitness & Wellness, Inc.

Stability Ball Exercises

EXERCISE 38 THE PLANK

Action: Place your knees or feet (increased difficulty) on the ball and raise your body off the floor to a horizontal position. Pull the abdominal muscles in and hold the body in a straight line for 5 to 10 seconds. Repeat the exercise 3 to 5 times.

Muscles Involved: Abdominals, erector spinae, lower back, hip flexors, gluteal, quadriceps, hamstrings, chest, shoulder, and triceps

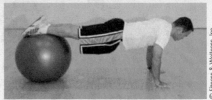

© Fitness & Wellness, Inc.

EXERCISE 39 ABDOMINAL CRUNCHES

Action: On your back and with the feet slightly separated, lie with the ball under your back and shoulder blades. Cross the arms over your chest (a). Press your lower back into the ball and crunch up 20 to 30°. Keep your neck and shoulders in line with your trunk (b). Repeat the exercise 10 to 20 times (you may also do an oblique crunch by rotating the ribcage to the opposite hip at the end of the crunch [c]).

Muscles Involved: Rectus abdominus, internal and external abdominal obliques

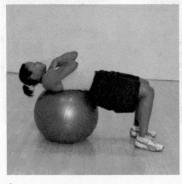

A

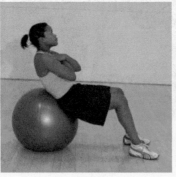

B

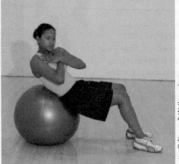

C

Photos © Fitness & Wellness, Inc.

EXERCISE 40 SUPINE BRIDGE

Action: With the feet slightly separated and knees bent, lie with your neck and upper back on the ball; hands placed on the abdomen. Gently squeeze the gluteal muscles while raising your hips off the floor until the upper legs and trunk reach a straight line. Hold this position for 5 to 10 seconds. Repeat the exercise 3 to 5 times.

Muscles Involved: Gluteal, abdominals, lower back, hip flexors, quadriceps, and hamstrings

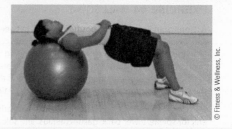

EXERCISE 41 REVERSE SUPINE BRIDGE

Action: Lie face up on the floor with the heels on the ball. Keeping the abdominal muscles tight, slowly lift the hips off the floor and squeeze the gluteal muscles until the body reaches a straight line. Hold the position for 5 to 10 seconds. Repeat the exercise 3 to 5 times.

Muscles Involved: Gluteal, abdominals, lower back, erector spinae, hip flexors, quadriceps, and hamstrings

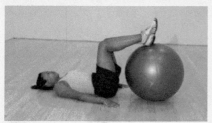

A

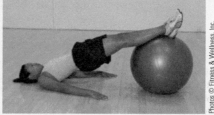

B

EXERCISE 42 PUSH-UPS

Action: Place the front of your thighs (knees or feet—more difficult) over the ball with the body straight, the arms extended, and the hands under your shoulders. Now bend the elbows and lower the upper body as far as possible. Return to the original position. Repeat the exercise 10 times.

Muscles Involved: Triceps, chest, shoulder, abdominals, erector spinae, lower back, hip flexors, quadriceps, and hamstrings

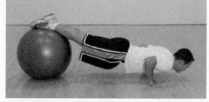

EXERCISE 43 BACK EXTENSION

Action: Lie face down with the hips over the ball. Keep the legs straight with the toes on the floor and slightly separated (a). Keep your arms to the sides and extend the trunk until the body reaches a straight position (b). Repeat the exercise 10 times.

Muscles Involved: Erector spinae, abdominals, and lower back

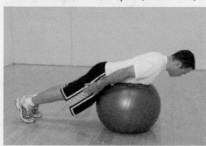

A

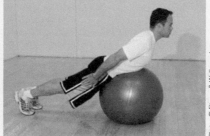

B

EXERCISE 44 WALL SQUAT

Action: Stand upright and position the ball between your lower back and a wall. Place your feet slightly in front of you, about a foot apart (a). Lean into the ball and lower your body by bending the knees until the thighs are parallel to the ground (b) (to avoid excessive strain on the knees, it is not recommended that you go beyond this point). Return to the starting position. Repeat the exercise 10 to 20 times.

Muscles Involved: Quadriceps, hip flexors, hamstrings, abdominals, erector spinae, lower back, gastrocnemius, and soleus

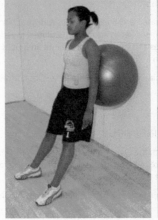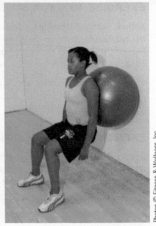

A   B

EXERCISE 45 JACKKNIVES

Action: Lie face down with the hips on the ball and walk forward with your hands until the thighs are over the ball. Keep the arms fully extended, hands on floor, and the body straight (a). Now, pull the ball forward with your legs by bending at the knees and raising your hips while keeping the abdominal muscles tight (b). Repeat the exercise 10 times.

Muscles Involved: Hip flexors, abdominals, erector spinae, lower back, quadriceps, hamstrings, chest, and shoulder

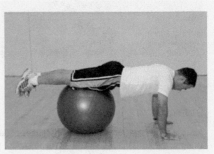

A

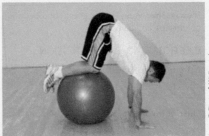

B

EXERCISE 46 HAMSTRING ROLL

Action: Lie on your back with your knees bent and the heels on the ball. Raise your hips off the floor, while keeping the knees bent (a). Tighten the abdominal muscles and roll the ball out with your feet to extend the legs (b). Now roll the ball back into the original position. Repeat the exercise 10 times.

Muscles Involved: Hamstrings, abdominals, erector spinae, lower back, hip flexors, quadriceps, and chest

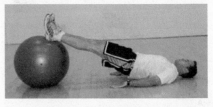

A

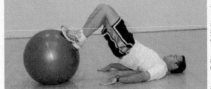

B

Muscular Flexibility

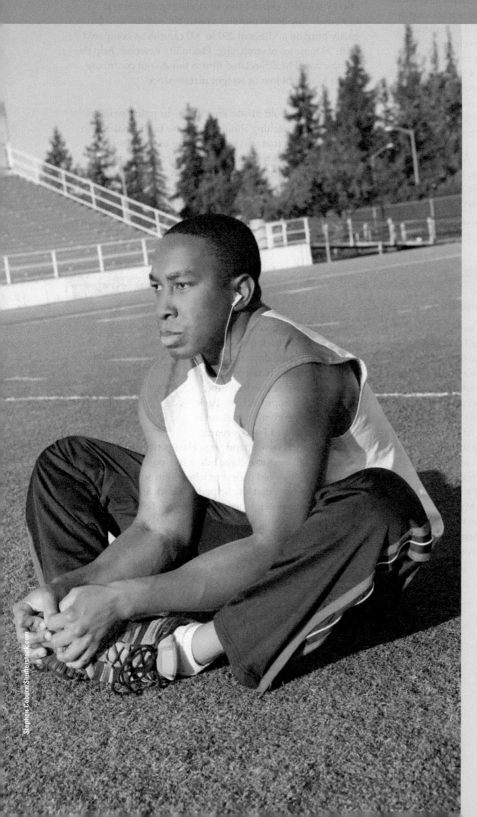

Stephen Coburn/Shutterstock.com

"Regrettably, most people neglect flexibility training, limiting freedom of movement, physical and mental relaxation, release of muscle tension and soreness, and injury prevention."

American Council on Exercise (ACE)

Objectives

▶ **Explain** the importance of muscular flexibility to adequate fitness.

▶ **Identify** the factors that affect muscular flexibility.

▶ **Explain** the health–fitness benefits of stretching.

▶ **Become** familiar with a battery of tests to assess overall body flexibility (Modified Sit-and-Reach Test, Total Body Rotation Test, Shoulder Rotation Test).

▶ **Be** able to interpret flexibility test results according to health–fitness and physical–fitness standards.

▶ **Learn** the principles that govern development of muscular flexibility.

▶ **List** some exercises that may cause injury.

▶ **Become** familiar with a program for preventing and rehabilitating low-back pain.

▶ **Create** your own personal flexibility profile.

CENGAGE**brain**.com

Visit www.cengagebrain.com to access course materials and companion resources for this text including quiz questions designed to check your understanding of the chapter contents. See the preface on page xv for more information.

Will stretching before exercise prevent injuries? The research on this subject is controversial. Some data suggest that intense stretching prior to physical activity modestly increases the risk for injuries and leads to a temporary decrease in muscle contraction velocity, strength, and power. Other studies, however, show no changes and even some improvement with intense pre-exercise stretching. The most important factor prior to vigorous exercise is to gradually increase the exercise intensity through mild calisthenics and light- to moderate-intensity aerobic exercise.

To prevent injuries while participating in activities that require flexibility, the American College of Sports Medicine recommends stretching following an appropriate warm-up phase. For activities that do not require much flexibility, you can perform the flexibility program following the aerobic and/or strength-training phase of your training.

Does strength training limit flexibility? A popular myth is that individuals with large musculature, frequently referred to as "muscle-bound," are inflexible. Data show that strength-training exercises, when performed through a full range of motion, do not limit flexibility. With few exceptions, most strength-training exercises can be performed from complete extension to complete flexion. Body builders and gymnasts, who train heavily with weights, have better than average flexibility.

Will stretching exercises help me lose weight? The energy (caloric) expenditure of stretching exercises is extremely low. In 30 minutes of aerobic exercise you can easily burn an additional 250 to 300 calories as compared with 30 minutes of stretching. Flexibility exercises help develop overall health-related fitness but do not contribute much to weight loss or weight maintenance.

How much should stretching "hurt" to gain flexibility? Proper stretching should not cause undue pain. Pain is an indication that you are stretching too aggressively. Stretching exercises should be performed to the point of "mild tension" or "limits of discomfort." It is best to decrease the degree of stretch to mild tension and hold the final position for a longer period of time (15 to 60 seconds).

Real Life Story — Gina's Experience

When I was younger, I was in ballet and we stretched all the time; so I was very flexible. After I stopped taking lessons, I also stopped stretching. I would exercise once in a while, but I wasn't interested in stretching because it doesn't burn that many calories and I was exercising just to lose weight. My second year of college, however, I was really stressed out. I was working a ton of hours, going to classes, keeping up with homework, and on top of that, I had back pain that I had to deal with. Sometimes I would be sitting and trying to do the reading for class, but my back would hurt and I could feel my heart speeding and my breathing rate accelerating really fast because I couldn't stop worrying about all the things that were going on in my life. My back pain was sometimes so bad that I considered taking medication, but I didn't really want to do that. Then my friend got me to go to a yoga class with her. I didn't think I would like it, but I

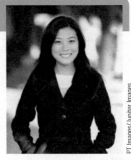

PT Images/Jupiter Images

was shocked by how much it helped me. My back pain improved that same day and after each class my body felt great and I was calm and relaxed! In time, my flexibility improved, my back pain disappeared, my usual anxiety was gone, and I was sleeping great at night. I now attend yoga classes two to three times a week. If I can't get to a class, I do a few poses in my room or even some of my old ballet stretches. I am so happy to have found something that has helped my back and also really helps calm me down when I am stressed. For me, stretching is the pain-killer and anti-anxiety medication that has no side effects!

My Personal Flexibility Health

I. Can you touch your toes without bending your knees while sitting on the floor? _____ Yes _____ No
How about the tips of your fingers behind your back with the preferred upper arm (hand) over your shoulder and the other hand coming up from behind your lower back? _____ Yes _____ No

II. The most important factor that determines range of motion about a joint is the degree of physical activity. _____ Yes _____ No

III. Vigorous stretching conducted prior to participating in athletic events that rely on force and power for peak performance enhances sports performance. _____ Yes _____ No

IV. Back pain can be reduced greatly through aerobic exercise, muscular flexibility exercise, and muscular strength and endurance training. _____ Yes _____ No

V. Have you ever experienced back pain episodes similar to Gina's and can you explain the probable cause of Gina's pain? _____ Yes _____ No

Very few people who exercise take the time to stretch, and only a few of those who stretch do so properly. When joints are not regularly moved through their entire range of motion, muscles and ligaments shorten in time, and flexibility decreases. Repetitive movement through regular/structured exercise, such as with running, cycling, or aerobics, without proper stretching also causes muscles and ligaments to tighten. Most fitness participants underestimate and overlook the contribution of good muscular flexibility to overall fitness.

Flexibility refers to the achievable range of motion at a joint or group of joints without causing injury. Some muscular/skeletal problems and injuries are thought to be related to a lack of flexibility. In daily life, we often have to make rapid or strenuous movements that we are not accustomed to making. Abruptly forcing a tight muscle beyond its achievable range of motion may lead to injury.

A decline in flexibility can cause poor posture and subsequent aches and pains that lead to limited and painful joint movement. Inordinate tightness is uncomfortable and debilitating. Approximately 80 percent of all low-back problems in the United States stem from improper alignment of the vertebral column and pelvic girdle, a direct result of inflexible and weak muscles. This backache syndrome costs U.S. industry billions of dollars each year in lost productivity, health services, and worker compensation.

Benefits of Good Flexibility

Improving and maintaining good range of motion in the joints enhances the quality of life. Good flexibility promotes healthy muscles and joints. Improving elasticity of muscles and connective tissue around joints enables greater freedom of movement and the individual's ability to participate in many types of sports and recreational activities. Adequate flexibility also makes activities of daily living such as turning, lifting, and bending much easier to perform. A person must take care, however, not to overstretch joints. Too much flexibility leads to unstable and loose joints, which may increase injury rate, including joint **subluxation** and dislocation.

Taking part in a regular **stretching** program increases circulation to the muscle(s) being stretched, prevents low-back and other spinal column problems, improves and maintains good postural alignment, promotes proper and graceful body movement, improves personal appearance and self-image, and helps to develop and maintain motor skills throughout life.

Flexibility exercises have been prescribed successfully to treat **dysmenorrhea**[1] (painful menstruation), general neuromuscular tension (stress), and knots (trigger points) in muscles and fascia. Regular stretching helps decrease the aches and pains caused by psychological stress and contributes to a decrease in anxiety, blood pressure, and breathing rate.[2] Stretching also helps relieve muscle cramps encountered at rest or during participation in exercise.

Key Terms

Flexibility The achievable range of motion at a joint or group of joints without causing injury.

Subluxation Partial dislocation of a joint.

Stretching Moving the joints beyond the accustomed range of motion.

Dysmenorrhea Painful menstruation.

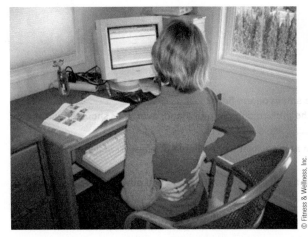

Excessive sitting and lack of physical activity lead to chronic back pain.

Mild stretching exercises in conjunction with calisthenics are helpful in warm-up routines to prepare for more vigorous aerobic or strength-training exercises, and in cool-down routines following exercise to facilitate the return to a normal resting state. Fatigued muscles tend to contract to a shorter-than-average resting length, and stretching exercises help fatigued muscles reestablish their normal resting length.

Flexibility in Older Adults

Similar to muscular strength, good range of motion is critical in older life (see "Exercise and Aging" in Chapter 9). Because of decreased flexibility, older adults lose mobility and may be unable to perform simple daily tasks such as bending forward or turning. Many older adults cannot turn their head or rotate their trunk to look over their shoulder but, rather, must step around 90° to 180° to see behind them. Adequate flexibility is also important in driving. Individuals who lose range of motion with age are unable to look over their shoulder to switch lanes or to parallel park, which increases the risk for automobile accidents.

Physical activity and exercise can be hampered severely by lack of good range of motion. Because of the pain during activity, older people who have tight hip flexors (muscles) cannot jog or walk very far. A vicious circle ensues, because the condition usually worsens with further inactivity. Lack of flexibility also may be a cause of falls and subsequent injury in older adults. A simple stretching program can alleviate

or prevent this problem and help people return to an exercise program.

Factors Affecting Flexibility

The total range of motion around a joint is highly specific and varies from one joint to another (hip, trunk, shoulder), as well as from one individual to the next. Muscular flexibility relates primarily to genetic factors. A regular stretching program helps maintain range of motion about a joint and can help improve it as well. Joint structure (shape of the bones), joint cartilage, ligaments, tendons, muscles, skin, tissue injury, and adipose tissue (fat)—all influence range of motion about a joint. Body temperature, age, and gender also affect flexibility.

The range of motion about a given joint depends mostly on the structure of that joint. Greater range of motion, however, can be attained through plastic and elastic elongation. **Plastic elongation** is the permanent lengthening of soft tissue. Even though joint capsules, ligaments, and tendons are basically nonelastic, they can undergo plastic elongation. This permanent lengthening, accompanied by increased range of motion, is best attained through proper stretching exercises.

Elastic elongation is the temporary lengthening of soft tissue. Muscle tissue has elastic properties and responds to stretching exercises by undergoing elastic or temporary lengthening. Elastic elongation increases extensibility, the ability to stretch the muscles.

Changes in muscle temperature can increase or decrease flexibility. Individuals who warm up properly have better flexibility than people who do not. Cool tem-

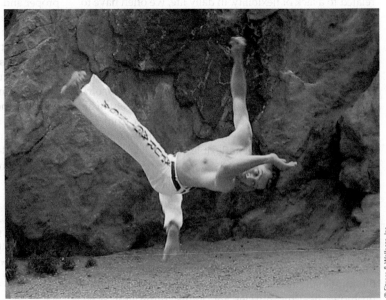

Adequate flexibility helps to develop and maintain sports skill throughout life.

| **Figure 8.1** | Procedure for the modified sit-and-reach test. |

To perform this test, you will need the Acuflex I* Sit-and-Reach Flexibility Tester, or you may simply place a yardstick on top of a box 12" high.

1. Warm up properly before the first trial.
2. Remove your shoes for the test. Sit on the floor with the hips, back, and head against a wall, the legs fully extended, and the bottom of the feet against the Acuflex I or sit-and-reach box.
3. Place the hands one on top of the other and reach forward as far as possible without letting the head and back come off the wall (the shoulders may be rounded as much as possible, but neither the head nor the back should come off the wall at this time). The technician then can slide the reach indicator on the Acuflex I (or yardstick) along the top of the box until the end of the indicator touches the participant's fingers. The indicator then must be held firmly in place throughout the rest of the test.

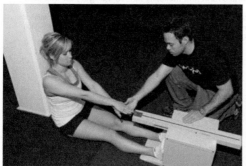

© Cengage Learning 2013

Determining the starting position for the Modified Sit-and-Reach Test.

4. Now your head and back can come off the wall. Gradually reach forward three times, the third time stretching forward as far as possible on the indicator (or yardstick) and holding the final position for at least 2 seconds. Be sure that during the test you keep the backs of the knees flat against the floor.
5. Record the final number of inches reached to the nearest half inch.

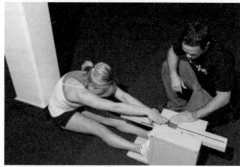

© Cengage Learning 2013

Modified Sit-and-Reach Test.

You are allowed two trials, and an average of the two scores is used as the final test score. The respective percentile ranks and fitness categories for this test are given in Tables 8.1 and 8.4.

*The Acuflex I Flexibility Tester for the Modified Sit-and-Reach Test can be obtained from Figure Finder Collection, Novel Products, P. O. Box 408, Rockton, IL 61072-0480. Phone: 800-323-5143, Fax 815-624-4866.

peratures have the opposite effect, impeding range of motion. Because of the effects of temperature on muscular flexibility, many people prefer to do their stretching exercises after the aerobic phase of their workout. Aerobic activities raise body temperature, facilitating plastic elongation.

Another factor that influences flexibility is the amount of adipose (fat) tissue in and around joints and muscle tissue. Excess adipose tissue will increase resistance to movement, and the added bulk also hampers joint mobility because of the contact between body surfaces.

On the average, women have better flexibility than men, and they seem to retain this advantage throughout life. Aging does decrease the extensibility of soft tissue, though, resulting in less flexibility in both sexes.

The most significant contributor to lower flexibility is sedentary living. With less physical activity, muscles lose their elasticity and tendons and ligaments tighten and shorten. Inactivity also tends to be accompanied by an increase in adipose tissue, which further decreases the range of motion around a joint. Finally, injury to muscle tissue and tight skin from excessive scar tissue have negative effects on range of motion.

Assessment of Flexibility

Because of the lack of practical flexibility tests, most health and fitness centers rely strictly on the Sit-and-Reach Test as an indicator of flexibility. This test measures flexibility of the hamstring muscles (back of the thigh) and, to a lesser extent, the lower back muscles.

Flexibility is joint specific. This means that a lot of flexibility in one joint does not necessarily indicate that other joints are just as flexible. Therefore, the Total Body Rotation Test and the Shoulder Rotation Test—indicators of the ability to perform everyday movements such as reaching, bending, and turning—are included to determine your flexibility profile.

The Sit-and-Reach Test has been modified from the traditional test to take length of arms and legs into consideration in determining the score (see Figure 8.1). In the original Sit-and-Reach Test, the 15-inch mark

Key Terms

Plastic elongation Permanent lengthening of soft tissue.
Elastic elongation Temporary lengthening of soft tissue.

| **Figure 8.2** | Procedure for the total body rotation test. |

An Acuflex II* Total Body Rotation Flexibility Tester or a measuring scale with a sliding panel is needed to administer this test. The Acuflex II or scale is placed on the wall at shoulder height and should be adjustable to accommodate individual differences in height. If you need to build your own scale, use two measuring tapes and glue them above and below the sliding panel centered at the 15" mark. Each tape should be at least 30" long. If no sliding panel is available, simply tape the measuring tapes onto a wall oriented in opposite directions as shown below. A line also must be drawn on the floor and centered with the 15" mark.

1. Warm up properly before beginning this test.
2. Stand with one side toward the wall, an arm's length away from the wall, with the feet straight ahead, slightly separated, and the toes touching the center line drawn on the floor. Hold out the arm away from the wall horizontally from the body, making a fist with the hand. The Acuflex II measuring scale (or tapes) should be shoulder height at this time.
3. Rotate the trunk, the extended arm going backward (always maintaining a horizontal plane) and making contact with the

panel, gradually sliding it forward as far as possible. If no panel is available, slide the fist alongside the tapes as far as possible. Hold the final position at least 2 seconds. Position the hand with the little finger side forward during the entire sliding movement. **Proper hand position is crucial. Many people attempt to open the hand, or push with extended fingers, or slide the panel with the knuckles—none of which is acceptable.** During the test the knees can be bent slightly, but **the feet cannot be moved or rotated**—they must be straight forward. The body must be kept as straight (vertical) as possible.

4. Conduct the test on either the right or the left side of the body. Perform two trials on the selected side. Record the farthest point reached, measured to the nearest half inch and held for at least 2 seconds. Use the average of the two trials as the final test score. Refer to Tables 8.2 and 8.4 to determine the percentile rank and flexibility fitness category for this test.

*The Acuflex II Flexibility Tester for the Total Body Rotation Test can be obtained from Figure Finder Collection, Novel Products, P.O. Box 408, Rockton, IL 61072-0408. Phone: 800-323-5143, Fax 815-624-4866.

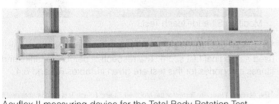

Acuflex II measuring device for the Total Body Rotation Test.

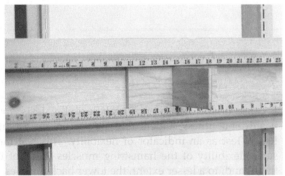

Homemade measuring device for the Total Body Rotation Test.

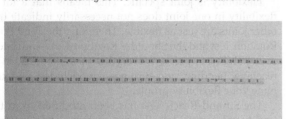

Measuring tapes for the Total Body Rotation Test.

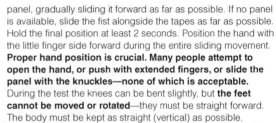

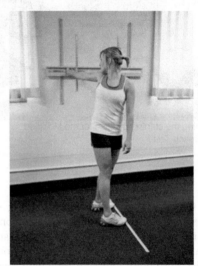

Total Body Rotation Test.

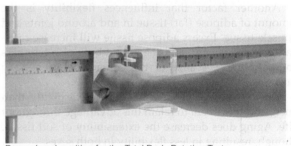

Proper hand position for the Total Body Rotation Test.

of the yardstick used to measure flexibility is always set at the edge of the box where the feet are placed. This does not take into consideration an individual with long arms and/or short legs or one with short arms and/or long legs.[3] All other factors being equal, an individual with longer arms or shorter legs, or both, receives a better rating because of the structural advantage.

The procedures and norms for the flexibility tests are described in Figures 8.1, 8.2, and 8.3 and Tables 8.1,

Figure 8.3	Procedure for the shoulder rotation test.

This test can be done using the Acuflex III* Flexibility Tester, which consists of a shoulder caliper and a measuring device for shoulder rotation. If this equipment is unavailable, you can construct your own device quite easily. The caliper can be built with three regular yardsticks. Nail and glue two of the yardsticks at one end at a 90° angle, and use the third one as the sliding end of the caliper. Construct the rotation device by placing a 60" measuring tape on an aluminum or wood stick, starting at about 6" or 7" from the end of the stick.

1. Warm up before the test.
2. Using the shoulder caliper, measure the biacromial width to the nearest fourth of an inch (use the top scale on the Acuflex III). Measure biacromial width between the lateral edges of the acromion processes of the shoulders.
3. Place the Acuflex III or homemade device behind the back and use a reverse grip (thumbs out) to hold on to the device. Place the index finger of the right hand next to the zero point of the scale or tape (lower scale on the Acuflex III) and hold it firmly in place throughout the test. Place the left hand on the other end of the measuring device wherever comfortable.

4. Standing straight up and extending both arms to full length, with elbows locked, slowly bring the measuring device over the head until it reaches about forehead level. For subsequent trials, depending on the resistance encountered when rotating the shoulders, move the left grip a half inch to one inch at a time, and repeat the task until you no longer can rotate the shoulders without undue strain or starting to bend the elbows. Always keep the right-hand grip against the zero point of the scale. Measure the last successful trial to the nearest half inch. Take this measurement at the inner edge of the left hand on the side of the little finger.
5. Determine the final score for this test by subtracting the biacromial width from the best score (shortest distance) between both hands on the rotation test. For example, if the best score is 35" and the biacromial width is 15", the final score is 20" (35 − 15 = 20). Using Tables 8.3 and 8.4, determine the percentile rank and flexibility fitness category for this test.

*The Acuflex III Flexibility Tester for the Shoulder Rotation Test can be obtained from Figure Finder Collection, Novel Products, Inc., P. O. Box 408, Rockton, IL 61072-0408. Phone: (800) 323-5143, Fax 815-624-4866.

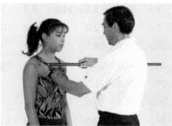

Measuring biacromial width.

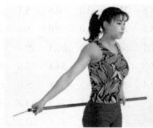

Starting position for the shoulder rotation test (note the reverse grip used for this test).

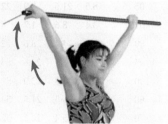

Shoulder rotation test.

© Cengage Learning 2013

Table 8.1	Percentile Ranks for the Modified Sit-and-Reach Test

Percentile Rank	Age Category—Men								Percentile Rank	Age Category—Women							
	≤18		19–35		36–49		≥50			≤18		19–35		36–49		≥50	
	in.	cm	in.	cm	in.	cm	in.	cm		in.	cm	in.	cm	in.	cm	in.	cm
99	20.8	52.8	20.1	51.1	18.9	48.0	16.2	41.1	99	22.6	57.4	21.0	53.3	19.8	50.3	17.2	43.7
95	19.6	49.8	18.9	48.0	18.2	46.2	15.8	40.1	95	19.5	49.5	19.3	49.0	19.2	48.8	15.7	39.9
90	18.2	46.2	17.2	43.7	16.1	40.9	15.0	38.1	90	18.7	47.5	17.9	45.5	17.4	44.2	15.0	38.1
80	17.8	45.2	17.0	43.2	14.6	37.1	13.3	33.8	80	17.8	45.2	16.7	42.4	16.2	41.1	14.2	36.1
70	16.0	40.6	15.8	40.1	13.9	35.3	12.3	31.2	70	16.5	41.9	16.2	41.1	15.2	38.6	13.6	34.5
60	15.2	38.6	15.0	38.1	13.4	34.0	11.5	29.2	60	16.0	40.6	15.8	40.1	14.5	36.8	12.3	31.2
50	14.5	36.8	14.4	36.6	12.6	32.0	10.2	25.9	50	15.2	38.6	14.8	37.6	13.5	34.3	11.1	28.2
40	14.0	35.6	13.5	34.3	11.6	29.5	9.7	24.6	40	14.5	36.8	14.5	36.8	12.8	32.5	10.1	25.7
30	13.4	34.0	13.0	33.0	10.8	27.4	9.3	23.6	30	13.7	34.8	13.7	34.8	12.2	31.0	9.2	23.4
20	11.8	30.0	11.6	29.5	9.9	25.1	8.8	22.4	20	12.6	32.0	12.6	32.0	11.0	27.9	8.3	21.1
10	9.5	24.1	9.2	23.4	8.3	21.1	7.8	19.8	10	11.4	29.0	10.1	25.7	9.7	24.6	7.5	19.0
05	8.4	21.3	7.9	20.1	7.0	17.8	7.2	18.3	05	9.4	23.9	8.1	20.6	8.5	21.6	3.7	9.4
01	7.2	18.3	7.0	17.8	5.1	13.0	4.0	10.2	01	6.5	16.5	2.6	6.6	2.0	5.1	1.5	3.8

▨ High physical fitness standard   ▢ Health fitness standard
© Cengage Learning 2013

Table 8.2	Percentile Ranks for the Total Body Rotation Test

		Age Category—Left Rotation								Age Category—Right Rotation							
	Percentile	**≤18**		**19–35**		**36–49**		**≥50**		**≤18**		**19–35**		**36–49**		**≥50**	
	Rank	in.	cm	in.	cm	in.	cm	in.	cm	in.	cm	in.	cm	in.	cm	in.	cm
	99	29.1	73.9	28.0	71.1	26.6	67.6	21.0	53.3	28.2	71.6	27.8	70.6	25.2	64.0	22.2	56.4
	95	26.6	67.6	24.8	63.0	24.5	62.2	20.0	50.8	25.5	64.8	25.6	65.0	23.8	60.5	20.7	52.6
	90	25.0	63.5	23.6	59.9	23.0	58.4	17.7	45.0	24.3	61.7	24.1	61.2	22.5	57.1	19.3	49.0
	80	22.0	55.9	22.0	55.9	21.2	53.8	15.5	39.4	22.7	57.7	22.3	56.6	21.0	53.3	16.3	41.4
	70	20.9	53.1	20.3	51.6	20.4	51.8	14.7	37.3	21.3	54.1	20.7	52.6	18.7	47.5	15.7	39.9
	60	19.9	50.5	19.3	49.0	18.7	47.5	13.9	35.3	19.8	50.3	19.0	48.3	17.3	43.9	14.7	37.3
Men	50	18.6	47.2	18.0	45.7	16.7	42.4	12.7	32.3	19.0	48.3	17.2	43.7	16.3	41.4	12.3	31.2
	40	17.0	43.2	16.8	42.7	15.3	38.9	11.7	29.7	17.3	43.9	16.3	41.4	14.7	37.3	11.5	29.2
	30	14.9	37.8	15.0	38.1	14.8	37.6	10.3	26.2	15.1	38.4	15.0	38.1	13.3	33.8	10.7	27.2
	20	13.8	35.1	13.3	33.8	13.7	34.8	9.5	24.1	12.9	32.8	13.3	33.8	11.2	28.4	8.7	22.1
	10	10.8	27.4	10.5	26.7	10.8	27.4	4.3	10.9	10.8	27.4	11.3	28.7	8.0	20.3	2.7	6.9
	05	8.5	21.6	8.9	22.6	8.8	22.4	0.3	0.8	8.1	20.6	8.3	21.1	5.5	14.0	0.3	0.8
	01	3.4	8.6	1.7	4.3	5.1	13.0	0.0	0.0	6.6	16.8	2.9	7.4	2.0	5.1	0.0	0.0
	99	29.3	74.4	28.6	72.6	27.1	68.8	23.0	58.4	29.6	75.2	29.4	74.7	27.1	68.8	21.7	55.1
	95	26.8	68.1	24.8	63.0	25.3	64.3	21.4	54.4	27.6	70.1	25.3	64.3	25.9	65.8	19.7	50.0
	90	25.5	64.8	23.0	58.4	23.4	59.4	20.5	52.1	25.8	65.5	23.0	58.4	21.3	54.1	19.0	48.3
	80	23.8	60.5	21.5	54.6	20.2	51.3	19.1	48.5	23.7	60.2	20.8	52.8	19.6	49.8	17.9	45.5
	70	21.8	55.4	20.5	52.1	18.6	47.2	17.3	43.9	22.0	55.9	19.3	49.0	17.3	43.9	16.8	42.7
	60	20.5	52.1	19.3	49.0	17.7	45.0	16.0	40.6	20.8	52.8	18.0	45.7	16.5	41.9	15.6	39.6
Women	50	19.5	49.5	18.0	45.7	16.4	41.7	14.8	37.6	19.5	49.5	17.3	43.9	14.6	37.1	14.0	35.6
	40	18.5	47.0	17.2	43.7	14.8	37.6	13.7	34.8	18.3	46.5	16.0	40.6	13.1	33.3	12.8	32.5
	30	17.1	43.4	15.7	39.9	13.6	34.5	10.0	25.4	16.3	41.4	15.2	38.6	11.7	29.7	8.5	21.6
	20	16.0	40.6	15.2	38.6	11.6	29.5	6.3	16.0	14.5	36.8	14.0	35.6	9.8	24.9	3.9	9.9
	10	12.8	32.5	13.6	34.5	8.5	21.6	3.0	7.6	12.4	31.5	11.1	28.2	6.1	15.5	2.2	5.6
	05	11.1	28.2	7.3	18.5	6.8	17.3	0.7	1.8	10.2	25.9	8.8	22.4	4.0	10.2	1.1	2.8
	01	8.9	22.6	5.3	13.5	4.3	10.9	0.0	0.0	8.9	22.6	3.2	8.1	2.8	7.1	0.0	0.0

☐ High physical fitness standard ☐ Health fitness standard

© Cengage Learning 2013

8.2, and 8.3. The flexibility test results in these three tables are provided in both inches and centimeters (cm). Be sure to use the proper column to read your percentile score based on your test results. For the flexibility profile, you should take all three tests. You will be able to assess your flexibility profile in Activity 8.1. Because of the specificity of flexibility, pinpointing an "ideal" level of flexibility is difficult. Nevertheless, flexibility is important to health and fitness and independent living, so an assessment will give an indication of your current level of flexibility.

Interpreting Flexibility Test Results

After obtaining your scores and fitness ratings for each test, you can determine the fitness category for each flexibility test using the guidelines given in Table 8.4. You also should look up the number of points assigned for each fitness category in this table. The overall flexibility fitness category is obtained by totaling the number of points from all three tests and using the ratings given in Table 8.5. Record your results in Activity 8.1 and Appendix A.

Table 8.3	Percentile Ranks for the Shoulder Rotation Test

Percentile Rank	Age Category—Men								Percentile Rank	Age Category—Women							
	≤18		19–35		36–49		≥50			≤18		19–35		36–49		≥50	
	in.	cm	in.	cm	in.	cm	in.	cm		in.	cm	in.	cm	in.	cm	in.	cm
99	2.2	5.6	−1.0	−2.5	18.1	46.0	21.5	54.6	99	2.6	6.6	−2.4	−6.1	11.5	29.2	13.1	33.3
95	15.2	38.6	10.4	26.4	20.4	51.8	27.0	68.6	95	8.0	20.3	6.2	15.7	15.4	39.1	16.5	41.9
90	18.5	47.0	15.5	39.4	20.8	52.8	27.9	70.9	90	10.7	27.2	9.7	24.6	16.8	42.7	20.9	53.1
80	20.7	52.6	18.4	46.7	23.3	59.2	28.5	72.4	80	14.5	36.8	14.5	36.8	19.2	48.8	22.5	57.1
70	23.0	58.4	20.5	52.1	24.7	62.7	29.4	74.7	70	16.1	40.9	17.2	43.7	21.5	54.6	24.3	61.7
60	24.2	61.5	22.9	58.2	26.6	67.6	29.9	75.9	60	19.2	48.8	18.7	47.5	23.1	58.7	25.1	63.8
50	25.4	64.5	24.4	62.0	28.0	71.1	30.5	77.5	50	21.0	53.3	20.0	50.8	23.5	59.7	26.2	66.5
40	26.3	66.8	25.7	65.3	30.0	76.2	31.0	78.7	40	22.2	56.4	21.4	54.4	24.4	62.0	28.1	71.4
30	28.2	71.6	27.3	69.3	31.9	81.0	31.7	80.5	30	23.2	58.9	24.0	61.0	25.9	65.8	29.9	75.9
20	30.0	76.2	30.1	76.5	33.3	84.6	33.1	84.1	20	25.0	63.5	25.9	65.8	29.8	75.7	31.5	80.0
10	33.5	85.1	31.8	80.8	36.1	91.7	37.2	94.5	10	27.2	69.1	29.1	73.9	31.1	79.0	33.1	84.1
05	34.7	88.1	33.5	85.1	37.8	96.0	38.7	98.3	05	28.0	71.1	31.3	79.5	33.4	84.8	34.1	86.6
01	40.8	103.6	42.6	108.2	43.0	109.2	44.1	112.0	01	32.5	82.5	37.1	94.2	34.9	88.6	35.4	89.9

▉ High physical fitness standard   ▢ Health fitness standard

© Cengage Learning 2013

Table 8.4	Flexibility Fitness Categories According to Percentile Ranks

Percentile Rank	Fitness Category	Points
≥90	Excellent	5
70–80	Good	4
50–60	Average	3
30–40	Fair	2
≤20	Poor	1

© Cengage Learning 2013

Table 8.5	Overall Flexibility Fitness Category

Total Points	Flexibility Category
≥13	Excellent
10–12	Good
7–9	Average
4–6	Fair
≤3	Poor

© Cengage Learning 2013

Principles of Muscular Flexibility Prescription

Even though genetics play a crucial role in body flexibility, the range of joint mobility can be increased and maintained through a regular stretching program. Because range of motion is highly specific to each body part (ankle, trunk, shoulder), a comprehensive stretching program should include all body parts and follow the basic guidelines for development of flexibility.

The overload and specificity of training principles (discussed in conjunction with strength development in Chapter 7) also apply to the development of muscular flexibility. To increase the total range of motion of a joint, the specific muscles surrounding that joint have to be stretched progressively beyond their accustomed length.

The principles of mode, intensity, repetitions, and frequency of exercise can also be applied to flexibility programs.

Modes of Training

There are several modes of stretching exercises and some modes are safer and more effective in terms of helping to increase flexibility:

1. Static (slow-sustained stretching)
2. Passive stretching
3. Ballistic stretching
4. Dynamic stretching
5. Controlled ballistic stretching
6. Proprioceptive neuromuscular facilitation (PNF) stretching

Static Stretching

With **static stretching** or slow-sustained stretching, muscles are lengthened gradually through a joint's complete range of motion and the final position is held for a few seconds. A slow-sustained stretch causes the muscles to relax and thereby achieve greater length. This type of stretch causes little pain and has a low risk for injury. In flexibility-development programs, slow-sustained stretching exercises are the most frequently used and recommended.

Passive Stretching

Although similar to static stretching, in **passive stretching**, the muscles are relaxed, that is, they are in a passive state; and an external force, provided by another person or apparatus, is applied to increase the range of motion.

Ballistic Stretching

Ballistic stretching requires the impetus of a moving body or body part to force a joint or group of joints beyond the normal range of motion. This type of stretching requires a fast and repetitive bouncing motion to achieve a greater degree of stretch. An example would be repeatedly bouncing down and up to touch the toes. Ballistic stretching is the least recommended form of stretching. Fitness professionals feel that it causes muscle soreness and increases the risk of injuries to muscles and nerves. Limited data, however, are available to corroborate such effects. This form of stretching should never be performed without a previous mild aerobic warm-up and only gentle bouncing actions are recommended for those who wish to use this mode of stretching.

Dynamic Stretching

Speed of movement, momentum, and active muscular effort are used in **dynamic stretching** to increase the range of motion about a joint or group of joints. Unlike ballistic stretching, it does not require bouncing motions. Exaggerating a kicking action, walking lunges, and arm circles are all examples of dynamic stretching. Research indicates that dynamic stretches are preferable to static stretches before competition because dynamic stretching does not seem to have a negative effect on the athlete's strength and power. Dynamic stretching is beneficial for athletes such as gymnasts, dancers, figure skaters, divers, hurdlers, whose sports activities require ballistic actions.

Precautions must be taken not to overstretch ligaments with ballistic and dynamic stretching. Ligaments undergo plastic or permanent elongation. If the stretching force cannot be controlled—as often occurs in fast, jerky movements—ligaments can easily be overstretched. This, in turn, leads to excessively loose joints, increasing the risk for injuries.

Controlled Ballistic Stretching

Controlled ballistic stretching, that is, exercises that are performed through slow, gentle, and controlled ballistic movements (instead of jerky, rapid, and bouncy movements) is quite effective in developing flexibility. Properly performed, this type of stretching can be done safely by most individuals.

Proprioceptive Neuromuscular Facilitation

Proprioceptive neuromuscular facilitation (PNF) stretching is based on a "contract-and-relax" method and requires the assistance of another person. The procedure is as follows:

1. The person assisting with the exercise provides initial force by pushing slowly in the direction of the desired stretch. This first stretch does not cover the entire range of motion.
2. The person being stretched then applies force in the opposite direction of the stretch, against the assistant, who tries to hold the initial degree of stretch as close as possible. This results in an isometric contraction at the angle of the stretch.
3. After 5 or 6 seconds of isometric contraction, the person being stretched relaxes the target muscle(s) completely. The assistant then increases the degree of stretch slowly to a greater angle and for the PNF technique the stretch is held for 10 to 30 seconds.
4. If a greater degree of stretch is achievable, the isometric contraction is repeated for another 5 or 6 seconds, after which the degree of stretch is slowly increased again and held for 10 to 30 seconds.

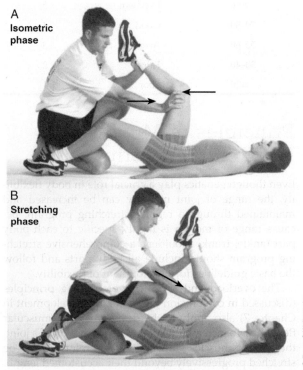

A
Isometric phase

B
Stretching phase

Proprioceptive neuromuscular facilitation (PNF) stretching technique (a) isometric phase (b) stretching phase.

If a progressive degree of stretch is used, steps 1 through 4 can be repeated up to five times. Each isometric contraction is held for about 6 seconds. The progressive stretches are held for 10 seconds, until the last trial, when the final stretched position is held for up to 30 seconds.

Theoretically, with the PNF technique, the isometric contraction helps relax the muscle being stretched, which results in lengthening the muscle. Some fitness leaders believe PNF is more effective than slow-sustained stretching. Another benefit of PNF is an increase in strength of the muscle(s) being stretched. Research has shown approximately 17 and 35 percent increases in absolute strength and muscular endurance, respectively, in the hamstring muscle group after 12 weeks of PNF stretching.[4] The results were consistent in both men and women and are attributed to the isometric contractions performed during PNF. Disadvantages of PNF are (1) more pain, (2) the need for a second person to assist, and (3) the need for more time to conduct each session.

Physiological Response to Stretching

Located within skeletal muscles are two sensory organs, also known as proprioceptors: The muscle spindle and the Golgi tendon organ. Their function is to protect muscles from injury during stretching.

Muscle spindles are located within the belly of the muscle and their primary function is to detect changes in muscle length. If overstretched or stretched too fast, the spindles send messages to the central nervous system, and through a feedback loop, motor neurons are activated and cause muscle contraction to resist muscle stretch. This mechanism is known as the stretch reflex. Muscle spindle action explains why injury rates are higher with ballistic stretching. Fast stretching speeds trigger the stretch reflex and cause muscles to contract and develop tension that can lead to injury.

Golgi tendon organs are located at the point where muscle fibers attach to the muscle tendon. When excessive force is generated by a muscle, these organs trigger a response opposite to that of the spindles; an inverse stretch reflex action that inhibits the muscle contraction and leads to muscle relaxation. The Golgi tendon organ prevents injury to the muscle by keeping it from generating too much tension while being stretched. This response explains the effectiveness of the PNF technique in increasing joint range of motion. The isometric contraction following the initial stretch triggers the inverse stretch reflex, thus lessening the tension and allowing the muscle to relax. At this point, the muscle tolerates a greater degree of stretch.

Intensity

The **intensity**, or degree of stretch, when doing flexibility exercises should be to only a point of mild discomfort or tightness at the end of the range of motion. Undue pain does not have to be part of the stretching routine.

All stretching should be done to slightly below the pain threshold. As participants reach this point, they should try to relax the muscle being stretched as much as possible. If you feel pain, the load is too high and may cause injury. After completing the stretch, the body part is brought back gradually to the starting point.

Repetitions

The time required for an exercise session for development of flexibility is based on the number of **repetitions** and the length of time each repetition is held in the final stretched position. As a general recommendation, a minimum of 15 minutes of flexibility exercise, including the major muscle/tendon units of the body, should be performed. Four or more repetitions per exercise should be done, holding the final position each time for 15 to 60 seconds.[5]

As flexibility increases, a person can gradually increase the time each repetition is held from 15 to about 60 seconds. Data indicate that stretching for 15 to 60 seconds is better to increase range of motion than stretching for shorter periods of time and is just as effective as stretching for longer durations.[6] Individuals who are susceptible to flexibility injuries should limit each stretch to 20 seconds. Pilates exercises are recommended for these individuals, as they increase joint stability (also see Chapter 7, pages 245–246).

Figure 8.4	Guidelines for flexibility development.
Mode:	Static, dynamic, or proprioceptive neuromuscular facilitation (PNF) stretching to include all major muscle/tendon groups of the body
Intensity:	To the point of mild tension or limits of discomfort
Repetitions:	Repeat each exercise 4 times, holding the final position between 15 and 30 seconds
Frequency:	At least 2 or 3 days per week
	Ideal, 5 to 7 days per week

© Cengage Learning 2013

Frequency of Exercise

Flexibility exercises should be conducted a minimum of two or three days per week, but ideally five to seven days per week. After six to eight weeks of almost daily stretching, flexibility can be maintained with two or three sessions per week, involving the major muscle/tendon groups of the body and doing four repetitions of 15 to 60 seconds for each exercise performed. Figure 8.4 summarizes the guidelines for flexibility development.

Over the years, people who lack adequate flexibility, and those who neglect stretching, can expect to see a decline in functional capacity and become more susceptible to injuries. Regular stretching increases not only range of motion by increasing muscular elongation but also by enhancing a person's level of stretch tolerance.

When to Stretch?

Many people do not differentiate a warm-up from stretching. Warming up means starting a workout slowly with walking, cycling, or slow jogging, followed by gentle stretching (not through the entire range of motion). Stretching implies movement of joints through their full range of motion and holding the final degree of stretch according to recommended guidelines.

A warm-up that progressively increases muscle temperature and mimics movement that will occur during training enhances performance. For some activities, gentle stretching is recommended in conjunction with warm-up routines. Before steady activities (walking, jogging, cycling), a warm-up of 3 to 5 minutes is recommended. The recommendation is up to 10 minutes before stop-and-go activities (e.g., racquet sports, basketball, and soccer) and athletic participation in general (e.g., football and gymnastics). Activities that require abrupt changes in direction are more likely to cause muscle strains if they are performed without proper warm-up that includes mild stretching.

Sports-specific/pre-exercise stretching can improve performance in sports that require a greater-than-average range of motion, such as gymnastics, dance, diving, and figure skating. A few studies suggest that intense stretching during warm-up can lead to a temporary short-term

(up to 60 minutes) decrease in strength and power. Thus, intense stretching conducted prior to participating in athletic events that rely on force and power for peak performance is not recommended.[7]

In terms of whether stretching before or after exercise is more effective for preventing injuries, the best time to stretch is controversial. In limited studies on athletic populations, the evidence is unclear. Additional research is necessary to clarify this issue.

In general, unless the activity requires extensive range of motion, a good time to stretch is after an aerobic workout. Higher body temperature in itself helps to increase the joint range of motion. Muscles also are fatigued following exercise, and a fatigued muscle tends to shorten, which can lead to soreness and spasms. Stretching exercises help fatigued muscles reestablish their normal resting length and prevent unnecessary pain.

Flexibility Exercises

To improve body flexibility, each major muscle group should be subjected to at least one stretching exercise. A complete set of exercises for developing muscular flexibility is presented on pages 292–294.

Although you may not be able to hold a final stretched position with some of these exercises (such as lateral head tilts and arm circles), you still should perform the exercise through the joint's full range of motion. Depending on the number and length of repetitions, a complete workout will last between 15 and 30 minutes.

Contraindicated Exercises

Most strength and flexibility exercises are relatively safe to perform, but even safe exercises can be hazardous if they are performed incorrectly. Some exercises may be safe to perform occasionally but, when executed repeatedly, may cause trauma and injury. Pre-existing muscle or joint conditions (old sprains or injuries) can further increase the risk of harm during certain exercises. As you develop your exercise program, you are encouraged to follow the exercise descriptions and guidelines given in this book.

A few exercises, however, are not recommended because of the potential high risk for injury. These exercises sometimes are done in videotaped workouts and some fitness classes. **Contraindicated exercises** may cause harm because of the excessive strain they place on muscles and joints, in particular the spine, lower back, knees, neck, or shoulders.

Illustrations of contraindicated exercises are presented in Figure 8.5. Safe alternative exercises are listed

Key Terms

Contraindicated exercises Exercises that are not recommended because they may cause injury to a person.

| Figure 8.5 | Contraindicated exercises. |

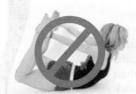
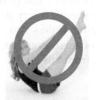
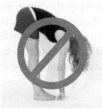

Double-Leg Lift   **Upright Double-Leg Lifts**   **V-Sits**   **Standing Toe Touch**
All three of these exercises cause excessive strain on the spine and may harm discs.
Excessive strain on the knee and lower back.
Alternatives: Strength Exercises 4 and 17, pages 255 and 259
Alternative: Flexibility Exercise 12, page 294

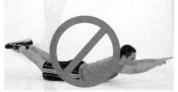
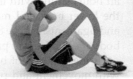
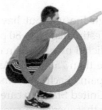
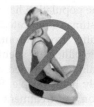

Swan Stretch
Excessive strain on the spine; may harm intervertebral discs.
Alternative: Flexibility Exercise 20, page 295

Cradle
Excessive strain on the spine, knees, and shoulders.
Alternatives: Flexibility Exercises 20 and 8, pages 295 and 293

Full Squat
Excessive strain on the knees.
Alternatives: Flexibility Exercise 8, page 293; Strength Exercises 1, 16, 28A and 28B, pages 254, 259, and 263

Head Rolls
May injure neck discs.
Alternative: Flexibility Exercise 1, page 292

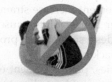

Knee to Chest
(with hands over the shin)
Excessive strain on the knee.
Alternative: Flexibility Exercises 15 and 16, page 294

Sit-Ups with Hands Behind the Head
Excessive strain on the neck.
Alternatives: Strength Exercises 4 and 17, pages 256 and 259

Yoga Plow
Excessive strain on the spine, neck, and shoulders.
Alternatives: Flexibility Exercises 12, 15, 16, 17, and 19, pages 294 and 295

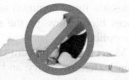
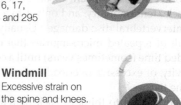

Windmill
Excessive strain on the spine and knees.
Alternatives: Flexibility Exercises 12 and 19, pages 294 and 295

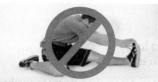
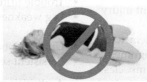
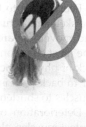

Hurdler Stretch
Excessive strain on the bent knee.
Alternatives: Flexibility Exercises 8 and 12, pages 293 and 294

The Hero
Excessive strain on the knees.
Alternatives: Flexibility Exercises 8 and 14, pages 293 and 294

Donkey Kicks
Excessive strain on the back, shoulders, and neck.
Alternatives: Flexibility Exercises 20, 14, and 1, pages 295, 294, and 292

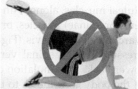

Straight-Leg Sit-Ups   **Alternating Bent-Leg Sit-Ups**
These exercises strain the lower back.
Alternatives: Strength Exercises 4 and 17, pages 256 and 259

below each contraindicated exercise and are illustrated in the exercises for strength (pages 254–258) and flexibility (pages 292–295). In isolated instances, a qualified physical therapist may select one or a few of the contraindicated exercises to treat a specific injury or disability in a carefully supervised setting. Unless you are specifically instructed to use one of these exercises, it is best that you select safe exercises from this book.

Preventing and Rehabilitating Low-Back Pain

Few people make it through life without having low-back pain at some point. An estimated 60 to 80 percent of the population has been afflicted by back pain or injury. Estimates indicate that more than 75 million Americans suffer from chronic back pain. Each year more than $86 billion are spent in the United States to care for back pain, with limited evidence that increased spending really helps people. When it comes to back pain, prevention and treatment through physical exercise are by far the best medicine.

It has been determined that backache syndrome is preventable more than 80 percent of the time, and is caused by (a) physical inactivity, (b) poor postural habits and body mechanics, (c) excessive body weight, and/or (d) psychological stress. Data also indicate that back injuries are more common among smokers because it reduces blood flow to the spine—increasing back pain susceptibility.

More than 95 percent of all back pain is related to muscle/tendon injury, and only 1 to 5 percent is related to intervertebral disc damage.[8] Usually, back pain is the result of repeated micro-injuries that occur over an extended time (sometimes years) until a certain movement, activity, or excessive overload causes a significant injury to the tissues.[9]

People tend to think of back pain as a problem with the skeleton. Actually, the spine's curvature, alignment, and movement are controlled by surrounding muscles. The most common reason for chronic low-back pain is a lack of physical activity. In particular, a major contributor to back pain is excessive sitting, which causes back muscles to shorten, stiffen, and become weaker.

Deterioration or weakening of the abdominal and gluteal muscles, along with tightening of the lower back (erector spinae) muscles, brings about an unnatural forward tilt of the pelvis (Figure 8.6). This tilt puts extra pressure on the spinal vertebrae, causing pain in the lower back. Accumulation of fat around the midsection of the body contributes to the forward tilt of the pelvis, which further aggravates the condition.

Low-back pain frequently is associated with faulty posture and improper body mechanics, or body positions. Incorrect posture and poor mechanics, such as

Figure 8.6 Incorrect and correct pelvic alignment.

© Cengage Learning 2013

prolonged static postures, repetitive bending and pushing, twisting a loaded spine, and prolonged (more than an hour) sitting with little movement increase strain on the lower back and many other bones, joints, muscles, and ligaments. Figure 8.7 provides a summary of proper body mechanics that promote back health.

In the majority of back injuries, pain is present only with movement and physical activity. According to the National Institutes of Health (NIH), most back pain goes away on its own in a few weeks. A physician should be consulted if any of the following conditions are present:

- Numbness in the legs
- Trouble urinating
- Leg weakness
- Fever
- Unintentional weight loss
- Persistent severe pain even at rest

A physician can rule out any disc damage, arthritis, osteoporosis, a slipped vertebrae, spinal stenosis (narrowing of the spinal canal), or other serious condition. For common back pain, he may prescribe proper bed rest using several pillows under the knees for leg support (Figure 8.7). This position helps relieve muscle spasms by stretching the muscles involved. He may also prescribe a muscle relaxant or anti-inflammatory medication (or both) and some type of physical therapy.

In most cases, an x-ray and MRI is not required unless pain lingers for more than four to six weeks. In the early stages of back pain, tight muscles and muscle spasms tend to compress the vertebrae, squeezing the intervertebral disks and revealing apparent disk problems on an x-ray. In these cases, the real problem is the tight muscles and

Figure 8.7   Your back and how to care for it.

Whatever the cause of low back pain, part of its treatment is the correction of faulty posture. But good posture is not simply a matter of "standing tall." It refers to correct use of the body at all times. In fact, for the body to function in the best of health it must be so used that no strain is put upon the muscles, joints, bones, and ligaments. To prevent low back pain, avoiding strain must become a way of life, practiced while lying, sitting, standing, walking, working, and exercising. When body position is correct, internal organs have enough room to function normally and blood circulates more freely.

With the help of this guide, you can begin to correct the positions and movements that bring on or aggravate backache. Particular attention should be paid to the positions recommended for resting, since it is possible to strain the muscles of the back and neck even while lying in bed. By learning to live with good posture, under all circumstances, you will gradually develop the proper carriage and stronger muscles needed to protect and support your hard-working back.

How to Stay on Your Feet Without Tiring Your Back

To prevent strain and pain in everyday activities, it is restful to change from one task to another before fatigue sets in. Housewives can lie down between chores; others should check body position frequently, drawing in the abdomen, flattening the back, bending the knees slightly.

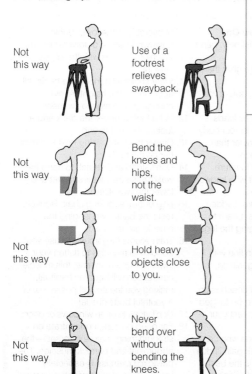

Not this way

Use of a footrest relieves swayback.

Not this way

Bend the knees and hips, not the waist.

Not this way

Hold heavy objects close to you.

Not this way

Never bend over without bending the knees.

Check Your Carriage Here

In correct, fully erect posture, a line dropped from the ear will go through the tip of the shoulder, middle of hip, back of kneecap, and front of anklebone.

Incorrect
Lower back is arched or hollow.

Incorrect
Upper back is stooped, lower back is arched, abdomen sags.

 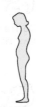

Incorrect
Note how, in strained position, pelvis tilts forward, chin is out, and ribs are down, crowding internal organs.

Correct
In correct position, chin is in, head up, back flattened, pelvis held straight.

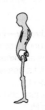 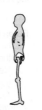

To find the correct standing position: Stand one foot away from wall. Now sit against wall, bending knees slightly. Tighten abdominal and buttock muscles. This will tilt the pelvis back and flatten the lower spine. Holding this position, inch up the wall to standing position, by straightening the legs. Now walk around the room, maintaining the same posture. Place back against wall again to see if you have held it.

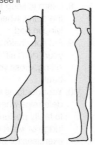

How to Sit Correctly

A back's best friend is a straight, hard chair. If you can't get the chair you prefer, learn to sit properly on whatever chair you get. *To correct sitting position from forward slump:* Throw head well back, then bend it forward to pull in the chin. This will straighten the back. Now tighten abdominal muscles to raise the chest. Check position frequently.

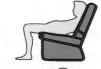
Use of footrest relieves swayback. Aim is to have knees higher than hips.

Correct way to sit while driving, close to pedals. Use seat belt or hard backrest, available commercially.

TV slump leads to "dowager's hump," strains neck and shoulders.

If chair is too high, swayback is increased.

Keep neck and back in as straight a line as possible with the spine. Bend forward from hips.

Driver's seat too far from pedals emphasizes curve in lower back.

Strained reading position. Forward thrusting strains muscles of neck and head.

(continued)

Figure 8.7   Your back and how to care for it.

How to Put Your Back to Bed

For proper bed posture, a firm mattress is essential. Bedboards, sold commercially, or devised at home, may be used with soft mattresses. Bedboards, preferably, should be made of 3/4-inch plywood. Faulty sleeping positions intensify swayback and result not only in backache but in numbness, tingling, and pain in arms and legs.

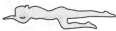

Incorrect:
Lying flat on back makes swayback worse.

Correct:
Lying on side with knees bent effectively flattens the back. Flat pillow may be used to support neck, especially when shoulders are broad.

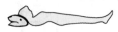

Use of high pillow strains neck, arms, shoulders.

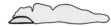

Sleeping on back is restful and correct when knees are properly supported.

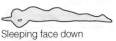

Sleeping face down exaggerates swayback, strains neck and shoulders.

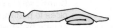

Raise the foot of the mattress eight inches to discourage sleeping on the abdomen.

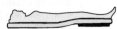

Bending one hip and knee does not relieve swayback.

Proper arrangement of pillows for resting or reading in bed.

A straight-back chair used behind a pillow makes a serviceable backrest.

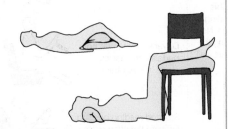

When Doing Nothing, Do it Right
- Rest is the first rule for the tired, painful back. The above positions relieve pain by taking all pressure and weight off the back and legs.
- Note pillows under knees to relieve strain on spine.
- For complete relief and relaxing effect, these positions should be maintained from 5 to 25 minutes.

Exercise Without Getting Out of Bed

Exercises to be performed while lying in bed are aimed not so much at strengthening muscles as at teaching correct positioning. But muscles used correctly become stronger and in time are able to support the body with the least amount of effort.

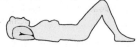

Do all exercises in this position. Legs should not be straightened.

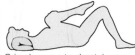

Bring knee up to chest. Lower slowly but do not straighten leg. Relax. Repeat with each leg 10 times.

Bring both knees slowly up to chest (place your hands on the lower thigh behind the knees). Tighten muscles of abdomen, press back flat against bed. Hold knees to chest 20 seconds, then lower slowly. Relax. Repeat 5 times. This exercise gently stretches the shortened muscles of the lower back, while strengthening abdominal muscles.

Exercise Without Attracting Attention

Use these inconspicuous exercises whenever you have a spare moment during the day, both to relax tension and improve the tone of important muscle groups.
1. Rotate shoulders, forward and backward.
2. Turn head slowly side to side.
3. Watch an imaginary plane take off, just below the right shoulder. Stretch neck, follow it slowly as it moves up, around and down, disappearing below the other shoulder. Repeat, starting on left side.
4. Slowly, slowly, touch left ear to left shoulder, right ear to right shoulder. Raise both shoulders to touch ears, drop them as far down as possible.
5. At any pause in the day—waiting for an elevator to arrive, for a specific traffic light to change—pull in abdominal muscles, tighten, hold it for the count of eight without breathing. Relax slowly. Increase the count gradually after the first week, practice breathing normally with the abdomen flat and contracted. Do this sitting, standing, and walking.

Rules to Live By—From Now On
1. Never bend from the waist only; bend the hips and knees.
2. Never lift a heavy object higher than your waist.
3. Always turn and face the object you wish to lift.
4. Avoid carrying unbalanced loads; hold heavy objects close to your body.
5. Never carry anything heavier than you can manage with ease.
6. Never lift or move heavy furniture. Wait for someone to do it who knows the principles of leverage.
7. Avoid sudden movements, sudden "overloading" of muscles. Learn to move deliberately, swinging the legs from the hips.
8. Learn to keep the head in line with the spine, when standing, sitting, lying in bed.
9. Put soft chairs and deep couches on your "don't sit" list. During prolonged sitting, cross your legs to rest your back.
10. Your doctor is the only one who can determine when low back pain is due to faulty posture and he is the best judge of when you may do general exercises for physical fitness. When you do, omit any exercise that arches or overstrains the lower back: backward bends, or forward bends, touching the toes with the knees straight.
11. Wear shoes with moderate heels, all about the same height. Avoid changing from high to low heels.
12. Put a footrail under the desk and a footrest under the crib.
13. Diaper the baby sitting next to him or her on the bed.
14. Don't stoop and stretch to hang the wash; raise the clothesbasket and lower the washline.
15. Beg or buy a rocking chair. Rocking rests the back by changing the muscle groups used.
16. Train yourself vigorously to use your abdominal muscles to flatten your lower abdomen. In time, this muscle contraction will become habitual, making you the envied possessor of a youthful body profile!
17. Don't strain to open windows or doors.
18. For good posture, concentrate on strengthening "nature's corset"—the abdominal and buttock muscles. The pelvic roll exercise is especially recommended to correct the postural relation between the pelvis and the spine.

subsequent muscle spasms. A daily physical activity and stretching program helps to decompress the spine, stretch tight muscles, strengthen weak muscles, and increases blood flow (promoting healing) to the back muscles.

Time is often the best treatment approach. Even with severe pain, most people feel better within days or weeks without being treated by health care professionals.[10] Up to 90 percent of people will heal on their own. To relieve symptoms, you may use over-the-counter pain relievers and hot or cold packs. You also should stay active to avoid further weakening of the back muscles. Low-impact activities such as walking, swimming, water aerobics, and cycling are recommended. Once you are pain free in the resting state, you need to start correcting the muscular imbalance by stretching the tight muscles and strengthening the weak ones. Stretching exercises always are performed first.

If there is no indication of disease or injury (such as leg numbness or pain), a herniated disc, or fractures, spinal manipulation by a chiropractor or other health care professional can provide pain relief. Spinal manipulation as a treatment modality for low back pain has been endorsed by the federal Agency for Health Care Policy and Research. The guidelines suggest that spinal manipulation may help to alleviate discomfort and pain during the first few weeks of an acute episode of low-back pain. Generally, benefits are seen in fewer than 10 treatments. People who have had chronic pain for more than 6 months should avoid spinal manipulation until they have been thoroughly examined by a physician.

Back pain is considered chronic if it persists longer than three months. Surgery is seldom the best option, as it often weakens the spine. Scar tissue and surgical alterations also decrease the success rate of a subsequent surgery. Only about 10 percent of people with chronic pain are candidates for surgery. If surgery is recommended, always seek a second opinion. And consider all other options. In many cases, pushing beyond the pain and participating in aggressive physical therapy ("exercise boot camps" for back pain) aimed at strengthening the muscles that support the spine are what's needed to overcome the condition. Data from the Physician's Neck & Back Clinic in Minneapolis showed that only 3 in 38 patients recommended for surgery needed such upon completion of a 10-week aggressive physical therapy program.[11]

Back pain can be reduced greatly through aerobic exercise, muscular flexibility exercise, and muscular strength and endurance training that includes specific exercises to strengthen the spine-stabilizing muscles. Exercise requires effort by the patient, and it may create discomfort initially, but exercise promotes circulation, healing, muscle size, and muscle strength and endurance. Many patients abstain from aggressive physical therapy because they are unwilling to commit the time required for the program.

In terms of alleviating back pain, *exercise is medicine*, but it needs to be the right type of exercise. Aerobic exercise is beneficial because it helps decrease body fat and psycho-logical stress. During an episode of back pain, however, people often avoid activity and cope by getting more rest. Rest is recommended if the pain is associated with a herniated disc, but if your physician rules out a serious problem, exercise is a better choice of treatment. Exercise helps restore physical function, and individuals who start and maintain an aerobic exercise program have back pain less frequently. Individuals who exercise also are less likely to require surgery or other invasive treatments.

Regular stretching exercises that help the hip and trunk go through a functional range of motion, rather than increasing the range of motion, are recommended. That is, for proper back care, stretching exercises should not be performed to the extreme range of motion. Individuals with a greater spinal range of motion also have a higher incidence of back injury. Spinal stability, instead of mobility, is desirable for back health.[12]

Yoga exercises are particularly beneficial to enhance flexibility; and **Iyegar yoga** in particular, has been shown to relieve chronic low back pain.[13] In fact yoga may help relieve chronic back pain better than conventional medicine. Following 24 weeks of biweekly classes, yoga participants had greater improvement in functional disability along with a decrease in pain intensity and low back pain–related depression. These benefits were still present six months after the end of class participation.

A strengthening program for a healthy back should be conducted around the endurance threshold—15 or more repetitions to near fatigue. Muscular endurance of the muscles that support the spine is more important than absolute strength because these muscles perform their work during the course of an entire day.

Critical Thinking

Consider your own low back health. Have you ever had episodes of low back pain? • If so, how long did it take you to recover, and what helped you recover from this condition?

Several exercises for preventing and rehabilitating the backache syndrome are given on pages 295–296. These exercises can be done twice or more daily when a person has back pain. Under normal circumstances, doing these exercises three or four times a week is enough to prevent the syndrome. Using some of the additional core exercises listed in Chapter 7 ("Core Strength Training," page 244) will further enhance your low-back management program. Back pain recurs more often in people who rely solely on medication, compared with people who use both medication and exercise therapy to recover.[14]

Key Terms

Iyegar yoga Form of yoga that aims to develop flexibility, strength, balance, and stamina using props (belts, blocks, blankets, and chairs) to aid in the correct performance of asanas or yoga postures.

Effects of Posture

Good posture enhances personal appearance, self-image, confidence, improves balance and endurance, protects against misalignment-related pains and aches, prevents falls, and enhances your overall sense of well-being.[15] The relationship between different body parts is the essence of posture.

Poor posture is a risk factor for musculoskeletal problems of the neck, shoulders, and lower back. Incorrect posture also strains hips and knees. Faulty posture and weak and inelastic muscles are also a leading cause of chronic low-back problems.

Adequate body mechanics also aid in reducing chronic low back pain. Proper body mechanics means using correct positions in all the activities of daily life, including sleeping, sitting, standing, walking, driving, working, and exercising. Because of the high incidence of low back pain, illustrations of proper body mechanics and a series of corrective and preventive exercises are shown in Figure 8.7 and Activity 8.2. Besides engaging in the recommended exercises you need to continually strive to maintain good posture. As posture improves, you frequently become motivated to change other aspects, such as muscular strength and flexibility and decreasing body fat.

Effects of Stress

Psychological stress, too, may lead to back pain.[16] The brain is "hardwired" to the back muscles. Excessive stress causes muscles to contract. Frequent tightening of the back muscles can throw the back out of alignment and constrict blood vessels that supply oxygen and nutrients to the back. Chronic stress also increases the release of hormones that have been linked to muscle and tendon injuries. Furthermore, people under stress tend to forget proper body mechanics, placing themselves at unnecessary risk for injury. If you are undergoing excessive stress and back pain at the same time, proper stress management (see Chapter 12) should be a part of your comprehensive back-care program.

Personal Flexibility and Low Back Conditioning Program

Activity 8.2 allows you to develop your own flexibility and low-back conditioning programs. Some of the exercises that help increase spinal stability and muscular strength endurance require isometric contractions. The recommendation calls for these contractions to be held for 2 to 20 seconds. The length of the hold will depend on your current fitness level and the difficulty of each exercise. For most exercises, you may start with a 2- to 5-second hold. Over the course of several weeks, you can increase the length of the hold up to 20 seconds.

Muscular Flexibility Assessment

Name: _____ Date: _____

Course: _____ Section: _____ Gender: _____ Age: _____

Test	Score	Fitness Category	Point
Modified Sit-and-Reach			
Total Body Rotation ☐ Right ☐ Left			
Shoulder Rotation			

Total Points: _____

Overall Flexibility Category: _____

Flexibility Development and Low Back Conditioning Programs

I. Stage of Change for Flexibility Training

Using Figure 2.5 (page 61) and Table 2.3 (page 60), identify your current stage of change for participation in a muscular stretching program:

_____

II. Instruction

Perform all of the recommended flexibility exercises given on pages 292–294. Use a combination of slow-sustained and proprioceptive neuromuscular facilitation stretching techniques. Indicate the technique(s) used for each exercise and, where applicable, the number of repetitions performed and the length of time that the final degree of stretch was held.

Stretching Exercises

Exercise	Stretching Technique	Repetitions	Length of Final Stretch
Lateral head tilt			NA*
Arm circles			NA
Side stretch			
Body rotation			
Chest stretch			
Shoulder hyperextension stretch			
Shoulder rotation stretch			NA
Quad stretch			
Heel cord stretch			
Adductor stretch			
Sitting adductor stretch			
Sit-and-reach stretch			
Triceps stretch			

*Not Applicable

Flexibility Development and Low Back Conditioning Programs (continued)

Stretching Schedule (Indicate days, time, and place where you will stretch):

Flexibility-training days: M ☐ T ☐ W ☐ Th ☐ F ☐ Sa ☐ Su ☐   Time of day: [____]   Place: [_____]

Low Back Conditioning Program

Perform all of the recommended exercises for the prevention and rehabilitation of low back pain given on pages 294–296. Indicate the number of repetitions performed for each exercise.

Flexibility Exercises	Repetitions	Strength/Endurance Exercises	Repetitions	Seconds Held
Hip flexors stretch	[ ]	Pelvic tilt	[ ]	[ ]
Single-knee-to-chest stretch	[ ]	The cat	[ ]	[ ]
Double-knee-to-chest stretch	[ ]	Abdominal crunch or abdominal curl-up	[ ]	[ ]
Upper and lower back stretch	[ ]	Reverse crunch	[ ]	[ ]
Sit-and-reach stretch	[ ]	Supine bridge	[ ]	[ ]
Gluteal stretch	[ ]	Pelvic clock	[ ]	[ ]
Back extension stretch	[ ]	Lateral bridge	[ ]	[ ]
Trunk rotation and lower back stretch	[ ]	Prone bridge	[ ]	[ ]
		Leg press	[ ]	[ ]
		Seated back	[ ]	[ ]
		Lat pull-down	[ ]	[ ]
		Back extension	[ ]	[ ]

Proper Body Mechanics

Perform the following tasks using the proper body mechanics given in Figure 8.7 (pages 285–286). Check off each item as you perform the task:

☐ Standing (carriage) position   ☐ Resting position for tired and painful back
☐ Sitting position   ☐ Lifting an object
☐ Bed posture

"Rules to Live By—From Now On"

Read the 18 "Rules to Live By—From Now On" given in Figure 8.7 (page 286) and indicate below those rules that you need to work on to improve posture and body mechanics and prevent low back pain.

_____
_____
_____
_____
_____
_____
_____

Assess Your Behavior

1. Do you give flexibility exercises the same priority in your fitness program as you do aerobic and strength training?

2. Are stretching exercises a part of your fitness program at least two times per week?

3. Do you include exercises to strengthen and enhance body alignment in your regular strength and flexibility program?

Assess Your Knowledge

Evaluate how well you understand the concepts presented in this chapter using the chapter-specific quizzing available in the online materials at www.cengagebrain.com.

1. Muscular flexibility is defined as
   a. the capacity of joints and muscles to work in a synchronized manner.
   b. the achievable range of motion at a joint or group of joints without causing injury.
   c. the capability of muscles to stretch beyond their normal resting length without injury to the muscles.
   d. the capacity of muscles to return to their proper length following the application of a stretching force.
   e. the limitations placed on muscles as the joints move through their normal planes.

2. Good flexibility
   a. promotes healthy muscles and joints.
   b. decreases the risk of injury.
   c. improves posture.
   d. decreases the risk of chronic back pain.
   e. All are correct choices.

3. Plastic elongation is a term used in reference to
   a. permanent lengthening of soft tissue.
   b. increased flexibility achieved through dynamic stretching.
   c. temporary elongation of muscles.
   d. the ability of a muscle to achieve a complete degree of stretch.
   e. lengthening of a muscle against resistance.

4. The most significant contributors to loss of flexibility are
   a. sedentary living and lack of physical activity.
   b. weight and power training.
   c. age and injury.
   d. muscular strength and endurance.
   e. excessive body fat and low lean tissue.

5. Which of the following is *not* a mode of stretching?
   a. proprioceptive neuromuscular facilitation
   b. elastic elongation
   c. ballistic stretching
   d. slow-sustained stretching
   e. All are modes of stretching.

6. PNF can help increase
   a. muscular strength.
   b. muscular flexibility.
   c. muscular endurance.
   d. range of motion.
   e. All are correct choices.

7. When performing stretching exercises, the degree of stretch should be
   a. through the entire arc of movement.
   b. to about 80 percent of capacity.
   c. to mild tension at the end of the range of motion.
   d. applied until the muscle(s) start shaking.
   e. progressively increased until the desired stretch is attained.

8. When stretching, the final stretch should be held for
   a. 1 to 10 seconds.
   b. 15 to 60 seconds.
   c. 30 to 90 seconds.
   d. 1 to 3 minutes.
   e. as long as the person is able to sustain the stretch.

9. Low back pain is associated primarily with
   a. physical inactivity.
   b. faulty posture.
   c. excessive body weight.
   d. improper body mechanics.
   e. All are correct choices.

10. The following exercise helps stretch the lower back and hamstring muscles:
    a. adductor stretch.
    b. cat stretch.
    c. back extension stretch.
    d. single-knee-to-chest stretch.
    e. quad stretch.

Correct answers can be found at the back of the book.

EXERCISE 1 NECK STRETCHES

Action: Gently tilt the head laterally (a). You may increase the degree of stretch by gently pulling with one hand (b). You may also stretch the neck by raising your head toward the ceiling (c—do not extend your head backward; look straight forward). You may also turn your head 30° and gradually bring the head forward until you feel an adequate stretch in the muscles on the back of the neck (d). The degree of stretch can again be increased by gently pulling forward with the hand (e). Perform the exercises on both the right and left sides. Repeat each exercise several times, and hold the final stretched position for several seconds.

Areas Stretched: Neck flexors and extensors; ligaments of the cervical spine

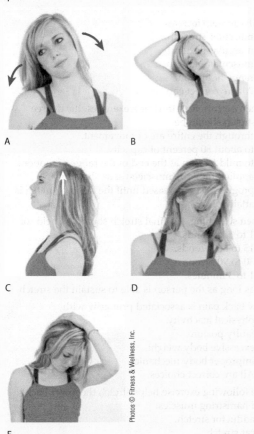

A   B

C   D

E

EXERCISE 2 ARM CIRCLES

Action: Gently circle your arms all the way around. Conduct the exercise in both directions.

Areas Stretched: Shoulder muscles and ligaments

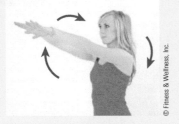

EXERCISE 3 SIDE STRETCH

Action: Stand straight up, feet separated to shoulder-width, and place your hands on your waist. Now move the upper body to one side and hold the final stretch for a few seconds. Repeat on the other side.

Areas Stretched: Muscles and ligaments in the pelvic region

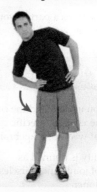

EXERCISE 4 BODY ROTATION

Action: Place your arms slightly away from the body and rotate the trunk as far as possible, holding the final position for several seconds. Conduct the exercise for both the right and left sides of the body. You also can perform this exercise by standing about 2 feet away from the wall (back toward the wall) and then rotating the trunk, placing the hands against the wall.

Areas Stretched: Hip, abdominal, chest, back, neck, and shoulder muscles; hip and spinal ligaments

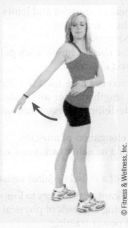

EXERCISE 5 CHEST STRETCH

Action: Place your hands on the shoulders of your partner, who in turn will push you down by your shoulders. Hold the final position for a few seconds.

Areas Stretched: Chest (pectoral) muscles and shoulder ligaments

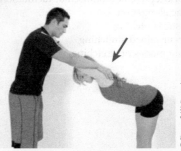

EXERCISE 6 SHOULDER HYPEREXTENSION STRETCH

Action: Have a partner grasp your arms from behind by the wrists and slowly push them upward. Hold the final position for a few seconds.

Areas Stretched: Deltoid and pectoral muscles; ligaments of the shoulder joint

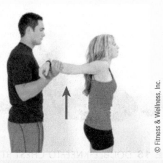

EXERCISE 7 SHOULDER ROTATION STRETCH

Action: With the aid of surgical tubing or an aluminum or wood stick, place the tubing or stick behind your back and grasp the two ends using a reverse (thumbs-out) grip. Slowly bring the tubing or stick over your head, keeping the elbows straight. Repeat several times (bring the hands closer together for additional stretch).

Areas Stretched: Deltoid, latissimus dorsi, and pectoral muscles; shoulder ligaments

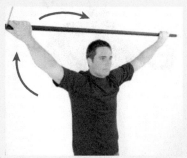

EXERCISE 8 QUAD STRETCH

Action: Lie on your side and move one foot back by flexing the knee. Grasp the front of the ankle and pull the ankle toward the gluteal region. Hold for several seconds. Repeat with the other leg.

Areas Stretched: Quadriceps muscle; knee and ankle ligaments

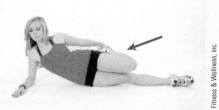

EXERCISE 9 HEEL CORD STRETCH

Action: Stand against the wall or at the edge of a step and stretch the heel downward, alternating legs. Hold the stretched position for a few seconds.

Areas Stretched: Heel cord (Achilles tendon); gastrocnemius and soleus muscles

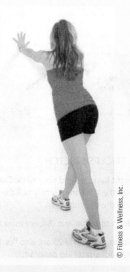

EXERCISE 10 ADDUCTOR STRETCH

Action: Stand with your feet about twice shoulder-width apart and place your hands slightly above the knees. Flex one knee and slowly go down as far as possible, holding the final position for a few seconds. Repeat with the other leg.

Areas Stretched: Hip adductor muscles

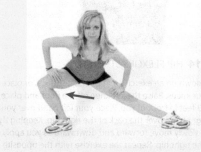

EXERCISE 11 SITTING ADDUCTOR STRETCH

Action: Sit on the floor and bring your feet in close to you, allowing the soles of the feet to touch each other. Now place your forearms (or elbows) on the inner part of the thigh and push the legs downward, holding the final stretch for several seconds.

Areas Stretched: Hip adductor muscles

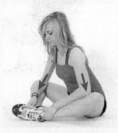

EXERCISE 12 SIT-AND-REACH STRETCH

Action: Sit on the floor with legs together and gradually reach forward as far as possible. Hold the final position for a few seconds. This exercise also may be performed with the legs separated, reaching to each side as well as to the middle.

Areas Stretched: Hamstrings and lower back muscles; lumbar spine ligaments

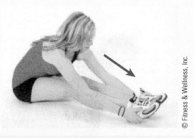

© Fitness & Wellness, Inc.

EXERCISE 13 TRICEPS STRETCH

Action: Place the right hand behind your neck. Grasp the right arm above the elbow with the left hand. Gently pull the elbow backward. Repeat the exercise with the opposite arm.

Areas Stretched: Back of upper arm (triceps muscle); shoulder joint

Note: Exercises 14 through 21 and 23 are also flexibility exercises and can be added to your stretching program.

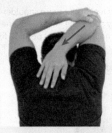

© Fitness & Wellness, Inc.

EXERCISE 14 HIP FLEXORS STRETCH

Action: Kneel down on an exercise mat or a soft surface, or place a towel under your knees. Raise the left knee off the floor and place the left foot about 3 feet in front of you. Place your left hand over your left knee and the right hand over the back of the right hip. Keeping the lower back flat, slowly move forward and downward as you apply gentle pressure over the right hip. Repeat the exercise with the opposite leg forward.

Areas Stretched: Flexor muscles in front of the hip joint

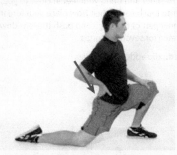

© Fitness & Wellness, Inc.

EXERCISE 15 SINGLE-KNEE-TO-CHEST-STRETCH

Action: Lie down flat on the floor. Bend one leg at approximately 100° and gradually pull the opposite leg toward your chest. Hold the final stretch for a few seconds. Switch legs and repeat the exercise.

Areas Stretched: Lower back and hamstring muscles; lumbar spine ligaments

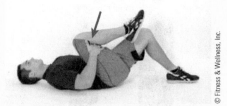

© Fitness & Wellness, Inc.

EXERCISE 16 DOUBLE-KNEE-TO-CHEST STRETCH

Action: Lie flat on the floor and then curl up slowly into a fetal position. Hold for a few seconds.

Areas Stretched: Upper and lower back and hamstring muscles; spinal ligaments

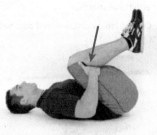

© Fitness & Wellness, Inc.

Exercises for the Prevention and Rehabilitation of Low Back Pain

EXERCISE 17 UPPER AND LOWER BACK STRETCH

Action: Sit on the floor and bring your feet in close to you, allowing the soles of the feet to touch each other. Holding on to your feet, bring your head and upper chest gently toward your feet.

Areas Stretched: Upper and lower back muscles and ligaments

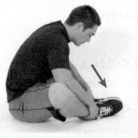

EXERCISE 18 SIT-AND-REACH STRETCH

(See Exercise 12 on page 294)

EXERCISE 19 GLUTEAL STRETCH

Action: Lie on the floor, bend the right leg, and place your right ankle slightly above the left knee. Grasp behind the left thigh with both hands and gently pull the leg toward the chest. Repeat the exercise with the opposite leg.

Areas Stretched: Buttock area (gluteal muscles)

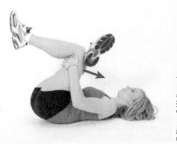

EXERCISE 20 BACK EXTENSION STRETCH

Action: Lie face down on the floor with the elbows by the chest, forearms on the floor, and the hands beneath the chin. Gently raise the trunk by extending the elbows until you reach an approximate 90° angle at the elbow joint. Be sure the forearms remain in contact with the floor at all times. Do NOT extend the back beyond this point. Hyperextension of the lower back may lead to or aggravate an existing back problem. Hold the stretched position for about 10 seconds.

Areas Stretched: Abdominal region

Additional Benefits: Restore lower back curvature

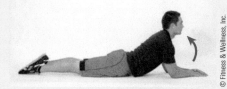

EXERCISE 21 TRUNK ROTATION AND LOWER BACK STRETCH

Action: Sit on the floor and bend the left leg, placing the left foot on the outside of the right knee. Place the right elbow on the left knee and push against it. At the same time, try to rotate the trunk to the left (counterclockwise). Hold the final position for a few seconds. Repeat the exercise with the other side.

Areas Stretched: Lateral side of the hip and thigh; trunk and lower back

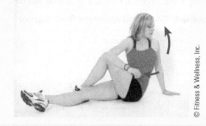

EXERCISE 22 PELVIC TILT

(See Exercise 12 in Chapter 7, page 257) This is perhaps the most important exercise for the care of the lower back. It should be included as a part of your daily exercise routine and should be performed several times throughout the day when pain in the lower back is present as a result of muscle imbalance.

EXERCISE 23 THE CAT

Action: Kneel on the floor and place your hands in front of you (on the floor) about shoulder-width apart. Relax the trunk and lower back (a). Now arch the spine and pull in your abdomen as far as you can and hold this position for a few seconds (b). Repeat the exercise 4–5 times.

Areas Stretched: Low back muscles and ligaments

Areas Strengthened: Abdominal and gluteal muscles

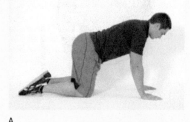

A

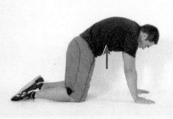

B

EXERCISE 24 ABDOMINAL CRUNCH OR ABDOMINAL CURL-UP

(See Exercise 4 in Chapter 7, page 255) It is important that you do not stabilize your feet when performing either of these exercises, because doing so decreases the work of the abdominal muscles. Also, remember not to "swing up" but, rather, to curl up as you perform these exercises.

EXERCISE 25 REVERSE CRUNCH

(See Exercise 11 in Chapter 7, page 257)

EXERCISE 26 SUPINE BRIDGE

Action: Lie face up on the floor with the knees bent at about 120°. Do a pelvic tilt (Exercise 12 in Chapter 7, page 257) and maintain the pelvic tilt while you raise the hips off the floor until the upper body and upper legs are in a straight line. Hold this position for several seconds.

Areas Strengthened: Gluteal and abdominal flexor muscles

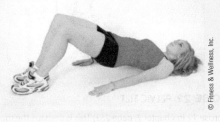

© Fitness & Wellness, Inc.

EXERCISE 27 PELVIC CLOCK

Action: Lie face up on the floor with the knees bent at about 120°. Fully extend the hips as in the supine bridge (Exercise 26). Now progressively rotate the hips in a clockwise manner (2 o'clock, 4 o'clock, 6 o'clock, 8 o'clock, 10 o'clock, and 12 o'clock), holding each position in an isometric contraction for about 1 second. Repeat the exercise counterclockwise.

Areas Strengthened: Gluteal, abdominal, and hip flexor muscles

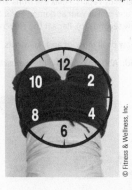

© Fitness & Wellness, Inc.

EXERCISE 28 LATERAL BRIDGE

(See Exercise 13 in Chapter 7, page 257)

EXERCISE 29 PRONE BRIDGE

(See Exercise 14 in Chapter 7, page 258)

EXERCISE 30 LEG PRESS

(See Exercise 16 in Chapter 7, page 259)

EXERCISE 31 SEATED BACK

(See Exercise 20 in Chapter 7, page 260)

EXERCISE 32 LAT PULL-DOWN

(See Exercise 24 in Chapter 7, page 261)

EXERCISE 33 BACK EXTENSION

(See Exercise 36 in Chapter 7, page 267)

EXERCISE 34 LATERAL TRUNK FLEXION

(See Exercise 37 in Chapter 7, page 268)

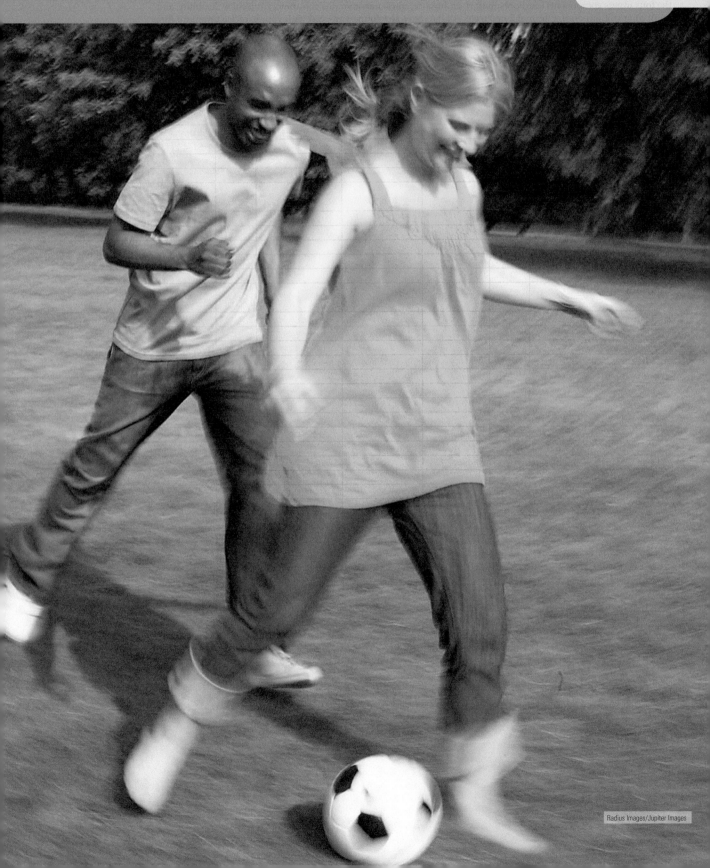

Physical Fitness and Wellness Profile

Figure A.1	Personal Fitness and Wellness Profile.

Fill out the following profile as you obtain the results for each fitness and wellness component. Attempt to determine the four fitness components (cardiorespiratory endurance, muscular strength/endurance, muscular flexibility, and body composition) during the first 2 or 3 weeks of the terms so you may proceed with your exercise program. After determining each component, discuss with your instructor the goals to be accomplished and the date of completion.

Name: _____ Course: _____ Section: _____ Gender: _____ Age: _____

Item	Pre-Assessment			Goal[a]	Post-Assessment		
	Date	Test Results	Category		Date	Test Results	Category
Cardiorespiratory Endurance							
VO_{2max}							
Daily min. of phys. activity							
Total daily steps							
Muscular Strength							
Muscular Flexibility							
Body Composition							
Body weight							
Percent body fat							
Lean body mass							
BMI							
Waist circumference							
Cardiovascular Risk							
Cancer Risk							
Lung							
Colorectal							
Skin							
Breast[b]							
Cervical[b]							
Endometrial[b]							
Prostate							
Testicular							
Pancreatic							
Kidney and Bladder							
Oral							
Esophageal and Stomach							
Ovarian							
Thyroid							
Liver							
Leukemia							
Lymphomas							
Stress							
Life Exp. Survey							
Vulnerability Scale							
Tobacco Use[c]							

INSTRUCTOR'S SIGNATURE: _____ STUDENT'S SIGNATURE: _____

[a]Indicate goal to complete by end of the term.
[b]Women only
[c]For test results, indicate type and amount smoked; for classification indicate smoker, ex-smoker, nonsmoker.

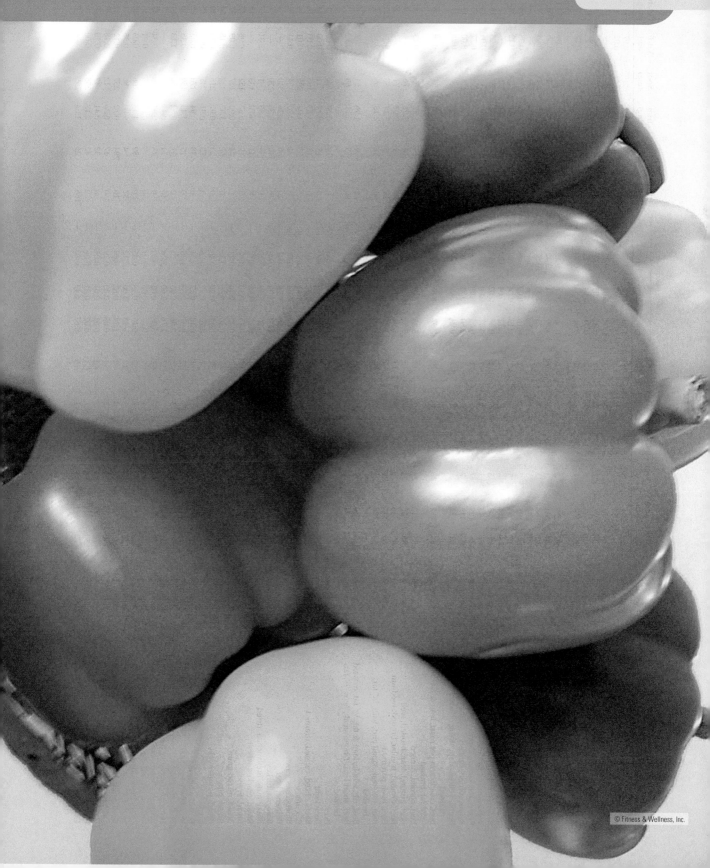

Nutritive Value of Selected Foods

Fat Breakdown (g) columns: Sat, Mono, Poly, Trans.

Food Description	Qty	Measure	Wt (g)	Ener (cal)	Prot (g)	Carb (g)	Dietary Fiber (g)	Fat (g)	Sat	Mono	Poly	Trans	Chol (mg)	Calc (mg)	Iron (mg)	Sodi (mg)	Vit E (mg)	Folate (mcg)	Vit C (mg)	Selenium (mcg)
Almonds, dry roasted, no salt added	¼	cup(s)	35	206	8	7	4	18	1.40	11.61	4.36	—	0	92	1.56	<1	8.97	11	0	1
Apple juice, unsweetened, canned	½	cup(s)	124	58	<1	14	<1	<1	0.02	0.01	0.04	—	0	8	0.46	4	0.01	0	1	<1
Apples, raw medium, w/peel	1	item(s)	138	72	<1	19	3	<1	0.04	0.01	0.07	—	0	8	0.17	1	—	4	6	0
Applesauce, sweetened, canned	½	cup(s)	128	97	<1	25	2	<1	0.04	0.01	0.07	—	0	5	0.45	4	0.27	1	2	<1
Apricot, fresh w/o pits	4	item(s)	140	67	2	16	3	1	0.04	0.24	0.11	—	0	18	0.55	1	1.25	13	14	<1
Apricot, halves w/skin, canned in heavy syrup	½	cup(s)	129	107	1	28	2	<1	0.01	0.04	0.02	—	0	12	0.39	5	0.77	3	4	<1
Asparagus, boiled, drained	½	cup(s)	90	20	2	4	2	0.19	0.06	0	0.12	—	0	20.7	0.81	12.6	1.35	134.1	6.92	5.48
Avocado, California, whole, w/o skin or pit	1	item(s)	170	284	3	15	12	26	3.59	16.61	3.42	0	0	22	1.00	14	3.35	105	15	1
Bacon, cured, broiled, pan fried, or roasted	2	slice(s)	13	68	5	<1	0	5	1.73	2.33	0.57	0	14	1	0.18	291	0.04	<1	0	8
Bagel chips, plain	3	item(s)	29	130	3	19	2	5	0.50	—	0.49	—	0	53	0.72	70	0.08	64	0	23
Bagel, plain, enriched, toasted	1	item(s)	66	195	7	38	2	1	0.16	0.09	0.09	—	0	53	2.52	379	0.12	128	0	1
Banana, fresh whole, w/o peel	1	item(s)	118	105	1	27	3	<1	0.13	0.04	0.20	—	0	6	0.31	1	—	24	11	1
Beans, black, boiled	½	cup(s)	86	114	8	20	7	<1	0.12	0.04	0.14	—	0	23	1.81	1	0.25	128	0	1
Beans, Fordhook lima, frozen, boiled, drained	½	cup(s)	85	88	5	16	5	<1	0.07	0.02	0.02	—	0	26	1.55	59	0.04	18	11	1
Beans, mung, sprouted, boiled, drained	½	cup(s)	62	13	1	3	<1	<1	0.02	0.00	0.03	—	0	7	0.40	6	0.77	18	7	<1
Beans, red kidney, canned	½	cup(s)	128	109	7	20	8	<1	0.06	0.03	0.24	—	0	31	1.61	436	0.00	65	1	1
Beans, refried, canned	½	cup(s)	127	119	7	20	8	2	0.60	0.71	0.19	—	10	44	2.10	378	0.28	14	8	2
Beans, yellow snap, string or wax, boiled, drained	½	cup(s)	62	22	1	5	2	<1	0.04	0.00	0.09	—	0	29	0.80	2	0.19	21	6	<1
Beef, chuck, arm pot roast, lean & fat, ¼" fat, braised	3	ounce(s)	85	282	23	0	0	20	7.97	8.68	0.77	—	84	9	2.64	51	0.13	8	0	21
Beef, corned, canned	3	ounce(s)	85	213	23	0	0	13	5.25	5.07	0.54	—	73	10	1.77	855	—	8	0	36
Beef, ground, lean, broiled, well	3	ounce(s)	85	238	24	0	0	15	5.89	6.56	0.56	—	86	10	2.08	76	0.39	9	0	22
Beef, ground, regular, broiled, medium	3	ounce(s)	85	246	20	0	0	18	6.91	7.70	0.65	0.17	77	9	2.07	71	0.12	8	0	16
Beef, liver, pan fried	3	ounce(s)	85	149	23	4	0	4	1.27	0.56	0.49	—	324	5	5.24	65	—	221	0	28
Beef, rib steak, small end, lean, ¼" fat, broiled	3	ounce(s)	85	188	24	0	0	10	3.84	4.01	0.27	—	68	11	2.18	59	0.12	7	0	19
Beef, rib, whole, lean & fat, ¼" fat, roasted	3	ounce(s)	85	320	19	0	0	27	10.71	11.42	0.94	—	72	9	1.96	54	0.00	6	0	19
Beef, short loin, T-bone steak, lean, ¼" fat, broiled	3	ounce(s)	85	174	23	0	0	9	3.05	4.23	0.26	—	50	5	3.11	65	0.00	7	0	9
Beer	12	fluid ounce(s)	356	118	1	6	<1	<1	0.00	0.00	0.00	0	0	18	0.07	14	0.00	21	0	2
Beer, light	12	fluid ounce(s)	354	99	1	5	1	0	0.00	0.00	0.00	0	0	18	0.14	11	0.00	14	0	2
Beets, sliced, canned, drained	½	cup(s)	85	26	1	6	1	<1	0.02	0.02	0.04	0	0	13	1.55	165	0.03	26	3	<1
Biscuits	1	item(s)	41	121	3	16	1	5	1.40	1.41	1.82	—	<1	33	1.01	205	0.01	26	<1	7
Blueberries, raw	½	cup(s)	72	41	1	10	2	<1	0.02	0.03	0.11	—	0	4	0.20	1	0.41	4	7	<1
Bologna, beef	1	slice(s)	28	90	3	1	0	8	3.50	4.26	0.31	—	20	0	0.36	310	—	4	<1	8
Bologna, turkey	1	slice(s)	28	50	3	1	0	4	1.00	1.09	0.98	—	20	40	0.36	270	—	—	0	—
Brazil nuts, unblanched, dried	¼	cup(s)	35	230	5	4	3	23	5.30	8.59	7.20	—	0	56	0.85	1	2.01	8	0	671
Bread, cracked wheat	1	slice(s)	25	65	2	12	1	1	0.23	0.48	0.17	—	0	11	0.70	135	—	15	0	6
Bread, French	1	slice(s)	25	69	2	13	1	1	0.16	0.30	0.17	—	0	19	0.63	152	0.08	37	0	8
Bread, mixed grain	1	slice(s)	26	65	2	12	2	1	0.21	0.40	0.24	—	0	24	0.90	127	0.09	31	0	8
Bread, pita	1	item(s)	60	165	5	33	1	1	0.10	0.06	0.32	—	0	52	1.57	322	0.18	64	0	16
Bread, pumpernickel	1	slice(s)	32	80	3	15	2	1	0.14	0.30	0.40	—	0	22	0.92	215	0.13	30	0	8
Bread, rye	1	slice(s)	32	83	2	15	2	1	0.20	0.42	0.26	—	0	23	0.91	211	0.11	35	0	10
Bread, white	1	slice(s)	25	67	2	13	1	1	0.18	0.17	0.34	—	0	38	0.94	170	0.05	28	0	4
Bread, whole wheat	1	slice(s)	46	128	4	24	3	2	0.37	0.53	1.35	—	0	15	1.43	159	0.35	30	0	18
Broccoli, chopped, boiled, drained	½	cup(s)	78	27	2	6	3	<1	0.06	0.03	0.13	—	0	31	0.52	32	1.13	84	51	1
Brownie, prepared from mix	1	item(s)	24	112	2	12	1	7	1.76	2.60	2.26	—	18	14	0.44	82	0.34	7	<1	3
Brussels sprouts, boiled, drained	½	cup(s)	78	28	2	6	2	1	0.08	0.03	0.20	—	0	28	0.94	16	0.85	47	48	1
Bulgur, cooked	½	cup(s)	91	76	3	17	4	<1	0.04	0.03	0.09	—	0	9	0.87	5	0.01	16	0	1
Buns, hamburger, plain	1	item(s)	43	120	4	21	1	2	0.47	0.48	0.85	—	0	59	1.43	206	0.35	48	0	8
Butter	1	tablespoon(s)	15	108	<1	<1	0	12	6.13	5.00	0.43	—	32	4	0.00	86	0.12	<1	0	<1
Buttermilk, low fat	1	cup(s)	245	98	8	12	0	2	1.34	0.62	0.08	—	10	284	0.12	257	0.18	12	2	5
Cabbage, boiled, drained, no salt added	1	cup(s)	150	33	1	7	3	1	0.08	0.05	0.29	—	0	47	0.26	12	0.10	30	30	1
Cabbage, raw, shredded	1	cup(s)	70	17	1	4	2	<1	0.01	0.01	0.04	—	0	33	0.41	13	0.00	30	23	1
Cake, angel food, from mix	1	slice(s)	50	129	3	29	<1	<1	0.02	0.01	0.06	—	0	42	0.12	255	0.00	10	0	8
Cake, butter pound, ready to eat, commercially prepared	1	slice(s)	75	291	4	37	<1	15	8.67	4.43	0.80	—	166	26	1.04	299	—	0	<1	—

Food	Amount	Unit																		
Cake, carrot, cream cheese frosting, from mix	1	slice(s)	111	484	5	52	1	29	5.43	7.24	15.10	—	60	28	1.39	273	—	13	1	—
Cake, chocolate, chocolate icing, commercially prepared	1	slice(s)	64	235	3	35	2	10	3.05	5.61	1.18	—	27	28	1.41	214	—	11	<1	2
Cake, devil's food cupcake, chocolate frosting	1	item(s)	35	120	2	20	1	4	1.80	1.60	0.60	—	19	21	0.70	92	—	2	0	2
Cake, white, coconut frosting, from mix	1	slice(s)	112	399	5	71	2	12	4.36	4.14	2.42	—	1	101	1.30	318	0.13	35	<1	12
Candy, Almond Joy bar	1	item(s)	49	240	2	29	2	13	9.00	3.63	0.74	0	3	20	0.36	70	—	2	0	—
Candy, Life Savers	1	item(s)	2	8	0	2	0	<1	0.00	—	0.04	—	0	<1	0.04	1	—	—	0	0
Candy, M & Ms peanut chocolate candy, small bag	1	item(s)	49	250	5	30	2	13	5.00	5.42	2.07	0	5	40	0.36	25	—	17	1	2
Candy, M & Ms plain chocolate candy, small bag	1	item(s)	48	240	2	34	1	10	6.00	3.30	0.30	—	5	40	0.36	30	—	3	1	1
Candy, milk chocolate bar	1	item(s)	91	483	8	53	2	28	16.69	7.20	0.63	—	22	228	0.83	92	—	11	2	—
Candy, Milky Way bar	1	item(s)	58	270	2	41	1	10	5.00	3.50	0.35	—	5	60	0.18	95	—	6	1	3
Candy, Reese's peanut butter cups	2	piece(s)	45	250	5	25	1	14	5.00	6.17	2.34	—	3	20	0.36	140	—	25	0	2
Candy, Special Dark chocolate bar	1	item(s)	41	220	2	24	3	13	8.00	4.59	0.41	—	3	0	0.72	0	—	1	0	<1
Candy, Starburst fruit chews, original fruits	1	package	59	240	0	48	0	5	1.00	2.10	1.83	—	0	10	0.18	0	—	0	30	<1
Candy, York peppermint patty	1	item(s)	42	170	1	34	1	3	2.00	1.32	0.12	—	0	0	0.36	10	0.04	2	0	<1
Cantaloupe	1/2	item(s)	80	27	1	7	1	<1	0.04	0.00	0.07	—	0	7	0.17	13	0.40	17	30	<1
Carrots, raw	1/2	cup(s)	61	25	1	6	2	<1	0.02	0.01	0.06	—	0	20	0.18	42	0.80	12	4	<1
Carrots, sliced, boiled, drained	1/2	cup(s)	78	27.29	1	6.41	2.33	0.14	0.02	0	0.08	—	0	23.39	0.26	45.24	—	10.92	2.8	0.54
Cashews, dry roasted	1/4	cup(s)	34	197	5	11	1	16	3.14	9.36	2.68	—	0	15	2.06	5	0.32	24	0	4
Catsup/ketchup	1	tablespoon(s)	15	14	<1	4	<1	<1	0.01	0.01	0.04	—	0	3	0.08	167	0.22	2	27	<1
Cauliflower, boiled, drained	1/2	cup(s)	62	14	1	3	2	<1	0.04	0.02	0.13	—	0	10	0.20	9	0.04	27	27	<1
Celery, stalk	2	item(s)	80	11	1	2	1	<1	0.03	0.03	0.06	—	0	32	0.16	64	0.22	29	2	6
Cereal, All-Bran	1	cup(s)	62	160	8	46	20	3	—	—	1.00	—	0	300	9.00	160	—	800	12	6
Cereal, All-Bran Buds	1	cup(s)	91	212	6	73	42	3	0.00	0.00	—	—	0	0	13.64	606	—	1212	18	26
Cereal, Bran Flakes, Post	1	cup(s)	40	133	4	32	7	1	0.00	0.39	0.71	—	0	0	10.77	293	—	133	0	—
Cereal, Cap'n Crunch	1	cup(s)	36	144	2	30	1	2	0.53	0.50	0.27	—	0	5	6.00	269	—	133	0	—
Cereal, Cheerios	1	cup(s)	30	110	3	22	3	2	0.00	0.00	0.50	—	0	100	8.10	280	—	200	6	7
Cereal, Complete wheat bran flakes	1	cup(s)	39	120	4	31	7	1	—	—	—	—	0	0	23.94	279	—	532	80	11
Cereal, Corn Flakes	1	cup(s)	28	100	2	24	1	0	0.00	0.00	0.00	—	0	0	8.10	200	—	100	6	4
Cereal, Corn Pops	1	cup(s)	31	120	1	28	0	0	0.00	0.00	0.00	—	0	0	1.80	120	—	100	6	1
Cereal, Cracklin' Oat Bran	1	cup(s)	65	266	5	47	7	9	2.70	4.70	1.33	—	0	27	2.38	186	—	218	20	2
Cereal, Cream of Wheat, instant, prepared	1/2	cup(s)	121	61	2	13	<1	<1	0.01	0.01	0.04	—	0	27	8.60	1	—	357	0	14
Cereal, Frosted Flakes	1	cup(s)	41	160	1	37	1	0	0.00	0.00	0.00	—	0	0	5.99	200	—	133	8	2
Cereal, Frosted Mini-Wheats	5	item(s)	51	180	5	41	5	1	0.00	0.00	0.50	—	0	0	15.30	5	—	100	0	2
Cereal, granola, prepared	1/2	cup(s)	61	299	9	32	5	15	2.76	4.7	6.53	—	0	48	2.59	13	3.59	51	1	16.95
Cereal, Kashi puffed	1	cup(s)	25	70	3	13	5	0	0.35	—	0.72	—	0	0	0.72	0	—	—	0	—
Cereal, Life	1	cup(s)	43	160	4	33	3	2	0.35	0.64	0.61	—	0	124	11.92	218	—	142	0	11
Cereal, Multi-Bran Chex	1	cup(s)	58	200	4	49	7	2	0.00	0.00	0.00	—	0	100	16.20	390	—	100	6	5
Cereal, Nutri-Grain golden wheat	1	cup(s)	40	133	3	31	5	1	0.19	0.37	0.67	—	0	9	1.46	279	—	133	20	9
Cereal, oatmeal, cooked w/water	1/2	cup(s)	117	74	3	13	2	1	0.00	0.00	0.44	—	0	9	0.80	1	0.12	5	0	9
Cereal, Product 19	1	cup(s)	30	100	2	25	1	0	0.00	0.00	0.00	—	0	0	18.00	210	—	400	60	4
Cereal, Raisin Bran	1	cup(s)	59	190	4	47	8	1	0.00	0.10	0.36	—	0	20	10.80	300	—	140	0	—
Cereal, Rice Chex	1	cup(s)	25	96	2	22	<1	0	0.00	0.00	0.00	—	0	80	7.20	232	—	160	5	5
Cereal, Rice Krispies	1	cup(s)	26	96	2	23	0	0	0.00	0.00	0.25	—	0	0	1.44	256	—	80	5	4
Cereal, Shredded Wheat	1	cup(s)	25	88	3	20	3	1	0.04	0.01	0.13	—	0	10	1.08	2	—	12	0	4
Cereal, Smacks	1	cup(s)	36	133	3	32	1	1	0.00	0.00	0.10	—	0	0	0.48	67	—	133	8	17
Cereal, Special K	1	cup(s)	31	110	7	22	1	0	0.00	0.00	0.00	—	0	0	8.70	220	—	400	15	7
Cereal, Total whole grain	1	cup(s)	40	146	3	31	4	1	0.00	0.00	0.00	0	0	1330	23.94	253	31.24	532	80	2
Cereal, Wheaties	1	cup(s)	30	110	3	24	3	1	0.00	0.00	0.00	—	0	0	8.10	220	2.26	200	6	1
Cheese, American, processed	1	ounce(s)	28	106	6	<1	0	9	5.58	2.54	0.28	—	27	156	0.05	422	0.08	2	0	4
Cheese, blue, crumbled	1	ounce(s)	28	100	6	1	0	8	5.29	2.21	0.23	—	21	150	0.09	395	0.07	10	0	4
Cheese, cheddar, shredded	1/4	cup(s)	28	114	7	<1	0	9	5.96	2.65	0.27	—	30	204	0.19	175	0.08	5	0	4
Cheese, feta	1	ounce(s)	28	74	4	1	0	6	4.18	1.29	0.17	—	25	138	0.18	312	0.05	9	0	4
Cheese, Monterey jack	1	ounce(s)	28	104	7	<1	0	8	5.34	2.45	0.25	—	25	209	0.20	150	0.07	5	0	4
Cheese, mozzarella, part skim milk	1	ounce(s)	28	71	7	1	0	4	2.83	1.26	0.13	—	18	219	0.06	173	0.04	3	0	1
Cheese, Parmesan, grated	1	tablespoon(s)	5	22	2	<1	0	1	0.87	0.42	0.06	—	4	55	0.05	76	0.01	1	0	—
Cheese, ricotta, part skim milk	1/4	cup(s)	62	85	7	3	0	5	3.03	1.42	0.16	—	19	167	0.27	77	0.04	8	0	10
Cheese, Swiss	1	ounce(s)	28	106	8	2	0	8	4.98	2.04	0.27	—	26	221	0.06	54	0.11	8	0	5
Cherries, sweet, raw	1/2	cup(s)	73	46	1	12	2	<1	0.03	0.03	0.04	—	0	9	0.26	0	0.05	3	5	0
Chicken, broiler breast, meat & skin, flour coated, fried	3	ounce(s)	85	189	27	1	<1	8	2.08	2.98	1.67	—	76	14	1.01	65	—	5	0	20

Food Description	Qty	Measure	Wt (g)	Ener (cal)	Prot (g)	Carb (g)	Dietary Fiber (g)	Fat (g)	Fat Breakdown (g) Sat	Mono	Poly	Trans	Chol (mg)	Calc (mg)	Iron (mg)	Sodi (mg)	Vit E (mg)	Folate (mcg)	Vit C (mg)	Selenium (mcg)
Chicken, broiler drumstick, meat & skin, flour coated, fried	3	ounce(s)	85	208	23	1	<.1	12	3.11	4.61	2.75	—	77	10	1.14	76	—	9	0	16
Chicken, light meat, roasted	3	ounce(s)	85	130	23	0	0	3	0.92	1.29	0.79	—	64	11	0.92	43	0.23	3	0	22
Chicken, roasted (meat only)	3	ounce(s)	85	142	21	0	0	6	1.54	2.13	1.28	—	64	10	1.03	64	—	4	0	21
Chickpeas or bengal gram, garbanzo beans, boiled	½	cup(s)	82	134	7	22	6	2	0.22	0.48	0.95	—	0	40	2.37	6	0.29	141	1	3
Chocolate milk, low fat	1	cup(s)	250	158	8	26	1	3	1.54	0.75	0.09	—	8	288	0.60	153	0.05	13	2	5
Cilantro	1	teaspoon(s)	2	<1	<.1	<.1	<.1	<.1	0.00	0.00	0.00	—	0	1	0.03	1	—	1	1	<.1
Cocoa, hot, prepared w/milk	1	cup(s)	250	193	9	27	3	6	3.58	1.69	0.09	0.18	20	263	1.20	110	0.08	13	1	7
Coconut, dried, not sweetened	¼	cup(s)	60	393	4	14	10	38	34.06	1.63	0.42	—	0	15	1.98	22	0.26	5	1	11
Cod, Atlantic cod or scrod, baked or broiled	3	ounce(s)	44	46	10	0	0	<1	0.07	0.05	0.13	—	24	6	0.22	35	—	5	<1	17
Coffee, brewed	8	fluid ounce(s)	237	9	<1	0	0	0	0.00	0.00	0.00	0	0	2	0.02	2	0.02	5	0	0
Collard greens, boiled, drained	½	cup(s)	95	25	2	5	3	<1	0.04	0.02	0.16	—	0	133	1.10	15	0.84	88	17	<1
Cookies, animal crackers	12	piece(s)	30	134	2	22	<1	4	1.03	2.29	0.56	—	0	13	0.82	1118	0.04	50	0	—
Cookies, chocolate chip	1	item(s)	30	140	2	16	1	8	2.09	3.26	2.09	0	13	11	0.70	109	0.54	16	<.1	4
Cookies, chocolate sandwich, extra crème filling	1	item(s)	13	65	<1	9	<1	3	0.50	1.39	1.22	1.10	0	3	0.37	64	0.25	6	0	<1
Cookies, Fig Newtons	1	item(s)	16	55	1	10	1	1	0.50	0.50	0.00	0.50	0	5	0.36	60	—	—	<1	—
Cookies, oatmeal	1	item(s)	69	234	6	45	3	4	0.70	1.28	1.85	0	<.1	26	1.94	311	0.23	30	<1	17
Cookies, peanut butter	1	item(s)	35	163	4	17	1	9	1.65	4.72	2.43	0	13	28	0.67	157	0.74	21	<.1	5
Cookies, sugar	1	item(s)	16	61	1	7	<1	3	0.63	1.27	0.87	0	18	5	0.32	50	0.28	8	<.1	3
Corn, yellow sweet, frozen, boiled, drained	½	cup(s)	82	66	2	16	2	1	0.08	0.16	0.26	—	0	2	0.39	1	0.06	29	3	1
Cornbread	1	piece(s)	55	141	5	18	1	5	2.09	1.44	1.50	0	21	88	1.01	209	0.33	36	2	6
Cornmeal, yellow whole grain	½	cup(s)	61	221	5	47	4	2	0.31	0.58	1.00	—	0	4	2.10	21	0.26	15	0	9
Cottage cheese, low fat, 1% fat	½	cup(s)	113	81	14	3	0	1	0.73	0.33	0.04	—	5	69	0.16	459	0.01	14	0	10
Cottage cheese, low fat, 2% fat	½	cup(s)	113	102	16	4	0	2	1.38	0.62	0.07	—	9	78	0.18	459	0.02	15	0	12
Crab, blue, canned	2	ounce(s)	57	56	12	0	0	1	0.14	0.12	0.25	—	50	57	0.48	189	1.04	24	2	18
Crackers, cheese (mini)	30	item(s)	30	151	3	17	1	8	2.81	3.63	0.74	—	4	45	1.43	299	0.66	46	0	3
Crackers, honey graham	4	item(s)	28	118	2	22	1	3	0.43	1.14	1.07	—	0	7	1.04	169	0.09	13	0	3
Crackers, matzo, plain	1	item(s)	28	112	3	24	1	<1	0.06	0.04	0.17	—	0	4	0.90	1	0.02	5	0	10
Crackers, Ritz	5	item(s)	16	80	1	10	1	4	0.50	1.50	0.00	—	0	20	0.72	135	—	10	1	—
Crackers, rye crispbread	1	item(s)	10	37	1	8	2	<1	0.01	0.02	0.06	—	0	3	0.24	26	0.08	5	0	4
Crackers, saltine	5	item(s)	15	65	1	11	<1	2	0.44	0.96	0.25	0.54	0	18	0.81	195	0.15	19	0	2
Crackers, wheat	10	item(s)	30	142	3	19	1	6	1.55	3.43	0.84	—	0	15	1.32	239	0.15	35	0	2
Cranberry juice cocktail	½	cup(s)	127	72	0	18	<1	<1	0.01	0.02	0.06	—	0	4	0.19	3	0.28	0	45	0
Cream cheese	2	tablespoon(s)	29	101	2	1	0	10	6.37	2.85	0.37	—	32	23	0.35	86	0.09	4	0	1
Cream, heavy whipping, liquid	1	tablespoon(s)	15	52	<1	<1	0	6	3.45	1.60	0.21	—	21	10	0.00	6	0.16	1	<.1	<.1
Cream, light whipping, liquid	1	tablespoon(s)	15	44	<1	<1	0	5	2.90	1.36	0.13	—	17	10	0.00	5	0.13	1	<.1	<.1
Croissant, butter	1	item(s)	57	231	5	26	1	12	6.59	3.15	0.62	—	38	21	1.16	424	—	35	<1	13
Cucumber	¼	item(s)	75	11	<1	3	<1	<.1	0.03	0.00	0.04	—	0	12	0.21	2	0.02	5	2	<1
Danish pastry, nut	1	item(s)	65	280	5	30	1	16	3.78	8.90	2.78	—	30	61	1.17	236	0.53	54	1	9
Dates, domestic, whole	¼	cup(s)	44.5	126	1	33	4	<1	0.01	0.01	0	—	0	17	0.45	1	0.02	9	<1	1
Distilled alcohol, 90 proof	1	fluid ounce(s)	28	73	0	0	0	0	0.00	0.00	0.00	0	0	0	0.01	<1	0.00	0	0	0
Doughnut, cake	1	item(s)	47	198	2	23	1	11	1.70	4.37	3.70	—	17	21	0.92	257	—	22	<.1	0
Doughnut, glazed	1	item(s)	60	242	4	27	1	14	3.49	7.72	1.74	—	4	26	0.36	205	—	13	<.1	5
Egg substitute, Egg Beaters	¼	cup(s)	61	30	6	1	0	0	0.00	0.00	0.00	0	0	20	1.08	115	—	60	0	—
Eggs, fried	1	item(s)	46	92	6	<1	0	7	1.98	2.92	1.22	—	210	27	0.91	94	0.56	23	0	16
Eggs, hard boiled	1	item(s)	50	78	6	1	0	5	1.63	2.04	0.71	—	212	25	0.60	62	0.51	22	0	15
Eggs, poached	1	item(s)	50	74	6	<1	0	5	1.54	1.90	0.68	—	211	27	0.92	147	0.48	24	0	16
Eggs, raw, white	1	item(s)	33	17	4	<1	0	<.1	0.00	0.00	0.00	—	0	2	0.03	55	0.00	1	0	7
Eggs, raw, whole	1	item(s)	50	74	6	<1	0	5	1.55	1.91	0.68	—	212	27	0.92	70	0.49	24	0	16
Eggs, raw, yolk	1	item(s)	17	53	3	1	0	4	1.59	1.95	0.70	—	205	21	0.45	8	0.43	24	0	9
Eggs, scrambled, prepared w/milk & butter	2	item(s)	122	203	14	3	0	15	4.49	5.82	2.62	—	429	87	1.46	342	1.04	37	<1	27
Figs, raw, medium	2	item(s)	101	74	1	19	3	<1	0.06	0.07	0.14	—	0	35	0.37	1	0.11	6	2	<1
Fish fillets, batter coated or breaded, fried	3	ounce(s)	85	197.19	12.46	14.42	0.42	10.44	2.39	2.19	5.32	—	28.89	15.3	1.79	452.2	—	17	0	7.73
Flounder, baked	3	ounce(s)	85	114	15	<1	<.1	6	1.15	2.17	1.44	0	44	19	0.35	281	0.41	7	3	34
Flour, all purpose, white, bleached, enriched	½	cup(s)	63	228	6	48	2	1	0.10	0.05	0.26	—	0	9	2.90	1	0.04	114	0	21
Flour, whole wheat	½	cup(s)	60	203	8	44	7	1	0.19	0.14	0.47	—	0	20	2.33	3	0.49	26	0	42

The following is a nutrient-composition data table (a continuation page of a food-composition appendix). No column headers are printed on this page; the columns, in order, are: Food / Amount / Unit / Weight (g) / Energy (cal) / Protein (g) / Carbohydrate (g) / Dietary Fiber (g) / Fat (g) / Saturated Fat (g) / Monounsaturated (g) / Polyunsaturated (g) / (sparse col) / Cholesterol (mg) / Calcium (mg) / Iron (mg) / Sodium (mg) / Vitamin E (mg) / Folate (µg) / Vitamin C (mg) / Selenium (µg).

Food	Amt	Unit	Wt (g)	Cal	Prot	Carb	Fiber	Fat	Sat	Mono	Poly		Chol	Calc	Iron	Sod	Vit E	Fol	Vit C	Sel
Frankfurter, beef & pork	1	item(s)	57	174	7	1	1	16	6.14	7.79	1.56	—	29	6	0.66	638	0.14	2	0	8
Frankfurter, beef	1	item(s)	45	149	5	2	2	13	5.26	6.44	0.53	—	24	6	0.68	513	0.09	2	0	4
Frankfurter, turkey	1	item(s)	45	102	6	1	1	8	2.65	2.51	2.25	—	48	48	0.83	642	0.28	4	0	7
Frozen yogurt, chocolate, soft serve	½	cup(s)	72	115	3	18	0	4	2.61	1.26	0.16	—	4	106	0.90	71	—	8	<1	2
Frozen yogurt, vanilla, soft serve	½	cup(s)	72	117	3	17	2	4	2.46	1.14	0.15	—	1	103	0.22	63	0.08	4	1	2
Fruit cocktail, canned in heavy syrup	½	cup(s)	119	91	<1	23	1	<1	0.01	0.02	0.04	—	0	7	0.36	7	0.50	4	2	1
Fruit cocktail, canned in juice	½	cup(s)	125	55	1	14	1	<1	0.00	0.00	0.00	—	0	9	0.25	5	0.47	6	3	1
Granola bar, plain, hard	1	item(s)	25	115	2	16	1	5	0.58	1.07	2.95	—	0	15	0.72	72	—	6	<1	4
Grape juice, sweetened, added vitamin C, from frozen concentrate	½	cup(s)	125	64	<1	16	<1	<1	0.04	0.01	0.03	—	0	5	0.13	3	0.00	1	30	<1
Grapefruit juice, pink, sweetened, canned	½	cup(s)	124	58	1	14	<1	<1	0.02	0.02	0.03	—	0	10	0.45	3	0.05	13	34	<1
Grapefruit juice, white	½	cup(s)	124	48	1	11	<1	<1	0.02	0.02	0.03	—	0	11	0.25	1	0.27	12	47	<1
Grapefruit, raw, pink or red	½	cup(s)	115	48	1	12	2	<1	0.02	0.02	0.04	—	0	25	0.09	0	0.15	15	36	<1
Grapes, European, red or green, adherent skin	½	cup(s)	80	55	1	14	1	<1	0.04	0.01	0.04	—	0	8	0.29	2	0.15	2	9	<.1
Haddock, baked or broiled	3	ounce(s)	85	50	11	0	0	<1	0.07	0.07	0.14	—	33	19	0.60	39	—	4	0	18
Halibut, Atlantic & Pacific, cooked, dry heat	3	ounce(s)	85	119	23	0	0	2	0.35	0.82	0.80	—	35	51	0.91	59	—	12	0	40
Ham, cured, boneless, 11% fat, roasted	3	ounce(s)	85	151	19	0	0	8	2.65	3.77	1.20	—	50	7	1.14	1275	0.26	3	0	17
Ham, deli sliced, cooked	1	slice(s)	28	30	5	1	0	1	0.50	0.39	0.11	—	15	0	0.00	240	—	1	—	—
Honey	1	tablespoon(s)	21	64	<1	17	<1	0	0.00	0.00	0.00	—	0	1	0.09	1	0.00	<1	<1	1
Honeydew melon	½	cup(s)	89	32	<1	8	1	<1	0.03	0.00	0.05	—	0	5	0.15	16	0.02	17	16	1
Ice cream, chocolate	½	cup(s)	66	143	3	19	1	7	4.49	2.12	0.27	—	22	72	0.61	50	0.20	11	<1	2
Ice cream, chocolate, soft serve	½	cup(s)	66	177	3	24	1	8	5.17	2.43	0.31	—	22	103	0.33	103	0.22	11	<1	—
Ice cream, light vanilla	½	cup(s)	66	109	4	18	<1	3	1.71	0.57	0.10	—	17	77	0.05	49	0.08	3	<1	1
Jams, jellies, preserves, all flavors	1	tablespoon(s)	20	56	<1	14	<1	<1	0.00	0.01	0.00	—	0	4	0.10	6	0.00	2	1.76	—
Jams, jellies, preserves, all flavors, low sugar	1	tablespoon(s)	18	25	<1	6	<1	<1	0.00	0.01	0.02	—	0	2	0.05	<1	0.01	1	4.93	—
Kale, frozen, chopped, boiled, drained	½	cup(s)	65	20	2	3	1	<1	0.04	0.02	0.15	—	0	90	0.61	10	0.60	9	16	1
Kiwifruit	1	item(s)	77	53	1	11	3	1	0.02	0.03	0.19	—	0	30	0.38	2	—	<1	74	—
Lamb, chop, loin, domestic, lean & fat, ¼" fat, broiled	3	ounce(s)	85	269	21	0	0	20	8.36	8.25	1.43	—	85	17	1.54	65	0.11	15	0	23
Lamb, leg, domestic, lean & fat, ¼" fat, cooked	3	ounce(s)	85	250	21	0	0	18	7.51	7.50	1.28	—	82	14	1.60	61	0.12	15	0	22
Lemon juice	1	tablespoon(s)	15	4	<1	1	<1	0	0.00	0.00	0.00	—	0	1	0.00	<1	0.02	2	7	<1
Lemonade, from frozen concentrate	8	fluid ounce(s)	248	131	<1	34	<1	<1	0.04	0.06	0.04	—	0	10	0.52	7	0.02	2	13	<1
Lentils, boiled	½	cup(s)	99	115	9	20	8	<1	0.05	0.08	0.17	—	0	19	3.30	2	0.11	179	1	3
Lentils, sprouted	1	cup(s)	77	82	7	17	7	<1	0.04	0.08	0.17	—	0	19	2.47	8	0.10	77	13	<1
Lettuce, butterhead, Boston, or bibb	1	cup(s)	55	7	1	1	1	<1	0.02	0.00	0.06	—	0	19	0.69	3	0.07	40	1	<1
Lettuce, romaine, shredded	1	cup(s)	56	10	1	2	1	<1	0.02	0.01	0.09	—	0	19	0.55	5	0.07	77	13	<1
Lobster, northern, cooked, moist heat	3	ounce(s)	85	83	17	1	0	1	0.09	0.14	0.08	—	61	52	0.33	323	0.85	9	0	36
Macadamias, dry roasted, no salt added	¼	cup(s)	34	241	3	4	3	25	4.00	19.86	0.50	—	0	23	0.89	1	0.19	3	<1	<1
Mayonnaise w/ soybean oil	1	tablespoon(s)	14	99	<1	<1	0	11	1.64	2.70	5.89	0.04	5	2	0.07	78	0.72	1	0	<1
Mayonnaise, low calorie	1	tablespoon(s)	16	37	<1	3	0	3	0.53	0.72	1.70	—	4	5	0.00	80	0.32	0	0	8
Milk, fat free, nonfat, or skim	1	cup(s)	245	83	8	12	0	<1	0.29	0.12	0.02	—	5	223	0.12	108	0.02	12	0	5
Milk, fat free, nonfat, or skim, w/ nonfat milk solids	1	cup(s)	245	91	9	12	0	<1	0.40	0.16	0.02	—	5	316	0.12	130	0.02	12	2	8
Milk, low fat, 1%	1	cup(s)	244	102	8	12	0	2	1.54	0.68	0.09	—	12	264	0.07	122	0.07	12	0	6
Milk, low fat, 1%, w/ nonfat milk solids	1	cup(s)	245	105	9	12	0	2	1.48	0.69	0.09	—	10	314	0.12	127	0.06	12	2	6
Milk, reduced fat, 2%	1	cup(s)	244	122	8	11	0	5	2.35	2.04	0.17	—	20	271	0.07	115	0.07	12	0	6
Milk, reduced fat, 2% w/ nonfat milk solids	1	cup(s)	244	125	9	12	0	5	2.93	1.36	0.17	—	20	314	0.12	127	0.15	12	1	9
Milk, whole, 3.3%	1	cup(s)	244	146	8	11	0	8	4.55	1.98	0.48	—	24	246	0.07	105	0.15	12	0	4
Milk, whole, evaporated, canned	2	tablespoon(s)	32	42	2	3	0	2	1.45	0.74	0.08	—	9	82	0.06	33	0.04	3	<1	—
Milkshakes, chocolate	1	cup(s)	227	270	7	48	1	6	3.81	0.17	0.51	—	25	299	0.70	252	0.11	11	0	17
Muffin, English, plain, enriched	1	item(s)	57	134	4	26	1	1	0.15	0.16	0.48	—	0	30	1.43	264	0.26	42	0	9
Muffin, English, wheat	1	item(s)	57	127	5	26	2	1	0.16	0.16	0.48	—	0	101	1.64	218	0.76	36	<1	3
Muffins, blueberry	1	item(s)	63	160	3	23	1	6	0.87	1.48	3.25	—	20	50	1.15	288	0.00	29	<1	<1
Mushrooms, raw	½	cup(s)	35	8	1	1	<1	<1	0.02	0.00	0.05	—	0	1	0.18	1	0.00	6	1	3
Mustard greens, frozen, boiled, drained	½	cup(s)	75	14	2	2	2	<1	0.01	0.08	0.04	—	0	76	0.84	19	1.01	53	10	<1
Oil, canola	1	tablespoon(s)	14	120	0	0	0	14	0.97	8.01	4.03	—	0	0	0.00	0	2.33	0	0	0
Oil, corn	1	tablespoon(s)	14	120	0	0	0	14	1.73	3.29	7.98	0.04	0	0	0.00	0	1.94	0	0	0
Oil, olive	1	tablespoon(s)	14	119	0	0	0	14	1.82	9.98	1.35	—	0	<1	0.09	<1	1.94	0	0	0
Oil, peanut	1	tablespoon(s)	14	119	0	0	0	14	2.28	6.24	4.32	—	0	0	0.00	0	2.12	0	0	0
Oil, safflower	1	tablespoon(s)	14	120	0	0	0	14	0.84	10.15	1.95	—	0	0	0.00	0	4.64	0	0	0
Oil, soybean w/ cottonseed oil	1	tablespoon(s)	14	120	0	0	0	14	2.45	4.01	6.54	—	0	0	0.00	0	1.65	0	0	0

Food Description	Qty	Measure	Wt (g)	Ener (cal)	Prot (g)	Carb (g)	Dietary Fiber (g)	Fat (g)	Fat Breakdown (g) Sat	Mono	Poly	Trans	Chol (mg)	Calc (mg)	Iron (mg)	Sodi (mg)	Vit E (mg)	Folate (mcg)	Vit C (mg)	Selenium (mcg)
Okra, sliced, boiled, drained	½	cup(s)	80	18	1	4	2	<1	0.04	0.02	0.04	—	0	62	0.22	5	0.22	37	13	<1
Onions, chopped, boiled, drained	½	cup(s)	106	47	1	11	1	<1	0.03	0.03	0.08	—	0	23	0.26	3	0.02	16	6	1
Orange juice, unsweetened, from frozen concentrate	½	cup(s)	125	56	1	13	<1	<.1	0.01	0.01	0.01	—	0	11	0.12	1	0.25	55	48	<1
Orange, raw	1	item(s)	131	62	1	15	3	<1	0.02	0.03	0.03	—	0	52	0.13	0	0.24	39	70	1
Oysters, eastern, farmed, raw	3	ounce(s)	85	50	4	5	0	1	0.38	0.13	0.50	—	21	37	4.91	151	—	15	4	54
Oysters, eastern, wild, cooked, moist heat	3	ounce(s)	85	116	12	7	0	4	1.31	0.53	1.65	—	89	77	10.19	359	—	12	5	61
Pancakes, blueberry, from recipe	3	item(s)	114	253	7	33	1	10	2.26	2.64	4.74	—	64	235	1.96	470	—	41	3	16
Pancakes, from mix w/egg & milk	3	item(s)	114	249	9	33	2	9	2.33	2.36	3.33	—	81	245	1.48	576	—	105	1	—
Papaya, raw	½	cup(s)	70	27	<1	7	1	<.1	0.03	0.03	0.02	—	0	17	0.07	2	0.51	27	43	<1
Pasta, egg noodles, enriched, cooked	½	cup(s)	80	106	4	20	1	1	0.25	0.34	0.33	0.02	26	10	1.27	6	0.14	51	0	17
Pasta, macaroni, enriched, cooked	½	cup(s)	70	99	3	20	1	<1	0.07	0.06	0.19	—	0	5	0.98	1	0.04	54	0	15
Pasta, spaghetti, al dente, cooked	½	cup(s)	65	95	4	20	1	1	0.05	0.05	0.15	—	0	7	1.00	1	0.04	8	0	40
Pasta, spaghetti, whole wheat, cooked	½	cup(s)	70	87	4	19	3	<1	0.07	0.05	0.15	—	0	11	0.74	2	0.21	4	0	18
Pasta, tricolor vegetable macaroni, enriched, cooked	½	cup(s)	67	86	3	18	3	<.1	0.01	0.01	0.03	—	0	7	0.33	4	0.06	44	0	13
Peach, halves, canned in heavy syrup	½	cup(s)	131	97	1	26	2	<1	0.01	0.05	0.06	—	0	4	0.35	8	0.64	4	4	<1
Peach, halves, canned in water	½	cup(s)	122	29	1	7	2	<.1	0.01	0.03	0.03	—	0	2	0.39	4	0.60	4	4	<1
Peach, raw, medium	1	item(s)	98	38	1	9	1	<1	0.02	0.07	0.08	—	0	6	0.25	0	0.72	4	6	<.1
Peanut butter, smooth	1	tablespoon(s)	16	96	4	3	1	8	1.60	3.96	2.38	—	0	8	0.30	80	1.44	12	0	1
Peanuts, oil roasted, salted	¼	cup(s)	36	216	10	5	3	19	3.12	9.33	5.49	—	0	22	0.54	115	2.50	43	<1	1
Pear, halves, canned in heavy syrup	½	cup(s)	133	98	<1	25	2	<1	0.01	0.04	0.04	—	0	7	0.29	7	0.11	1	1	0
Pear, raw	1	item(s)	166	96	1	26	5	<1	0.01	0.04	0.05	—	0	15	0.28	2	0.20	12	7	<1
Peas, green, canned, drained	½	cup(s)	85	59	4	11	3	<1	0.05	0.03	0.14	—	0	17	0.81	214	0.03	37	8	1
Peas, green, frozen, boiled, drained	½	cup(s)	80	62	4	11	4	<1	0.04	0.02	0.10	—	0	19	1.22	58	0.02	47	8	1
Pecans, dry roasted, no salt added	¼	cup(s)	57	403	5	8	5	42	3.56	24.92	11.66	—	0	41	1.59	1	0.74	9	<1	2
Pepperoni, beef & pork	1	slice(s)	11	55	2	<1	0	5	1.77	2.32	0.48	—	9	1	0.15	224	—	<1	0	—
Peppers, green bell or sweet, raw	½	cup(s)	75	15	1	3	1	<1	0.04	0.01	0.05	—	0	7	0.25	2	0.28	8	60	0
Pickle relish, sweet	1	tablespoon(s)	15	20	<.1	5	<1	<.1	0.01	0.03	0.02	—	0	<1	0.13	122	0.06	<1	<1	0
Pickle, dill	1	ounce(s)	28	5	<1	1	<1	<.1	0.01	0.00	0.02	—	0	3	0.15	363	0.03	<1	1	0
Pie crust, frozen, ready to bake, enriched, baked	1	slice(s)	16	82	1	8	<1	5	1.69	2.51	0.65	—	0	3	0.36	104	0.42	9	0	<1
Pie crust, prepared w/water, baked	1	slice(s)	20	100	1	10	<1	6	1.54	3.46	0.77	—	0	12	0.43	146	—	20	0	—
Pie, apple, from home recipe	1	slice(s)	155	411	4	58	2	19	4.73	8.36	5.17	—	0	11	1.74	327	—	37	3	12
Pie, pecan, from home recipe	1	slice(s)	122	503	6	64	0	27	4.87	13.64	6.97	—	106	39	1.81	320	—	32	<1	15
Pie, pumpkin, from home recipe	1	slice(s)	155	316	7	41	0	14	4.92	5.73	2.81	—	65	146	1.97	349	—	33	3	11
Pineapple, canned in extra heavy syrup	½	cup(s)	130	108	<1	28	1	<1	0.01	0.02	0.05	—	0	18	0.49	1	—	7	9	—
Pineapple, canned in juice	½	cup(s)	125	75	1	20	1	<.1	0.01	0.01	0.04	—	0	17	0.35	1	0.01	6	12	<1
Pineapple, raw, diced	½	cup(s)	78	37	<1	10	1	<.1	0.01	0.01	0.03	—	0	10	0.22	1	0.02	12	28	<.1
Pinto beans, boiled, drained, no salt added	½	cup(s)	114	25	2	5	0	<1	0.04	0.03	0.21	—	0	17	0.75	58	—	146	7	1
Pomegranate	1	item(s)	154	105	1	26	1	<1	0.06	0.07	0.10	—	0	5	0.46	5	0.92	9	9	1
Popcorn, air popped	1	cup(s)	8	31	1	6	1	<1	0.05	0.09	0.15	—	0	1	0.22	<1	0.02	2	0	1
Popcorn, popped in oil	1	cup(s)	33	165	3	19	3	9	1.61	2.70	4.43	—	0	3	0.92	292	—	6	<.1	2
Pork, ribs, loin, country style, lean & fat, roasted	3	ounce(s)	85	279	20	0	0	22	7.83	9.36	1.71	—	78	21	0.90	44	—	4	<1	32
Potato chips, salted	20	item(s)	28	152	2	15	1	10	3.11	2.79	3.46	—	0	7	0.46	169	1.91	13	9	2
Potatoes, au gratin mix, prepared w/water, whole milk, & butter	½	cup(s)	114	106	3	15	1	5	2.94	1.34	0.15	—	17	94	0.36	499	—	8	4	3
Potatoes, baked, flesh & skin	1	item(s)	202	220	5	51	4	<1	0.05	0.00	0.09	—	0	20	2.75	16	—	22	26	2
Potatoes, baked, flesh only	½	cup(s)	61	57	1	13	1	<.1	0.02	0.00	0.03	—	0	3	0.21	3	0.02	5	8	<1
Potatoes, hashed brown	½	cup(s)	78	207	2	27	2	10	1.11	3.13	2.78	—	0	11	0.43	267	0.01	12	10	<1
Potatoes, mashed, from dehydrated granules w/milk, water, & margarine	½	cup(s)	105	122	2	17	1	5	1.27	2.05	1.41	—	2	34	0.22	181	0.54	8	7	6
Pretzels, plain, hard, twists	5	item(s)	30	114	3	24	1	1	0.23	0.41	0.37	—	0	11	1.30	515	—	51	0	2
Prune juice, canned	1	cup(s)	256	182	2	45	3	<.1	0.01	0.05	0.02	—	0	31	3.02	10	0.31	0	10	2

Prunes, dried	2	item(s)	17	40	<1	11	1	<.1	0.01	0.06	0.02	—	0	9	0.42	1	0.00	1	1	<1
Pudding, chocolate	½	cup(s)	144	154	5	23	1	5	2.78	1.94	0.23	0	35	138	1.04	135	0.00	7	<1	5
Pudding, tapioca, ready to eat	1	item(s)	142	169	3	28	<1	5	0.85	2.24	1.93	—	1	119	0.33	226	0.43	4	1	2
Pudding, vanilla	½	cup(s)	136	116	5	17	<.1	3	1.31	1.21	0.16	0	35	133	0.25	134	0.00	6	<1	5
Quinoa, dry	½	cup(s)	85	318	11	59	5	5	0.50	1.30	1.99	—	0	51	7.86	18	—	42	0	—
Raisins, seeded, packed	¼	cup(s)	41	122	1	32	3	<1	0.07	0.01	0.07	—	0	12	1.07	12	—	1	2	<1
Raspberries, raw	½	cup(s)	62	32	1	7	4	<1	0.01	0.04	0.23	—	0	15	0.42	1	0.54	13	16	<1
Raspberries, red, sweetened, frozen	½	cup(s)	125	129	1	33	6	<1	0.01	0.02	0.11	—	0	19	0.81	1	0.90	33	21	<1
Rice, brown, long grain, cooked	½	cup(s)	98	108	3	22	2	1	0.18	0.32	0.31	—	0	10	0.41	5	0.03	4	0	10
Rice, white, long grain, boiled	½	cup(s)	79	103	2	22	<1	<1	0.06	0.07	0.06	—	0	8	0.95	1	0.03	46	0	6
Rice, wild brown, cooked	½	cup(s)	82	82.81	3.27	17.49	1.47	0.27	0.04	0.04	0.17	—	0	2.46	0.49	2.46	—	21.31	0	0.65
Roll, hard	1	item(s)	57	167	6	30	1	2	0.35	0.65	0.98	—	0	54	1.87	310	0.24	54	0	22
Salad dressing, blue cheese	2	tablespoon(s)	31	154	1	2	0	16	3.03	3.76	8.51	—	5	25	0.06	335	1.84	9	1	<1
Salad dressing, French	2	tablespoon(s)	31	143	<1	5	0	14	1.76	2.63	6.56	—	0	7	0.25	261	1.56	0	0	0
Salad dressing, French, low fat	2	tablespoon(s)	33	76	<1	10	<1	4	0.36	1.92	1.64	—	0	4	0.28	262	0.10	1	0	1
Salad dressing, Italian	2	tablespoon(s)	29	86	<1	3	0	8	1.32	1.86	3.80	—	0	2	0.19	486	1.47	0	0	1
Salad dressing, Italian, diet	2	tablespoon(s)	30	23	<1	1	0	2	0.14	0.66	0.51	—	2	3	0.20	410	0.06	0	0	2
Salad dressing, ranch	2	tablespoon(s)	30	146	<1	2	<.1	16	2.32	3.85	8.92	—	1	4	0.03	354	1.85	<1	<.1	—
Salad dressing, thousand island	2	tablespoon(s)	31	115	<1	5	<1	11	1.59	2.46	5.68	—	8	5	0.37	269	1.25	0	0	<1
Salad dressing, thousand island, low calorie	2	tablespoon(s)	31	62	<1	7	<1	4	0.23	1.98	0.82	—	<1	5	0.28	254	0.31	0	0	0
Salami, pork, dry or hard	1	slice(s)	13	52	3	<1	0	4	1.52	2.05	0.48	—	10	2	0.17	289	—	<1	0	3
Salmon, broiled or baked w/butter	3	ounce(s)	85	155	23	0	0	6	1.16	2.29	2.33	—	40	15	1.02	99	1.15	4	2	41
Salmon, smoked chinook (lox)	2	ounce(s)	57	66	10	0	0	2	0.52	1.14	0.56	—	13	6	0.48	1134	—	1	0	22
Salsa	2	tablespoon(s)	16	4	<1	1	<1	<.1	0.00	0.00	0.02	—	0	5	0.16	69	0.19	3	2	<.1
Sardines, Atlantic, with bones, canned in oil	2	item(s)	24	50	6	0	0	3	0.36	0.92	1.23	—	34	108	0.70	121	0.49	3	0	13
Sauerkraut, canned	½	cup(s)	114	22	1	5	3	<1	0.04	0.01	0.07	—	0	34	1.67	751	0.11	27	17	1
Sausage, Italian, pork, cooked	1	item(s)	68	220	14	1	0	17	6.14	8.13	2.23	—	53	16	1.02	627	—	3	1	15
Sausage, smoked, pork link	1	piece(s)	76	295	17	2	—	24	8.58	11.09	2.85	—	52	23	0.88	1137	—	4	0	16
Scallops, mixed species, breaded, fried	3	item(s)	47	100	8	5	0	5	1.24	2.09	1.32	—	28	20	0.38	216	—	23	1	13
Seaweed, spirulina, dried	½	cup(s)	8	22	4	2	<1	1	0.20	0.05	0.16	—	0	9	2.14	79	0.38	7	1	1
Shrimp, mixed species, breaded, fried	3	ounce(s)	85	205.69	18.18	9.74	0.34	10.43	1.77	3.24	4.32	—	150.44	56.95	1.07	292.39	—	20.39	1.27	35.44
Shrimp, mixed species, cooked, moist heat	3	ounce(s)	85	84	18	0	0	1	0.25	0.17	0.37	—	166	33	2.63	190	1.17	3	2	34
Soda, Coca-Cola Classic cola	12	fluid ounce(s)	360	146	0	41	0	0	0.00	0.00	0.00	0	0	—	—	50	—	—	0	—
Soda, Coke diet cola	12	fluid ounce(s)	360	2	0	<1	0	0	0.00	0.00	0.00	0	0	—	—	42	—	—	0	—
Soda, cola	12	fluid ounce(s)	426	179	<1	46	0	0	0.00	0.00	0.00	—	0	13	0.09	17	0.00	0	0	<1
Soda, ginger ale	12	fluid ounce(s)	366	124	0	32	0	0	0.00	0.00	0.00	0	0	11	0.66	26	0.00	0	0	<1
Soda, lemon lime	12	fluid ounce(s)	368	147	0	38	0	0	0.00	0.00	0.00	—	0	7	0.26	41	0.00	0	0	0
Soda, root beer	12	fluid ounce(s)	370	152	0	39	0	0	0.00	0.00	0.00	0	0	18	0.18	48	0.00	0	0	<1
Sour cream	2	tablespoon(s)	24	51	1	1	0	5	3.13	1.45	0.19	—	11	28	0.01	13	0.14	3	<1	1
Sour cream, fat free	2	tablespoon(s)	32	24	1	5	0	0	0.00	0.00	0.00	0	3	40	0.00	45	0.00	4	0	—
Soy sauce	1	tablespoon(s)	18	10	1	2	0	<.1	0.00	0.00	0.01	—	0	3	0.36	1029	0.00	3	0	—
Spinach, canned, drained	½	cup(s)	108	25	3	4	3	1	0.09	0.02	0.23	—	0	138	2.49	29	2.10	106	16	2
Spinach, chopped, boiled, drained	½	cup(s)	90	21	3	3	2	<1	0.04	0.01	0.10	—	0	122	3.21	63	1.87	131	9	1
Spinach, raw, chopped	1	cup(s)	30	7	1	1	1	<1	0.02	0.00	0.05	—	0	30	0.81	24	0.61	58	8	<1
Squash, acorn, baked	½	cup(s)	103	57	1	15	5	<1	0.03	0.01	0.06	—	0	45	0.95	4	—	19	11	1
Squash, summer, all varieties, sliced, boiled, drained	½	cup(s)	90	18	1	4	1	<1	0.06	0.02	0.12	—	0	24	0.32	1	0.13	18	5	<1
Squash, winter, all varieties, baked, mashed	½	cup(s)	103	38	1	9	3	<1	0.13	0.05	0.27	—	0	23	0.45	1	0.12	21	10	<1
Squid, mixed species, fried	3	ounce(s)	85	149	15	7	0	6	1.60	2.34	1.82	—	221	33	0.86	260	—	12	4	44
Strawberries, raw	½	cup(s)	72	23	<1	6	1	<1	0.01	0.03	0.11	—	0	12	0.30	1	0.21	17	42	<1
Strawberries, sweetened, frozen, thawed	½	cup(s)	128	99	1	27	2	<1	0.01	0.02	0.09	—	0	14	0.60	1	0.31	5	50	1
Sugar, brown, packed	1	teaspoon(s)	5	17	0	4	0	0	0.00	0.00	0.00	0	0	4	0.09	2	0.00	<.1	0	<.1
Sugar, white, granulated	1	teaspoon(s)	4	15	0	4	0	0	0.00	0.00	0.00	—	0	<.1	0.00	0	0.00	0	0	<.1
Sweet potatoes, baked, peeled	½	cup(s)	100	90	2	21	3	<1	0.03	0.00	0.06	—	0	38	0.69	36	0.71	6	20	<1
Syrup, maple	¼	cup(s)	80	209	0	54	0	<1	0.03	0.05	0.08	—	0	54	0.96	7	0.00	0	0	<1
Taco shell, hard	1	item(s)	13	62	1	8	1	3	0.43	1.19	1.13	—	0	21	0.33	49	0.22	17	0	2
Tangerine, raw	1	item(s)	84	37	1	9	2	<1	0.02	0.03	0.03	—	0	12	0.08	1	0.17	17	26	<1
Tea, decaffeinated, prepared	8	fluid ounce(s)	237	2	0	1	0	0	0.00	0.00	0.01	0	0	0	0.05	7	0.00	12	0	0
Tea, herbal, prepared	8	fluid ounce(s)	237	2	0	<1	0	0	0.00	0.00	0.01	0	0	5	0.19	2	0.00	2	0	0
Tea, prepared	8	fluid ounce(s)	237	2	0	1	0	0	0.00	0.00	0.01	0	0	0	0.05	7	0.00	12	0	0
Teriyaki sauce	1	tablespoon(s)	18	15	1	3	<.1	0	0.00	0.00	0.00	0	0	5	0.31	690	0.00	4	0	<1
Tofu, firm	3	ounce(s)	79	80	8	2	1	4	0.50	0.87	2.17	—	0	60	1.08	0	—	—	0	—
Tomato juice, canned	½	cup(s)	122	21	1	5	<1	<.1	0.01	0.01	0.03	—	0	12	0.52	328	0.39	24	22	<1

Food Description	Qty	Measure	Wt (g)	Ener (cal)	Prot (g)	Carb (g)	Dietary Fiber (g)	Fat (g)	Fat Breakdown (g)				Chol (mg)	Calc (mg)	Iron (mg)	Sodi (mg)	Vit E (mg)	Folate (mcg)	Vit C (mg)	Selenium (mcg)
									Sat	Mono	Poly	Trans								
Tomato sauce	½	cup(s)	112	46	2	8	2	1	0.18	0.29	0.72	0	0	21	1.08	199	0.39	15	15	1
Tomatoes, fresh, ripe, red	1	item(s)	123	22.13	1.08	4.82	1.47	0.24	0.05	0.06	0.16	—	0	12.3	0.33	6.15	0.66	18.45	15.62	0
Tomatoes, stewed, canned, red	½	cup(s)	128	33	1	8	—	<1	0.03	0.04	0.10	—	0	43	1.70	282	1.06	6	10	1
Tortilla chips, plain	6	item(s)	28	142	2	18	2	7	1.43	4.39	1.03	—	0	44	0.43	150	1	3	0	2
Tortillas, corn, soft	1	item(s)	26	58	2	12	1	1	0.09	0.17	0.29	—	0	46	0.36	42	0.07	26	0	1
Tortillas, flour	1	item(s)	32	104	3	18	1	2	0.56	1.21	0.34	—	0	40	1.06	153	0.06	33	0	7
Tuna, light, canned in oil, drained	2	ounce(s)	57	113	17	0	0	5	0.87	1.68	1.64	—	10	7	0.79	202	0.50	3	0	43
Tuna, light, canned in water, drained	2	ounce(s)	57	66	14	0	0	<1	0.13	0.09	0.19	—	17	6	0.87	192	0.19	2	0	46
Turkey, breast, processed, oven roasted, fat free	1	slice(s)	28	25	4	1	0	0	0.00	0.00	0.00	0	10	0	0.00	330	—	—	0	—
Turkey, breast, processed, traditional carved	2	slice(s)	45	40	9	0	0	1	0.00	0.07	0.14	—	20	0	0.72	540	—	—	0	—
Turkey, roasted, dark meat, meat only	3	ounce(s)	85	159	24	0	0	6	2.06	1.39	1.84	—	72	27	1.98	67	0.54	8	0	35
Turkey, roasted, light meat, meat only	3	ounce(s)	85	133	25	0	0	3	0.88	0.48	0.73	—	59	16	1.15	54	0.08	5	0	27
Turnip greens, chopped, boiled, drained	½	cup(s)	72	14	1	3	3	<1	0.04	0.01	0.07	—	0	99	0.58	21	1.35	85	20	1
Turnips, cubed, boiled, drained	½	cup(s)	78	17	1	4	2	<.1	0.01	0.00	0.03	—	0	26	0.14	12	0.02	7	9	<1
Vegetables, mixed, canned, drained	½	cup(s)	82	40	2	8	2	<.1	0.04	0.01	0.10	—	0	22	0.86	121	0.28	20	4	<1
Vinegar, balsamic	1	tablespoon(s)	15	10	0	2	0	0	0.00	—	—	—	0	0	0.00	0	—	0	0	0
Waffle, plain, frozen, toasted	2	item(s)	66	174	4	27	2	5	0.95	2.12	1.84	—	16	153	2.95	519	0.65	36	0	11
Walnuts, dried black, chopped	¼	cup(s)	31	193	8	3	2	18	1.05	4.69	10.96	—	0	19	0.98	1	0.56	10	1	5
Watermelon	½	cup(s)	77	23	<1	6	<1	<1	0.01	0.03	0.04	—	0	5	0.19	1	0.04	2	6	<1
Wheat germ, crude	2	tablespoon(s)	14	52	3	7	2	1	0.24	0.20	0.86	—	0	6	0.90	2	0.02	40	0	11
Wine cooler	10	fluid ounce(s)	300	150	<1	18	<.1	<.1	0.01	0.00	0.02	0	0	17	0.81	25	0.00	5	<.1	—
Wine, red, California	5	fluid ounce(s)	150	125	<1	4	0	0	0.00	0.00	0.00	0	0	12	1.43	15	0.00	1	0	—
Wine, sparkling, domestic	5	fluid ounce(s)	150	105	<1	4	0	0	0.00	0.00	0.00	—	0	13	0.47	7	—	0	0	<1
Wine, white	5	fluid ounce(s)	148	100	<1	1	0	0	0.00	0.00	0.00	0	0	—	0.00	—	—	0	0	—
Yogurt, custard style, fruit flavors	6	ounce(s)	170	190	7	32	0	4	2.00	—	—	—	15	200	0.00	90	—	—	0	—
Yogurt, fruit, low fat	1	cup(s)	245	243	10	46	0	3	1.82	0.77	0.08	—	12	338	0.15	130	0.05	22	1	7
Yogurt, fruit, nonfat, sweetened w/low calorie sweetener	1	cup(s)	241	122	11	19	1	<1	0.21	0.10	0.04	—	3	370	0.62	139	0.17	26	1	7
Yogurt, plain, low fat	1	cup(s)	245	154	13	17	0	4	2.45	1.04	0.11	—	15	448	0.20	172	0.05	27	2	8
VEGETARIAN FOODS																				
Prepared																				
Macaroni & cheese (lacto)	8	ounce(s)	226	181	8	17	<1	9	4.37	2.88	0.89	—	22	187	0.77	768	0.29	39	<1	16
Steamed rice & vegetables (vegan)	8	ounce(s)	228	265	5	40	3	10	1.84	3.91	4.07	—	0	41	1.43	1403	3.05	28	13	8
Vegan spinach enchiladas (vegan)	1	piece(s)	82	93	5	15	2	2	0.34	0.55	1.27	—	0	117	1.13	134	—	46	1	5
Vegetable chow mein (vegan)	8	ounce(s)	227	166	6	22	2	6	0.65	2.66	2.47	—	0	190	3.65	371	0.06	47	7	6
Vegetable lasagna (lacto)	8	ounce(s)	225	177	12	25	2	4	1.92	0.93	0.74	—	10	144	1.91	637	0.05	64	15	19
Vegetarian chili (vegan)	8	ounce(s)	227	116	6	21	7	2	0.24	0.29	0.34	—	1	68	2.42	383	0.15	58	16	5
Vegetarian vegetable soup (vegan)	8	ounce(s)	226	92	3	14	2	4	0.77	1.67	1.30	—	0	37	1.32	503	0.55	38	24	1
Boca burger																				
All American flamed grilled patty	1	item(s)	71	110	14	6	4	4	1.00	—	—	—	3	150	1.80	370	—	—	0	—
Boca meatless ground burger	½	cup(s)	57	70	11	7	4	1	0.00	—	—	—	0	80	1.44	220	—	—	0	—
Breakfast links	2	item(s)	45	100	10	6	6	4	0.00	—	—	—	0	60	1.44	330	—	—	0	—
Breakfast patties	1	item(s)	38	80	8	5	3	4	0.00	—	—	—	0	60	1.44	260	—	—	0	—
Vegan original patty	1	item(s)	71	90	13	4	0	1	0.00	—	—	0	0	80	1.80	350	—	1	1	—
Gardenburger																				
Black bean burger	1	item(s)	71	80	8	11	4	2	0.00	—	—	—	0	40	1.44	330	—	—	0	—
Chik'n grill	1	item(s)	71	100	13	5	3	3	0.00	—	—	—	0	60	3.60	360	—	—	0	—
Meatless breakfast sausage	1	item(s)	43	50	5	2	2	4	0.00	—	—	—	0	20	0.72	120	—	—	0	—
Meatless meatballs	6	item(s)	85	110	12	8	4	5	1.00	—	—	—	0	60	1.80	400	—	—	0	—
Original	3	ounce(s)	85	132	7	19	4	4	1.80	1.80	0.60	—	24	72	0.00	672	—	12	1	8
Morningstar Farms																				
America's Original Veggie Dog links	1	item(s)	57	80	11	6	1	1	0.00	0.00	0.00	—	0	0	0.72	580	—	—	0	—
Better n Eggs egg substitute	¼	cup(s)	57	20	5	0	0	0	0.00	0.00	0.00	—	0	20	0.63	90	—	24	0	—
Breakfast links	2	item(s)	45	80	9	3	2	3	0.50	0.50	2.00	—	0	0	1.44	320	—	—	0	—
Breakfast strips	2	item(s)	16	60	2	2	1	5	0.50	1.00	3.00	—	0	0	0.27	220	—	—	0	—
Garden veggie patties	1	item(s)	67	100	10	9	4	3	0.50	0.50	1.50	—	0	40	0.72	350	—	—	0	—
Spicy black bean veggie burger	1	item(s)	78	150	11	16	5	5	0.50	1.50	2.50	—	0	40	1.80	470	—	—	0	—

MIXED FOODS, SOUPS, SANDWICHES

Mixed Dishes

Food	Amt	Unit																	
Bean burrito	1	item(s)	149	327	17	33	6	15	8.30	4.73	0.85	0	38	331	2.95	514	0.01	115	4	18
Beef & vegetable fajita	1	item(s)	223	397	23	35	3	18	5.50	7.53	3.45	—	45	84	3.74	757	0.80	23	27	—
Chicken & vegetables w/broccoli, onion, bamboo shoots in soy based sauce	1	cup(s)	162	287	22	6	1	19	5.13	7.65	4.68	—	84	22	1.38	962	1.12	13	8	—
Chicken cacciatore	1	cup(s)	230	266	28	5	1	14	3.98	5.78	3.11	0	103	45	2.21	451	0.00	15	8	22
Chicken Waldorf salad	½	cup(s)	100	178	14	6	1	11	1.76	3.18	5.05	0	42	20	0.78	246	0.62	15	2	11
Fettucine alfredo	1	cup(s)	222	247	11	42	1	3	1.61	0.79	0.43	0	9	153	1.88	386	0.00	103	1	35
Hummus	½	cup(s)	123	218	6	25	5	11	1.38	6.04	2.56	0	0	60	1.93	298	0.92	73	10	3
Lasagna w/ ground beef	1	cup(s)	237	288	18	22	2	15	7.47	4.84	0.84	—	68	222	2.33	493	0.22	50	10	22
Macaroni & cheese	1	cup(s)	200	393	15	40	1	19	8.18	6.72	2.66	0	30	323	2.26	800	0.72	12	<1	—
Meat loaf	1	slice(s)	115	244	17	7	<1	16	6.15	6.89	0.83	—	85	54	2.09	423	0.00	20	<1	17
Potato salad	½	cup(s)	125	179	3	14	2	10	1.79	3.10	4.67	—	85	24	0.81	661	—	9	13	5
Spaghetti & meatballs w/ tomato sauce, prepared	1	cup(s)	248	330	19	39	3	12	3.90	4.40	2.20	—	89	124	3.70	1009	—	—	22	22

Soups

Food	Amt	Unit																	
Spicy thai noodles (pad thai)	8	ounce(s)	231	222	9	36	3	6	0.83	3.33	1.83	0	37	32	1.58	598	0.36	44	22	3
Sushi w/ vegetables in seaweed	6	piece(s)	156	182	3	41	1	<1	0.10	0.11	0.11	—	0	20	1.54	153	0.12	10	2	—
Tuna salad	½	cup(s)	103	192	16	10	0	9	1.58	2.96	4.23	—	13	17	1.03	412	0.00	8	2	42
Chicken noodle, condensed, prepared w/water	1	cup(s)	241	75	4	9	1	2	0.65	1.11	0.55	0	7	17	0.77	1106	0.10	22	<1	6
Cream of chicken, condensed, prepared w/milk	1	cup(s)	248	191	7	15	<1	11	4.64	4.46	1.64	—	27	181	0.67	1047	—	7	1	8
Cream of mushroom, condensed, prepared w/milk	1	cup(s)	248	203	6	15	<1	14	5.13	2.98	4.61	—	20	179	0.60	918	1.24	10	2	4
Manhattan clam chowder, condensed, prepared w/water	1	cup(s)	244	78	2	12	1	2	0.38	0.38	1.29	—	2	27	1.63	578	0.34	10	4	9
Minestrone, condensed, prepared w/water	1	cup(s)	241	82	4	11	1	3	0.55	0.70	1.11	—	2	34	0.92	911	—	36	1	8
New England clam chowder, condensed, prepared w/milk	1	cup(s)	248	164	9	17	1	7	2.95	2.26	1.09	—	22	186	1.49	992	0.45	10	3	13
Split pea	1	cup(s)	165	85	4	19	2	<1	0.07	0.03	0.18	0	0	30	1.25	608	0.00	61	9	<1
Tomato, condensed, prepared w/milk	1	cup(s)	248	161	6	22	3	6	2.90	1.61	1.12	—	17	159	1.81	744	1.24	17	68	2
Tomato, condensed, prepared w/water	1	cup(s)	244	85	2	17	<1	2	0.37	0.44	0.95	—	0	12	1.76	695	2.32	15	66	<1
Vegetable beef, condensed, prepared w/water	1	cup(s)	244	78	6	10	<1	2	0.85	0.81	0.12	—	5	17	1.12	791	0.37	10	2	4
Vegetarian vegetable, condensed, prepared w/water	1	cup(s)	241	72	2	12	2	2	0.29	0.82	0.72	0	0	22	1.08	822	—	10	1	4

Sandwiches

Food	Amt	Unit																	
Bacon, lettuce, & tomato w/ mayonnaise	1	item(s)	164	349	11	34	2	19	4.54	7.22	6.07	—	20	76	2.54	837	1.16	31	15	—
Cheeseburger, large, plain	1	item(s)	185	609	30	47	0	33	14.84	12.74	2.44	—	96	91	5.46	1589	—	74	0	39
Cheeseburger, large, w/bacon, vegetables, & condiments	1	item(s)	195	608	32	37	2	37	16.24	14.49	2.71	—	111	162	4.74	1043	—	86	2	33
Club w/bacon, chicken, tomato, lettuce, & mayonnaise	1	item(s)	246	555	31	48	3	26	5.94	—	—	—	72	116	4.05	855	1.53	48	9	—
Cold cut submarine w/cheese & vegetables	1	item(s)	228	456	22	51	2	19	6.81	8.23	2.28	—	36	189	2.51	1651	—	87	12	31
Egg salad	1	item(s)	126	278	10	29	1	13	2.96	3.97	4.79	—	217	107	2.60	494	0.13	82	1	24
Hamburger, double patty, large, w/ condiments & vegetables	1	item(s)	226	540	34	40	0	27	10.52	10.33	2.80	—	122	102	5.85	791	—	77	1	26
Hamburger, large, plain	1	item(s)	137	426	23	32	2	23	8.38	9.88	2.14	—	71	74	3.58	474	—	60	0	27
Hot dog w/ bun, plain	1	item(s)	98	242	10	18	2	15	5.11	6.85	1.71	—	44	24	2.31	670	—	48	<.1	26
Pastrami	1	item(s)	134	331	14	27	2	18	6.18	8.74	1.02	—	51	68	2.64	1335	0.27	21	2	—
Peanut butter & jelly	1	item(s)	93	330	11	42	3	15	3.00	6.87	3.82	—	1	68	2.11	409	2.02	37	<1	—

FAST FOOD

Arby's

Food	Amt	Unit																	
Au jus sauce	1	serving(s)	85	5	<1	1	<1	<1	0.02	—	—	—	0	0	0.00	386	—	—	0	—
Beef 'n cheddar sandwich	1	item(s)	198	480	23	43	2	24	8.00	—	—	—	90	100	3.60	1240	—	—	1	—
Curly fries, medium	1	serving(s)	128	400	5	50	4	20	5.00	—	—	—	0	0	1.80	990	—	—	15	—
Market Fresh grilled chicken Caesar salad w/o dressing	1	serving(s)	338	230	33	8	3	8	3.50	—	—	—	80	200	1.80	920	—	—	42	—
Roast beef deluxe sandwich, light	1	item(s)	182	296	18	33	6	10	3.00	5.00	2.00	—	42	130	4.50	826	—	—	8	—
Roast beef sandwich, giant	1	item(s)	228	480	32	41	3	23	10.00	—	—	—	110	60	5.40	1440	—	—	0	—

Food Description	Qty	Measure	Wt (g)	Ener (cal)	Prot (g)	Carb (g)	Dietary Fiber (g)	Fat (g)	Sat	Mono	Poly	Trans	Chol (mg)	Calc (mg)	Iron (mg)	Sodi (mg)	Vit E (mg)	Folate (mcg)	Vit C (mg)	Selenium (mcg)
									| Fat Breakdown (g)											
FAST FOOD (continued)																				
Roast beef sandwich, regular	1	item(s)	157	350	21	34	2	16	6.00	—	—	—	85	60	3.60	950	—	—	0	—
Roast chicken deluxe sandwich, light	1	item(s)	194	260	23	33	3	5	1.00	—	—	—	40	100	2.70	1010	—	—	2	—
Burger King																				
BK Broiler chicken sandwich	1	item(s)	258	550	30	52	3	25	5.00	—	—	—	105	60	3.60	1110	—	—	6	—
Croissanwich w/sausage, egg, & cheese	1	item(s)	157	520	19	24	1	39	14.00	—	—	1.93	210	300	4.50	1090	—	—	0	—
Fish Fillet sandwich	1	item(s)	185	520	18	44	2	30	8.00	—	—	1.12	55	150	2.70	840	—	—	1	—
French fries, medium, salted	1	item(s)	117	360	4	46	4	18	5.00	—	—	4.50	0	20	0.72	640	—	—	9	—
Onion rings, medium	1	serving(s)	91	320	4	40	3	16	4.00	—	—	3.50	0	97	0.00	460	—	—	0	—
Whopper	1	item(s)	291	710	31	52	4	43	13.00	—	—	1	85	150	6.30	980	—	—	9	—
Whopper w/cheese	1	item(s)	316	800	36	53	4	50	18.00	—	—	2	110	250	6.30	1420	—	—	9	—
Chick Fil-A																				
Chargrilled chicken garden salad	1	item(s)	275	180	22	9	3	6	3.00	—	—	0	70	150	0.72	660	—	—	30	—
Chargrilled deluxe chicken sandwich	1	item(s)	195	290	27	31	3	7	1.50	—	—	0	70	80	1.80	990	—	—	5	—
Chicken biscuit w/cheese	1	item(s)	151	450	19	43	2	23	7.00	—	—	2.85	45	150	2.70	1430	—	—	0	—
Chicken salad sandwich	1	item(s)	153	350	20	32	5	15	3.00	—	—	0	65	150	1.80	880	—	—	0	—
Chick-n-Strips	4	item(s)	127	290	29	14	1	13	2.50	—	—	0	65	20	0.36	730	—	—	1	—
Coleslaw	1	item(s)	105	210	1	14	2	17	2.50	—	—	0	20	40	0.36	180	—	—	27	—
Dairy Queen																				
Banana split	1	item(s)	369	510	8	96	3	12	8.00	3.00	0.50	0	30	250	1.80	180	—	—	15	—
Chocolate chip cookie dough blizzard, small	1	item(s)	319	720	12	105	0	28	14.00	—	—	2.50	50	350	2.70	370	—	—	1	—
Chocolate malt, small	1	item(s)	418	650	15	111	0	16	10.00	—	—	0.50	55	450	1.80	370	—	—	2	—
Vanilla soft serve	½	cup(s)	94	140	3	22	0	5	3.00	—	—	0	15	150	0.72	70	—	—	0	—
Domino's																				
Classic hand tossed pizza																				
America's favorite feast, 12"	2	slice(s)	205	508	22	57	4	22	9.20	—	—	—	49	202	3.70	1221	—	—	1	—
Pepperoni feast, extra pepperoni & cheese, 12"	2	slice(s)	196	534	24	56	3	25	10.92	—	—	—	57	279	3.36	1349	—	—	<1	—
Vegi feast, 12"	2	slice(s)	203	439	19	57	4	16	7.09	—	—	—	34	279	3.44	987	—	—	1	—
Thin crust pizza																				
Extravaganzza, 12"	¼	item(s)	159	425	20	34	3	24	9.41	—	—	—	53	245	1.95	1408	—	—	1	—
Pepperoni, extra pepperoni & cheese, 12"	¼	item(s)	159	420	20	32	2	24	10.46	—	—	—	54	316	1.34	1362	—	—	<1	—
Ultimate deep dish pizza																				
America's favorite, 12"	2	slice(s)	235	617	26	59	4	33	12.88	—	—	—	58	334	4.43	1573	—	—	1	—
Pepperoni, extra pepperoni & cheese, 12"	2	slice(s)	235	629	26	57	4	34	13.57	—	—	—	61	332	4.25	1650	—	—	1	—
Vegi, 12"	2	slice(s)	235	547	22	59	4	26	10.19	—	—	—	41	333	4.33	1334	—	—	2	—
In-n-Out Burger																				
Cheeseburger w/mustard & ketchup	1	item(s)	268	400	22	41	3	18	9.00	—	—	—	55	200	3.60	1080	—	—	15	—
Chocolate shake	1	item(s)	425	690	9	83	0	36	24.00	—	—	—	95	300	0.72	350	—	—	0	—
Double-Double cheeseburger w/mustard & ketchup	1	item(s)	328	590	37	42	3	32	17.00	—	—	—	115	350	5.40	1510	—	—	15	—
French fries	1	item(s)	125	400	7	54	2	18	5.00	—	—	—	0	20	1.80	245	—	—	0	—
Hamburger w/mustard & ketchup	1	item(s)	243	310	16	41	3	10	4.00	—	—	—	35	40	3.60	720	—	—	15	—
Jack in the Box																				
Chicken club salad	1	item(s)	535	310	28	15	5	16	6.00	—	—	0	65	300	3.60	890	—	—	54	—
Hamburger	1	item(s)	104	250	12	30	2	9	3.50	—	—	0.88	30	100	3.60	610	—	—	0	—
Jack's Spicy Chicken sandwich	1	item(s)	253	580	24	53	3	31	6.00	—	—	2.81	60	150	1.80	950	—	—	9	—
Jumbo Jack hamburger w/cheese	1	item(s)	294	690	26	60	3	38	16.00	—	—	1.55	75	250	4.50	1360	—	—	9	—
Sourdough Jack	1	item(s)	244	700	30	36	3	49	16.00	—	—	2.98	80	200	4.50	1220	—	—	9	—
Jamba Juice																				
Banana berry smoothie	24	fluid ounce(s)	719	470	5	112	5	2	0.50	—	—	—	5	200	1.08	85	0.32	33	15	0
Chocolate mood smoothie	24	fluid ounce(s)	612	690	16	142	2	8	4.50	—	—	—	25	500	1.08	280	0.00	9	6	4
Jamba powerboost smoothie	24	fluid ounce(s)	730	440	6	103	7	2	0.00	—	—	—	0	1100	1.44	40	17.71	640	294	70

Orange juice, freshly squeezed	16	fluid ounce(s)	496	220	3	52	1	1	0.00	—	—	—	0	60	1.08	0	—	160	246	0
Protein berry pizzaz smoothie	24	fluid ounce(s)	710	440	20	92	6	2	0.00	—	—	—	0	1100	2.62	240	0.31	58	60	4
Kentucky Fried Chicken (KFC)																				
Extra Crispy chicken, breast	1	item(s)	162	470	34	19	0	28	8.00	—	—	4.50	135	19	1.44	1230	—	—	1	—
Hot & spicy chicken, whole wing	1	item(s)	55	180	11	9	0	11	3.00	—	—	0	60	10	0.72	420	—	—	1	—
Original Recipe chicken, drumstick	1	item(s)	59	140	14	4	0	8	2.00	—	—	1	75	10	0.70	440	—	—	1	—
Long John Silver's																				
Baked cod	1	serving(s)	101	120	22	1	0	5	1.00	—	—	—	90	20	0.72	240	—	—	0	—
Batter dipped fish sandwich	1	item(s)	177	440	17	48	3	20	5.00	—	—	—	35	60	3.60	1120	—	—	9	—
Clam chowder	1	item(s)	227	220	9	23	0	10	4.00	—	—	—	25	150	0.72	810	—	—	0	—
Crunchy shrimp basket	21	item(s)	114	340	12	32	2	19	5.00	—	—	—	105	500	1.80	720	—	—	1	—
McDonald's																				
Big Mac hamburger	1	item(s)	216	590	24	47	3	34	11.00	—	—	1.48	85	300	4.50	1090	—	—	4	—
Cheeseburger	1	item(s)	121	330	15	36	2	14	6.00	—	—	1.02	45	250	2.70	830	—	—	2	—
Chicken McNuggets	4	item(s)	72	210	10	12	1	13	2.50	—	—	1.13	35	20	0.72	460	—	—	1	—
Egg McMuffin	1	item(s)	138	300	18	29	2	12	4.50	—	—	0.42	235	300	2.70	830	0.72	—	1	—
Filet-o-fish sandwich	1	item(s)	156	470	15	45	1	26	5.00	—	—	1.11	50	200	1.80	890	—	—	1	—
French fries, small	1	serving(s)	68	210	3	26	2	10	1.50	—	—	2.30	0	10	0.36	135	—	—	9	—
Fruit n' yogurt parfait	1	item(s)	338	380	10	76	2	5	2.00	—	—	0.18	15	300	1.80	240	—	—	24	—
Hash browns	1	item(s)	53	130	1	14	1	8	1.50	—	—	2	0	10	0.36	330	—	—	2	—
Honey sauce	1	item(s)	14	45	0	12	0	0	0.00	0.00	0.00	—	0	10	0.18	0	—	—	1	—
McSalad Shaker garden salad	1	item(s)	149	100	7	4	2	6	3.00	—	—	—	75	150	1.08	120	—	—	15	—
McSalad Shaker grilled chicken caesar salad	1	item(s)	163	100	17	3	2	3	1.50	—	—	—	40	100	1.08	240	—	—	12	—
Newman's Own creamy Caesar salad dressing	1	item(s)	59	190	2	4	0	18	3.50	—	—	0.29	20	60	0.18	500	15.40	—	1	—
Plain hotcakes w/syrup & margarine	3	item(s)	228	600	9	104	0	17	3.00	—	—	4	20	100	4.50	770	—	—	1	—
Quarter Pounder hamburger	1	item(s)	172	430	23	37	2	21	8.00	—	—	1.01	70	200	4.50	840	—	—	2	—
Quarter Pounder hamburger w/cheese	1	item(s)	200	530	28	38	2	30	13.00	—	—	1.51	95	350	4.50	1310	—	—	2	—
Sausage McMuffin w/egg	1	item(s)	164	450	20	29	2	28	10.00	—	—	0.59	255	300	2.70	930	0.72	—	1	—
Vanilla milkshake	8	fluid ounce(s)	227	254	9	40	0	7	4.28	1.98	0.26	—	27	331	0.23	215	0.11	16	0	5
Pizza Hut																				
Pepperoni Lovers stuffed crust pizza	1	slice(s)	171	480	23	44	3	24	11.00	—	—	1.05	65	300	2.70	1300	—	—	4	—
Pepperoni Lovers thin 'n crispy pizza	1	slice(s)	94	270	13	22	2	14	7.00	—	—	0.51	40	200	1.44	700	—	—	2	—
Personal Pan supreme pizza	1	slice(s)	73	170	8	19	1	7	3.00	—	—	0.95	15	80	1.86	400	—	—	4	—
Veggie Lovers stuffed crust pizza	1	slice(s)	181	370	17	45	3	14	7.00	—	—	0.53	35	250	2.70	980	—	—	12	—
Veggie Lovers thin 'n crispy pizza	1	slice(s)	110	190	8	23	2	7	3.00	—	—	0.54	15	150	1.44	480	—	—	12	—
Starbucks																				
Cappuccino, tall	12	fluid ounce(s)	360	120	7	10	0	6	4.00	—	—	—	25	250	0.00	95	—	—	1	—
Cinnamon spice mocha, tall nonfat w/o whipped cream	12	fluid ounce(s)	360	170	11	32	0	0	0.50	0.00	0.00	0	5	300	0.72	150	—	—	0	—
Frappuccino, tall chocolate	12	fluid ounce(s)	360	290	13	52	1	5	1.00	—	—	—	3	400	1.80	300	—	—	5	—
Latte, tall w/nonfat milk	12	fluid ounce(s)	360	123	12	17	0	1	0.40	0.16	0.02	0	6	420	0.18	174	—	18	4	—
Latte, tall w/whole milk	12	fluid ounce(s)	360	212	11	17	0	11	6.90	3.24	0.42	—	46	400	0.18	165	—	17	3	—
Macchiato, tall caramel w/whole milk	12	fluid ounce(s)	360	190	6	27	0	7	4.00	—	—	—	25	200	0.36	105	—	—	1	—
Tazo chai black tea, tall nonfat	12	fluid ounce(s)	360	170	6	37	0	0	0.00	0.00	0.00	0	5	200	0.36	95	—	—	0	—
Subway																				
Chocolate chip cookie	1	item(s)	48	209	3	29	1	10	3.50	—	—	1.07	12	0	1.00	135	—	—	0	—
Classic Italian B.M.T. sandwich, 6″, white bread	1	item(s)	250	453	21	40	3	24	8.00	—	—	0	56	100	2.70	1740	—	—	24	—
Meatball sandwich, 6″, white bread	1	item(s)	284	501	23	46	4	25	10.00	—	—	0.75	56	100	3.60	1350	—	—	24	—
Roast beef sandwich, 6″, white bread	1	item(s)	220	264	18	39	3	5	1.00	—	—	0	20	40	3.60	840	—	—	24	—
Roasted chicken breast sandwich, 6″, white bread	1	item(s)	234	311	25	40	3	6	1.50	—	—	0	48	60	3.60	880	—	—	24	—
Tuna sandwich, 6″, white bread	1	item(s)	252	419	18	39	3	21	5.00	—	—	—	42	100	2.70	1180	—	—	24	—
Turkey breast sandwich, 6″, white bread	1	item(s)	220	254	16	39	3	4	1.00	—	—	0	15	40	2.70	1000	—	—	24	—
Taco Bell																				
7-layer burrito	1	item(s)	283	530	18	67	10	22	8.00	—	—	3	25	300	3.59	1360	—	—	5	—
Beef burrito supreme	1	item(s)	248	440	18	51	7	18	8.00	—	—	2	40	200	2.70	1330	—	—	9	—
Grilled chicken burrito	1	item(s)	198	390	19	49	3	13	4.00	—	—	—	40	151	1.44	1240	—	—	2	—
Taco	1	item(s)	78	170	8	13	3	10	4.00	—	—	0.50	25	60	1.08	350	—	—	2	—
Veggie fajita wrap supreme	1	item(s)	255	470	11	55	3	22	7.00	—	—	—	30	150	1.44	990	—	—	6	—

CONVENIENCE MEALS

Food Description	Qty	Measure	Wt (g)	Ener (cal)	Prot (g)	Carb (g)	Dietary Fiber (g)	Fat (g)	Sat	Mono	Poly	Trans	Chol (mg)	Calc (mg)	Iron (mg)	Sodi (mg)	Vit E (mg)	Folate (mcg)	Vit C (mg)	Selenium (mcg)
Budget Gourmet																				
Cheese manicotti w/meat sauce	1	item(s)	284	420	18	38	4	22	11.00	6.00	1.34	—	85	300	2.70	810	—	31	0	—
Chicken w/fettuccine	1	item(s)	284	380	20	33	3	19	10.00	—	—	—	85	100	2.70	810	—	—	0	—
Light beef stroganoff	1	item(s)	248	290	20	32	3	7	4.00	—	—	—	35	40	1.80	580	—	19	2	—
Light sirloin of beef in herb sauce	1	item(s)	269	260	19	30	5	7	4.00	2.30	0.31	—	30	40	1.80	850	—	38	6	—
Light vegetable lasagna	1	item(s)	298	290	15	36	5	9	1.79	0.89	0.60	—	15	283	3.03	780	—	75	59	—
Healthy Choice																				
Chicken enchilada suprema meal	1	item(s)	320	360	13	59	8	7	3.00	2.00	2.00	—	30	40	1.44	580	—	—	4	—
Lemon pepper fish meal	1	item(s)	303	280	11	49	5	5	2.00	1.00	2.00	—	30	40	0.36	580	—	—	30	—
Traditional salisbury steak meal	1	item(s)	354	360	23	45	5	9	3.50	4.00	1.00	—	45	80	2.70	580	—	—	21	—
Traditional turkey breasts meal	1	item(s)	298	330	21	50	4	5	2.00	1.50	1.50	—	35	40	1.44	600	—	—	0	—
Zucchini lasagna	1	item(s)	383	280	13	47	5	4	2.50	—	—	—	10	200	1.80	310	—	—	0	—
Stouffers																				
Cheese enchiladas with mexican rice	1	serving(s)	276	370	12	48	5	14	5.00	—	—	—	25	200	1.44	890	—	—	12	—
Chicken pot pie	1	item(s)	284	740	23	56	4	47	18.00	12.41	10.48	—	65	150	2.70	1170	—	—	2	—
Homestyle beef pot roast & potatoes	1	item(s)	252	270	16	25	3	12	4.50	—	—	—	35	20	1.80	820	—	—	6	—
Homestyle roast turkey breast w/stuffing & mashed potatoes	1	item(s)	273	300	16	34	2	11	3.00	—	—	—	35	40	0.72	1190	—	—	0	—
Lean Cuisine Everyday Favorites chicken chow mein w/rice	1	item(s)	255	210	12	33	2	3	1.00	1.00	0.50	0	30	20	0.36	620	—	—	0	—
Lean Cuisine Everyday Favorites lasagna w/meat sauce	1	item(s)	291	300	19	41	3	8	4.00	2.00	0.50	0	30	200	1.08	650	—	—	5	—
Weight Watchers																				
Smart Ones chicken enchiladas suiza entree	1	serving(s)	255	270	15	33	2	9	3.50	—	—	—	50	250	1.08	660	—	—	4	—
Smart Ones garden lasagna entree	1	item(s)	312	270	14	36	5	7	3.50	—	—	—	30	350	1.80	610	—	—	6	—
Smart Ones pepperoni pizza	1	item(s)	158	390	23	46	4	12	4.00	—	—	—	45	450	1.80	650	—	—	5	—
Smart Ones spicy penne pasta & ricotta	1	item(s)	289	280	11	45	4	6	2.00	—	—	—	5	150	2.70	400	—	—	6	—
Smart Ones spicy Szechuan style vegetables & chicken	1	item(s)	255	220	11	39	3	2	0.50	—	—	—	10	150	1.80	730	—	—	2	—

Notes and Suggested Readings

Chapter 1:

Notes

1. World Health Organization, *Global Strategy on Diet, Physical Activity, and Health,* http://who.int/dietphysicalactivity/en/, downloaded June 4, 2009.
2. U.S. Department of Health and Human Services, Office of the Surgeon General, *Disease Prevention,* http://surgeongeneral .gov/publichealthpriorities.html#disease, downloaded June 5, 2009.
3. U.S. Department of Health and Human Services, Centers for Disease Control and Prevention, National Center for Health Statistics, *National Vital Statistics Reports, Deaths: Preliminary Data for 2008,* 59, no. 2 (December 9, 2010).
4. American Heart Association, *Heart Disease & Stroke Statistics—2010 Update* (Dallas: American Heart Association, 2010).
5. American Cancer Society, *2010 Cancer Facts and Figures* (New York: ACS, 2010).
6. American College of Sports Medicine, *ACSM's Guidelines for Exercise Testing and Prescription* (Philadelphia: Wolters Kluwer/ Lippincott Williams & Wilkins, 2010).
7. National Academy of Sciences, Institute of Medicine, *Dietary Reference Intakes for Energy, Carbohydrates, Fiber, Fat, Fatty Acids, Cholesterol, Protein and Amino Acids (Macronutrients)* (Washington, DC: National Academy Press, 2005).
8. U.S. Department of Health and Human Services and Department of Agriculture, *Dietary Guidelines for Americans, 2005* (Washington, DC: DHHS, 2005).
9. W. L. Haskell, et al., "Physical Activity and Public Health: Updated Recommendation for Adults from the American College of Sports Medicine and the American Heart Association," *Medicine & Science in Sports & Exercise* 39 (2007): 1423-1434.
10. U.S. Department of Health and Human Services, *Physical Activity and Health: A Report of the Surgeon General* (Atlanta, GA: Centers for Disease Control and Prevention, National Center for Chronic Disease Prevention and Health Promotion, 1996).
11. U.S. Department of Health and Human Services, *2008 Physical Activity Guidelines for Americans,* http://health.gov/paguidelines, downloaded October 15, 2008.
12. See Haskell, et al., note 9.
13. American College of Sports Medicine, *Exercise Is Medicine,* http://www.exerciseismedicine.org/, downloaded March 4, 2011.
14. U.S. Department of Health and Human Services, *Healthy People 2020* (Washington, DC, 2010).
15. W. W. K. Hoeger, L. Bond, L. Ransdell, J. M. Shimon, and S. Merugu, "One-Mile Step Count at Walking and Running Speeds," *ACSM Health & Fitness Journal,* 11, no. 1 (2008): 14-19.
16. L. Sax et al., *The American Freshman: National Norms for Fall 2000* (Los Angeles: University of California-Los Angeles, Higher Education Research Institute, 2000).
17. H. G. Koenig, "The Healing Power of Faith," *Bottom Line/ Health* 18 (May 2004): 3-4.
18. L. Dossey, "Can Spirituality Improve Your Health?" *Bottom Line/Health* 15 (July 2001): 11-13.
19. R. S. Paffenbarger, Jr., R. T. Hyde, A. L. Wing, and C. H. Steinmetz, "A Natural History of Athleticism and Cardiovascular Health," *Journal of the American Medical Association* 252 (1984): 491-495.
20. S. N. Blair, H. W. Kohl III, R. S. Paffenbarger, Jr., D. G. Clark, K. H. Cooper, and L. W. Gibbons, "Physical Fitness and All-Cause Mortality: A Prospective Study of Healthy Men and Women," *Journal of the American Medical Association* 262 (1989): 2395-2401.
21. S. Mandic, et al., "Characterizing Differences in Mortality at the Low End of the Fitness Spectrum," *Medicine & Science in Sports & Exercise* 41 (2009): 1573-1579.
22. E. S. Ford, et al., "Healthy Living is Better Revenge," *Archives of Internal Medicine,* 169 (2009): 1355-1362.
23. S. Kodama, et al., "Cardiorespiratory Fitness as a Quantitative Predictor of All-Cause Mortality and Cardiovascular Events in Healthy Men and Women," *Journal of the American Medical Association* 301 (2010): 2024-2035.
24. D. P. Swain, "Moderate- or Vigorous-Intensity Exercise: What Should We Prescribe?" *ACSM's Health & Fitness Journal* 10, no. 5 (2007): 7-11.
25. P. T. Williams, "Physical Fitness and Activity as Separate Heart Disease Risk Factors: A Meta-analysis," *Medicine & Science in Sports & Exercise* 33 (2001): 754-761.
26. D. P. Swain and B. A. Franklin, "Comparative Cardioprotective Benefits of Vigorous vs. Moderate Intensity Aerobic Exercise," *American Journal of Cardiology* 97 (2006): 141-147.
27. Cooper Institute, Texas Youth Fitness Study (Dallas, TX), http://www.cooperinstitute.org/youth/documents/Texas %20Youth%20Fitness%20Study%20—%20Charts.pdf, downloaded March 9, 2011.
28. J. J. Ratey and E. Hagerman, *Spark: The Revolutionary New Science of Exercise and the Brain* (New York: Little, Brown and Company, 2008).
27. "Wellness Facts," *University of California at Berkeley Wellness Letter* (Palm Coast, FL: The Editors, April 1995).

Suggested Readings

Bouchard, C., S. N. Blair, and W. Haskell. *Physical Activity and Health.* Champaign, IL: Human Kinetics, 2007.

Hoeger, W. W. K., and S. A. Hoeger. *Principles and Labs for Fitness and Wellness.* Belmont, CA: Wadsworth/Cengage Learning, 2012.

Hoeger, W. W. K., and S. A. Hoeger. *Fitness and Wellness.* Belmont, CA: Wadsworth/Cengage Learning, 2013.Hoeger, W. W. K., L. W. Turner, and B. Q. Hafen. *Wellness: Guidelines for a Healthy Lifestyle.* Belmont, CA: Wadsworth/ Thomson Learning, 2007.

National Academy of Sciences, Institute of Medicine. *Dietary Reference Intakes for Energy, Carbohydrates, Fiber, Fat, Fatty Acids, Cholesterol, Protein and Amino Acids (Macronutrients).* Washington, DC: National Academy Press, 2005.

Haskell, W. L., et al., "Physical Activity and Public Health: Updated Recommendation for Adults from the American College of Sports Medicine and the American Heart Association," *Medicine & Science in Sports & Exercise* 39 (2007): 1423-1434.

U.S. Department of Health and Human Services. *2008 Physical Activity Guidelines for Americans,* available at http://www .health.gov/paguidelines.

U.S. Department of Health and Human Services, Public Health Service. *Healthy People 2020,* available at http://www .healthypeople.gov.

Chapter 2

Notes

1. J. Annesi, "Using Emotions to Empower Members for Long-Term Exercise Success," *Fitness Management* 17 (2001): 54-58.
2. P. T. Katzmarzyk, et al., "Sitting Time and Mortality from All Causes, Cardiovascular Disease, and Cancer," *Medicine and Science in Sports and Exercise* 41 (2009): 998-1005.
3. D. W. Dunstan, et al., "Television Viewing Time and Mortality: The Australian Diabetes, Obesity, and Lifestyle Study (AusDiab)," *Circulation* 121 (2010): 384-391.
4. Television Bureau of Advertising, "Time Spent Viewing per TV Home: Per Day Annual Averages," available at http://www.tvb.org/nav/build_frameset.asp?url=/rcentral/index.asp, accessed March 26, 2005.
5. R. Boynton-Jarret, T. N. Thomas, K. E. Peterson, J. Wiecha, A. M. Sobol, and S. L. Gortmaker, "Impact of Television Viewing Patterns on Fruit and Vegetable Consumption among Adolescents," *Pediatrics* 113 (2003): 1321-1326.
6. League of California Cities Planners Institute, Pasadena Conference Center (April 13-15, 2005).
7. J. Pucher and C. Lefevre, *The Urban Transport Crisis in Europe and North America* (London: Macmillan Press Ltd., 1996).
8. S. Gerrior, L. Bente, and H. Hiza, "Nutrient Content of the U.S. Food Supply, 1909-2000," *Home Economics Research Report No. 56* (U.S. Department of Agriculture, Center for Nutrition Policy and Promotion, 2004): 74, available at http://www.usda.gov/cnpp/nutrient_content.html, accessed April 18, 2005.
9. Marion Nestle, *Food Politics* (Berkeley: University of California Press, 2002), 1, 8, 22.
10. "Food Prepared Away from Home Is Increasing and Found to Be Less Nutritious," *Nutrition Research Newsletter* 21, no. 8 (August 2002): 10(2); A. Clauson, "Shares of Food Spending for Eating Reaches 47 Percent," *Food Review* 22 (1999): 20-22.
11. "A Diner's Guide to Health and Nutrition Claims on Restaurant Menus" (Washington, DC: Center for Science in the Public Interest, 1997), available at http://www.cspinet.org/reports/dinersgu.html, accessed March 25, 2005.
12. L. R. Young and M. Nestle, "Expanding Portion Sizes in the U.S. Marketplace: Implications for Nutrition Counseling," *Journal of the American Dietetic Association* 103, no. 2 (February 2003): 231.
13. American Institute for Cancer Research, "As Restaurant Portions Grow, Vast Majority of Americans Still Belong to 'Clean Plate Club,' New Survey Finds," AICR News Release, January 15, 2001.
14. T. V. E. Kral, L. S. Roe, J. S. Meengs, and D. E. Wall, "Increasing the Portion Size of a Packaged Snack Increases Energy Intake," *Appetite* 39 (2002): 86.
15. J. A. Ello-Martin, L. S. Roe, J. S. Meengs, D. E. Wall, and B. J. Rolls, "Increasing the Portion Size of a Unit Food Increases Energy Intake" *Appetite* 39 (2002): 74.
16. B. Wansink, "Can Package Size Accelerate Usage Volume?" *Journal of Marketing* 60 (1996): 1-14.
17. National Alliance for Nutrition and Activity (NANA), "From Wallet to Waistline: The Hidden Costs of Super Sizing," available at http://www.preventioninstitute.org/portionsizerept.html (accessed June 10, 2010).
18. S. H. A. Holt, N. Sandona, and J. C. Brand-Miller, "The Effects of Sugar-Free vs. Sugar-Rich Beverages on Feelings of Fullness and Subsequent Food Intake," *International Journal of Food Sciences and Nutrition* 51, no. 1 (January 2000): 59.
19. "Wellness Facts," *University of California at Berkeley Wellness Letter* (Palm Coast, FL: The Editors, May 2004).
20. G. S. Howard, D. W. Nance, and P. Myers, *Adaptive Counseling and Therapy* (San Francisco: Jossey-Bass, 1987).
21. J. O. Prochaska, J. C. Norcross, and C. C. DiClemente, *Changing for Good* (New York: William Morrow, 1994).

Suggested Readings

Brehm, B. *Successful Fitness Motivation Strategies*. Champaign, IL: Human Kinetics, 2004.

Burgand, M., and K. Gallagher. "Self-Monitoring: Influencing Effective Behavior Change in Your Clients." *ACSM's Health & Fitness Journal* 10, no. 1 (2006): 14-19.

Hagger, M. S., and N. L. D. Chatzisarantis, editors. *Intrinsic Motivation and Self-Determination in Exercise and Sport*. Champaign, IL: Human Kinetics, 2007.

Prochaska, J. O., J. C. Norcross, and C. C. DiClemente. *Changing for Good*. New York: William Morrow, 1994.

Rodgers, W. M., and C. C. Loitz. The Role of Motivation in Behavior Change. *ACSM's Health & Fitness Journal* 13, no 1 (2009): 7-12.

White, M. W., E. L. Mailey, and E. McAuley. Leading a Physically Active Lifestyle. *ACSM's Health & Fitness Journal* 14, no. 1 (2010): 8-15.

Chapter 3

Notes

1. S. Park, A., F. Subar, A. Hollenbeck, and A. Schatzkin, "Dietary Fiber Intake and Mortality in the NIH-AARP Diet and Health Study," Online *Archives of Internal Medicine* (February 14, 2011).
2. National Academy of Sciences, Institute of Medicine, *Dietary Reference Intakes for Energy, Carbohydrates, Fiber, Fat, Protein and Amino Acids (Macronutrients)* (Washington, DC: National Academy Press, 2002).
3. "Saturated Fat: Not Quite so Bad After All?," *University of California at Berkeley Wellness Letter* (June 2010).
4. Editors of Environmental Nutrition. *Healthy Eating: Essential Information for Living Longer and Living Better* (Norwalk, CT: Belvoir Media Group LLC, 2008).
5. J. L. Breslow, "n-3 Fatty Acids and Cardiovascular Disease," *American Journal of Clinical Nutrition* 83 (2006): 1477S-1482S.
6. P. E. Bowen, "Evaluating the Health Claim of Flaxseed and Cancer Prevention," *Nutrition Today* 36 (2001): 144-158; "Flax Facts," *University of California at Berkeley Wellness Letter* (May 2002).
7. See note 2.
8. "Soy and Breast Cancer," *University of California at Berkeley Wellness Letter* (June 2007).
9. A. Trichopoulou, et al., "Adherence to a Mediterranean Diet and Survival in a Greek Population," *New England Journal of Medicine* 348 (2003): 2599-2608.
10. G. Kojda and R. Hambrecht, "Molecular Mechanism of Vascular Adaptations to Exercise: Physical Activity as an Effective Antioxidant Therapy?"" *Cardiovascular Research* 67 (2005): 187-197.
11. G. Bjelakovic, et al., "Mortality in Randomized Trials of Antioxidant Supplements for Primary and Secondary Prevention," *Journal of the American Medical Association* 297 (2007): 842-857.
12. M. L. Neuhouser, et al., "Multivitamin Use and Risk of Cancer and Cardiovascular Disease in the Women's Health Initiative Cohorts," *Archives of Internal Medicine* 169 (2009): 294-304.
13. "Ride the D Train: Research Finds Even More Reasons to Get Vitamin D," *Environmental Nutrition* 28, no. 9 (2005): 1, 4.
14. "Vitamin D May Help You Dodge Cancer: How To Be Sure You Get Enough," *Environmental Nutrition* 30, no. 6 (2007): 1, 4.
15. "Understanding Vitamin D Cholecalciferol," Vitamin D Council, http://www.vitamindcouncil.org, downloaded June 19, 2009.
16. "A Busy B—Maybe Too Busy," *University of California at Berkeley Wellness Letter* 25, no. 12 (2009): 1-2.
17. American Dietetic Association, "Position of the American Dietetic Association: Nutrient Supplementation," *Journal of the American Dietetic Association* 109 (2009): 2073-2085.

18. Writing Group for the Women's Health Initiative, "Risks and Benefits of Combined Estrogen and Progestin in Healthy Postmenopausal Women: Principal Results from the Women's Health Initiative Randomized Controlled Trial," *Journal of the American Medical Association* 288 (2002): 321-333.

19. U.S. Department of Health and Human Services and U.S. Department of Agriculture, *Dietary Guidelines for Americans 2010* (Washington, DC: U.S. Government Printing Office, 2010).

Suggested Readings

Clark, N. *Nancy Clark's Sports Nutrition Guidebook.* Champaign, IL: Human Kinetics, 2008.

Editors of Environmental Nutrition. *Healthy Eating: Essential Information for Living Longer and Living Better.* Norwalk, CT: Belvoir Media Group LLC, 2008.

Editors of Tufts University Nutrition Letter. "Most Multivitamin Extras Don't Add Up." Norwalk, CT, February 2010.

McArdle, W. D., F. I. Katch, and V. L. Katch. *Sports & Exercise Nutrition.* Baltimore: Lippincott Williams & Wilkins, 2008.

National Academy of Sciences, Institute of Medicine. *Dietary Reference Intakes for Energy, Carbohydrates, Fiber, Fat, Protein and Amino Acids (Macronutrients).* Washington, DC: National Academy Press, 2002.

Rolfes, S. R., K. Pinna, and E. N. Whitney. *Understanding Normal and Clinical Nutrition.* Belmont, CA: Wadsworth/Cengage Learning, 2011.

Sizer, F. S., and E. N. Whitney. *Nutrition: Concepts and Controversies.* Belmont, CA: Wadsworth/Cengage Learning, 2011.

Whitney, E. N., and S. R. Rolfes. *Understanding Nutrition.* Belmont, CA: Wadsworth/Cengage Learning, 2011.

Chapter 4

Notes

1. J. Stevens, J. Cai, E. R. Pamuk, D. F. Williamson, M. J. Thun, and J. L. Wood, "The Effect of Age on the Association Between Body Mass Index and Mortality," *New England Journal of Medicine* 338 (1998): 1-7.

2. E. E. Calle, M. J. Thun, J. M. Petrelli, C. Rodriguez, and C. W. Heath, "Body-Mass Index and Mortality in a Prospective Cohort of U.S. Adults," *New England Journal of Medicine* 341 (1999): 1097-1105.

3. K. M. Flegal, et al., "Cause-Specific Excess Deaths Associated with Underweight, Overweight, and Obesity," *Journal of the American Medical Association* 298 (2007): 2028-2037.

4. K. M. Flegal, M. D. Carrol, R. J. Kuczmarski, and C. L. Johnson, "Overweight and Obesity in the United States: Prevalence and Trends, 1960-1994," *International Journal of Obesity and Related Metabolic Disorders* 22 (1998): 39-47.

5. C. Bouchard, G. A. Bray, and V. S. Hubbard, "Basic and Clinical Aspects of Regional Fat Distribution," *American Journal of Clinical Nutrition* 52 (1990): 946-950; G. Hu, et al., "Joint Effects of Physical Activity, Body Mass Index, Waist Circumference, and Waist-to-Hip Ratio on the Risk of Heart Failure," *Circulation* 121 (2010): 237-244; D. Canoy, et al., "Body Fat Distribution and Risk of Coronary Heart Disease in Men and Women in the European Prospective Investigation Into Cancer and Nutrition in Norfolk Cohort," *Circulation* 116 (2007): 2933-2943; J. P. Després, I. Lemieux, and D. Prudhomme, "Treatment of Obesity: Need to Focus on High Risk Abdominally Obese Patients," *British Medical Journal* 322 (2001): 716-720.

6. T. Pischon, et al., "General and Abdominal Adiposity and Risk of Death in Europe," *New England Journal of Medicine* 359 (2008): 2105-2120.

7. National Heart, Lung, and Blood Institute, National Institutes of Health, *The Practical Guide: Identification, Evaluation, and Treatment of Overweight and Obesity in Adults* (NIH Publication no. 00-4084) (Washington DC: Government Printing Office, 2000).

8. M. B. Snijder, et al., "The Prediction of Visceral Fat by Dual-Energy X-ray Absorptiometry in the Elderly: A Comparison with Computed Tomography and Anthropometry," *International Journal of Obesity* 26 (2002): 984-993.

9. I. Janssen, P. T. Katzmarzyk, and R. Ross, "Waist Circumference and Not Body Mass Index Explains Obesity-Related Health Risk," *American Journal of Clinical Nutrition* 79 (2004): 379-384.

Suggested Readings

Heymsfield, S. B., T. G. Lohman, Z. Wang, and S. B. Going. *Human Body Composition.* Champaign, IL: Human Kinetics, 2005.

Heyward, V. H., and D. Wagner. *Applied Body Composition Assessment.* Champaign, IL: Human Kinetics, 2004.

Parr, R., and S. Haight. "Abdominal Visceral Fat: The New Direction in Body Composition," *ACSM's Health & Fitness Journal* 10, no. 4 (2006): 26-30.

Chapter 5:

Notes

1. "Wellness Facts," *University of California at Berkeley Wellness Letter* (Palm Coast, FL: The Editors, May 2004).

2. C. L. Ogden, et al., "Prevalence of Overweight and Obesity in the U.S.," *Journal of the American Medical Association* 295 (2006): 1549-1555.

3. J. Stein, "The Epidemic of Obesity," *Journal of Clinical Endocrinology & Metabolism* 89 (2004): 2522-2525.

4. A. H. Mokdad, J. S. Marks, D. F. Stroup, and J. L. Gerberding, "Actual Causes of Death in the United States, 2000," *Journal of the American Medical Association* 291 (2004): 1238-1241.

5. R. Sturm and K. B. Wells, "Does Obesity Contribute as Much to Morbidity as Poverty or Smoking?" *Public Health* 115 (2001): 229-235.

6. E. E. Calle, et al., "Overweight, Obesity, and Mortality from Cancer in a Prospectively Studied Cohort of U.S. Adults," *New England Journal of Medicine* 348 (2003): 1625-1638.

7. A. Peeters, et al., "Obesity in Adulthood and Its Consequences for Life Expectancy: A Life-Table Analysis," *Annals of Internal Medicine* 138 (2003): 2432.

8. K. R. Fontaine, et al., "Years of Life Lost Due to Obesity," *Journal of the American Medical Association* 289 (2003): 187-193.

9. American College of Sports Medicine, "Position Stand: Appropriate Physical Activity Intervention Strategies for Weight Loss and Prevention of Weight Regain for Adults," *Medicine and Science in Sports and Exercise* 41 (2009): 459-471.

10. S. Thomsen, "A Steady Diet of Images," *BYU Magazine* 57, no. 3 (2003): 20-21.

11. S. Lichtman et al., "Discrepancy Between Self-Reported and Actual Caloric Intake and Exercise in Obese Subjects," *New England Journal of Medicine* 327 (1992): 1893-1898.

12. J. H. Wilmore, D. L. Costill, and W. L. Kenney, *Physiology of Sport and Exercise* (Champaign, IL: Human Kinetics, 2008).

13. C. D. Gardner, et al., "Comparison of the Atkins, Zone, Ornish, and LEARN Diets for Change in Weight and Related Risk Factors among Overweight Premenopausal Women," *Journal of the American Medical Association* 297 (2007): 969-977; G. D. Foster, et al., "A Randomized Trial of a Low-Carbohydrate Diet for Obesity," *New England Journal of Medicine* 348 (2003): 2082-2090.

14. American Psychiatric Association, *Diagnostic and Statistical Manual of Mental Disorders* (Washington, DC: APA, 1994).

15. See note 14.

16. R. L. Leibel, M. Rosenbaum, and J. Hirsh, "Changes in Energy Expenditure Resulting from Altered Body Weight," *New England Journal of Medicine* 332 (1995): 621-628.

17. R. J. Shepard, *Alive Man: The Physiology of Physical Activity* (Springfield, IL: Charles C. Thomas, 1975): 484-488.

18. A. Eliasson, et al., "Sleep Is a Critical Factor in the Maintenance of Healthy Weight," paper presented at American Thoracic Society International Conference (2009).

19. S. Pattel, et al., "Sleep Your Way to Weight Loss?" paper presented at American Thoracic Society International Conference (2006).

20. K. Knutson, "Impact of Sleep and Sleep Loss on Glucose Homeostasis and Appetite Regulation," *Sleep Medicine Clinic* 2 (2007): 187-197.

21. S. Taheri et al., "Short Sleep Duration is Associated with Reduced Leptin, Elevated Ghrelin, and Increased Body Mass Index," *PLoS Medicine* 1 (2004): e62, doi:10.1371/journal .pmed.0010062.

22. W. C. Miller, D. M. Koceja, and E. J. Hamilton, "A Meta-Analysis of the Past 25 Years of Weight Loss Research Using Diet, Exercise, or Diet Plus Exercise Intervention," *International Journal of Obesity* 21 (1997): 941-947.

23. National Academy of Sciences, Institute of Medicine, *Dietary Reference Intakes for Energy, Carbohydrates, Fiber, Fat, Protein and Amino Acids (Macronutrients)* (Washington, DC: National Academy Press, 2002).

24. J. G. Thomas, et al., "The National Weight Control Registry: A Study of Successful Losers," *ACSM Health & Fitness Journal* 15, no. 2 (2011): 8-12.

25. E. T. Poehlman, et al., "Effects of Endurance and Resistance Training on Total Daily Energy Expenditure in Young Women: A Controlled Randomized Trial," *Journal of Clinical Endocrinology and Metabolism* 87 (2002): 1004-1009; L. M. Van Etten, et al., "Effect of an 18-Wk Weight-Training Program on Energy Expenditure and Physical Activity," *Journal of Applied Physiology* 82 (1997): 298-304; W. W. Campbell, M. C. Crim, V. R. Young, and W. J. Evans, "Increased Energy Requirements and Changes in Body Composition with Resistance Training in Older Adults," *American Journal of Clinical Nutrition* 60 (1994): 167-175; Z. Wang, et al., "Resting Energy Expenditure: Systematic Organization and Critique of Prediction Methods," *Obesity Research* 9 (2001): 331-336.

26. J. R. Karp and W. L. Wescott, "The Resting Metabolic Rate Debate," *Fitness Management* 23, no. 1 (2007): 44-47.

27. A. Tremblay, J. A. Simoneau, and C. Bouchard, "Impact of Exercise Intensity on Body Fatness and Skeletal Muscle Metabolism," *Metabolism* 43 (1994): 814-818.

28. T. S. Church, et al. "Changes in Weight, Waist Circumference and Compensatory Responses with Different Doses of Exercise Among Sedentary, Overweight Postmenopausal Women," *PLoS ONE* 4, no. 2 (2009): e4515, doi:10.1371/journal.pone .0004515.

29. I. Lee, et al., "Physical Activity and Weight Gain Prevention," *Journal of the American Medical Association* 303 (2010): 1173-1179.

30. T. A. Hagobian and B. Braun, "Physical Activity and Hormonal Regulation of Appetite: Sex Differences and Weight Control," *Exercise and Sport Sciences Reviews*," 38 (2010): 25-30.

31. M. L. Klem, R. R. Wing, M. T. McGuire, H. M. Seagle, and J. O. Hill, "A Descriptive Study of Individuals Successful at Long-Term Maintenance of Substantial Weight Loss," *American Journal of Clinical Nutrition* 66 (1997): 239-246.

32. See note 24; U.S. Department of Health and Human Services, Department of Agriculture, *Dietary Guidelines for Americans 2005* (Washington, DC: DHHS, 2005).

33. W. W. K. Hoeger, C. Harris, E. M. Long, and D. R. Hopkins, "Four-Week Supplementation with a Natural Dietary Compound Produces Favorable Changes in Body Composition," *Advances in Therapy* 15, no. 5 (1998): 305-313; W. W. K. Hoeger, et al., "Dietary Supplementation with Chromium Picolinate/ L-Carnitine Complex in Combination with Diet and Exercise Enhances Body Composition," *Journal of the American Nutraceutical Association* 2, no. 2 (1999): 40-45.

34. D. Mozaffarian, et. al., "Changes in Diet and Lifestyle and Long-Term Weight Gain in Women and Men," *New England Journal of Medicine* 364 (2011): 2392-2404.

35. N. A. Christakis and J. H. Fowler, "The Spread of Obesity in a Large Social Network over 32 Years," *New England Journal of Medicine* 357 (2007): 370-379.

Suggested Readings

American College of Sports Medicine. "Position Stand: Appropriate Physical Activity Intervention Strategies for Weight Loss and Prevention of Weight Regain for Adults." *Medicine and Science in Sports and Exercise* 41 (2009): 459-471.

American Diabetes Association and American Dietetic Association. *Exchange Lists for Meal Planning*. Chicago: American Dietetic Association and American Diabetes Association, 2008.

National Academy of Sciences, Institute of Medicine. *Dietary Reference Intakes for Energy, Carbohydrates, Fiber, Fat, Protein and Amino Acids (Macronutrients)*. Washington, DC: National Academy Press, 2002.

Chapter 6:

Notes

1. R. B. O'Hara, et al., "Increased Volume Resistance Training: Effects upon Predicted Aerobic Fitness in a Select Group of Air Force Men," *ACSM's Health & Fitness Journal* 8, no. 4 (2004): 16-25.

2. American College of Sports Medicine, *ACSM's Guidelines for Exercise Testing and Prescription* (Philadelphia: Wolters Kluwer/ Lippincott Williams & Wilkins, 2010).

3. U.S. Department of Health and Human Services, *Physical Activity and Health: A Report of the Surgeon General* (Atlanta, GA: Centers for Disease Control and Prevention, National Center for Chronic Disease Prevention and Health Promotion, 1996).

4. U.S. Department of Health and Human Services, Centers for Disease Control and Prevention, National Center for Health Statistics, *Physical Activity Among Adults: United States, 2000*, no. 15 (Atlanta, GA: CDC, May 14, 2003).

5. American College of Sports Medicine, "Position Stand: Quantity and Quality of Exercise for Developing and Maintaining Cardiorespiratory, Musculoskeletal, and Neuromotor Fitness in Apparently Healthy Adults: Guidance for Prescribing Exercise" *Medicine and Science in Sports and Exercise* 43 (2011): 1334-1359.

6. See note 2.

7. See note 2.

8. S. E. Gormley, et al., "Effect of Intensity of Aerobic Training on VO_{2max}," *Medicine and Science in Sports and Exercise* 40 (2008): 1336-1343.

9. R. L. Gellish, et al., "Longitudinal Modeling of the Relationship Between Age and Maximal Heart Rate," *Medicine and Science in Sports and Exercise* 39 (2007): 822-829.

10. See note 3.

11. D. P. Swain, "Moderate or Vigorous Intensity Exercise: Which Is Better for Improving Aerobic Fitness?" *Preventive Cardiology* 8, no. 1 (2005): 55-58.

12. P. T. Williams, "Physical Fitness and Activity as Separate Heart Disease Risk Factors: A Meta-analysis," *Medicine and Science in Sports and Exercise* 33 (2001): 754-761.

13. D. P. Swain and B. A. Franklin, "Comparative Cardioprotective Benefits of Vigorous vs. Moderate Intensity Aerobic Exercise," *American Journal of Cardiology* 97, no. 1 (2006): 141-147.

14. R. F. DeBusk, U. Stenestrand, M. Sheehan, and W. L. Haskell, "Training Effects of Long versus Short Bouts of Exercise in Healthy Subjects," *American Journal of Cardiology* 65 (1990): 1010-1013.

15. National Academy of Sciences, Institute of Medicine, *Dietary Reference Intakes for Energy, Carbohydrates, Fiber, Fat, Protein*

and Amino Acids (Macronutrients) (Washington, DC: National Academy Press, 2002).

16. U.S. Department of Health and Human Services, Department of Agriculture, *Dietary Guidelines for Americans 2005* (Washington, DC: DHHS, 2005).

17. "Summary Statement: Workshop on Physical Activity and Public Health," *Sports Medicine Bulletin* 28 (1993): 7.

18. W. Dunstan, et al., "Television Viewing Time and Mortality: The Australian Diabetes, Obesity, and Lifestyle Study (AusDiab)," *Circulation* 121 (2010): 384-391.

19. P. T. Katzmarzyk, et al., "Sitting time and mortality from all causes, cardiovascular disease, and cancer," *Medicine and Science in Sports and Exercise* 41 (2009): 998-1005.

20. See note 2.

Suggested Readings

ACSM's Guidelines for Exercise Testing and Prescription. Philadelphia: Wolters Kluwer/Lippincott Williams & Wilkins, 2010.

ACSM's Resource Manual for Guidelines for Exercise Testing and Prescription. Philadelphia: Wolters Kluwer/Lippincott Williams & Wilkins, 2010.

Hoeger, W. W. K., and S. A. Hoeger. *Fitness & Wellness.* Belmont, CA: Wadsworth/Cengage Learning, 2013.

Hoeger, W. W. K., and S. A. Hoeger. *Principles and Labs for Fitness & Wellness.* Belmont, CA: Wadsworth/Cengage Learning, 2012.

Karvonen, M. J., E. Kentala, and O. Mustala. "The Effects of Training on the Heart Rate: A Longitudinal Study." *Annales Medicinae Experimetalis et Biologiae Fenniae* 35 1957: 307-315.

McArdle, W. D., F. I. Katch, and V. L. Katch. *Exercise Physiology: Energy, Nutrition, and Human Performance*, 5th ed. Philadelphia: Wolters Kluwer/Lippincott Williams & Wilkins, 2010.

Nieman, D. C. *Exercise Testing and Prescription: A Health-Related Approach.* Boston: McGraw-Hill, 2006.

Wilmore, J. H., and D. L. Costill. *Physiology of Sport and Exercise.* Champaign, IL: Human Kinetics, 2008.

Chapter 7:

Notes

1. C. Castaneda et al., "A Randomized Controlled Trial of Resistance Exercise Training to Improve Glycemic Control in Older Adults with Type 2 Diabetes," *Diabetes Care* 25 (2002): 2335-2341.

2. W. W. Campbell, M. C. Crim, V. R. Young, and W. J. Evans, "Increased Energy Requirements and Changes in Body Composition with Resistance Training in Older Adults," *American Journal of Clinical Nutrition* 60 (1994): 167-175.

3. W. J. Evans, "Exercise, Nutrition and Aging," *Journal of Nutrition* 122 (1992): 796-801.

4. P. E. Allsen, *Strength Training: Beginners, Body Builders and Athletes* (Dubuque, IA: Kendall/Hunt, 2009).

5. See note 2.

6. American College of Sports Medicine, "Progression Models in Resistance Training for Healthy Adults," *Medicine and Science in Sports and Exercise* 41 (2009): 687-708.

7. J. K. Kraemer and N. A. Ratamess, "Fundamentals of Resistance Training: Progression and Exercise Prescription," *Medicine and Science in Sports and Exercise* 36 (2004): 674-688.

8. B. M. Hather, P. A. Tesch, P. Buchanan, and G. A. Dudley, "Influence of Eccentric Actions on Skeletal Muscle Adaptations to Resistance Training," *Acta Physiologica Scandinavica* 143 (1991): 177-185; C. B. Ebbeling and P. M. Clarkson, "Exercise-Induced Muscle Damage and Adaptation," *Sports Medicine* 7 (1989): 207-234.

9. See note 6.

10. W. W. K. Hoeger, D. R. Hopkins, S. L. Barette, and D. F. Hale, "Relationship Between Repetitions and Selected Percentages of One Repetition Maximum: A Comparison Between Untrained and Trained Males and Females," *Journal of Applied Sport Science Research* 4, no. 2 (1990): 47-51.

11. American College of Sports Medicine, *ACSM's Guidelines for Exercise Testing and Prescription* (Baltimore: Wolters Kluwer/Lippincott Williams & Wilkins, 2010).

12. W. J. Kraemer and M. S. Fragala, "Personalize It: Program Design in Resistance Training," *ACSM's Health and Fitness Journal* 10, no. 4 (2006): 7-17.

13. See note 6.

Suggested Readings

American College of Sports Medicine, "Progression Models in Resistance Training for Healthy Adults." *Medicine and Science in Sports and Exercise* 41 (2009): 687-708.

Hesson, J. L. *Weight Training for Life.* Belmont, CA: Wadsworth/Cengage Learning, 2012.

Heyward, V. H. *Advanced Fitness Assessment and Exercise Prescription.* Champaign, IL: Human Kinetic Press, 2010.

Hoeger, W. W. K., and S. A. Hoeger. Principles and Labs for Fitness and Wellness. Belmont, CA: Wadsworth/Cengage, 2012.

Kraemer, J. K., and N. A. Ratamess. "Fundamentals of Resistance Training: Progression and Exercise Prescription." *Medicine and Science in Sports and Exercise* 36 (2004): 674-688.

Kraemer, W. J., and S. J. Fleck. *Optimizing Strength Training.* Champaign, IL: Human Kinetic Press, 2007.

Volek, J. "Influence of Nutrition on Responses to Resistance Training." *Medicine and Science in Sports and Exercise* 36 (2004): 689-696.

Chapter 8:

Notes

1. American College of Obstetricians and Gynecologists, *Guidelines for Exercise During Pregnancy*, 2003.

2. "Stretch Yourself Younger," *Consumer Reports on Health* 11 (August 1999): 6-7.

3. W. W. K. Hoeger and D. R. Hopkins, "A Comparison between the Sit and Reach and the Modified Sit and Reach in the Measurement of Flexibility in Women," *Research Quarterly for Exercise and Sport* 63 (1992): 191-195; W. W. K. Hoeger, D. R. Hopkins, S. Button, and T. A. Palmer, "Comparing the Sit and Reach with the Modified Sit and Reach in Measuring Flexibility in Adolescents," *Pediatric Exercise Science* 2 (1990): 156-162; D. R. Hopkins and W. W. K. Hoeger, "A Comparison of the Sit and Reach and the Modified Sit and Reach in the Measurement of Flexibility for Males," *Journal of Applied Sports Science Research* 6 (1992): 7-10.

4. J. Kokkonen and S. Lauritzen, "Isotonic Strength and Endurance Gains through PNF Stretching," *Medicine and Science in Sports and Exercise* 27 (1995): S22, 127.

5. American College of Sports Medicine, *ACSM's Guidelines for Exercise Testing and Prescription* (Baltimore: Wolters Kluwer/Lippincott Williams & Wilkins, 2010).

6. K. B. Fields, C. M. Burnworth, and M. Delaney, "Should Athletes Stretch before Exercise?" *Gatorade Sports Science Institute: Sports Science Exchange* 30, no. 1 (2007): 1-5.

7. S. B. Thacker, J. Gilchrist, D. F. Stroup, and C. D. Kimsey, Jr., "The Impact of Stretching on Sports Injury Risk: A Systematic Review of the Literature," *Medicine and Science in Sports and Exercise* 36 (2004): 371-378.

8. D. B. J. Andersson, L. J. Fine, and B. A. Silverstein, "Musculoskeletal Disorders," *Occupational Health: Recognizing and Preventing Work-Related Disease*, edited by B. S. Levy and D. H. Wegman (Boston: Little, Brown, 1995).

9. M. R. Bracko, "Can We Prevent Back Injuries?" *ACSM's Health & Fitness Journal* 8, no. 4 (2004): 5-11.

10. R. Deyo, "Chiropractic Care for Back Pain: The Physician's Perspective," *HealthNews* 4 (September 10, 1998).

11. B. W. Nelson et al., "Can Spinal Surgery Be Prevented by Aggressive Strengthening Exercise? A Prospective Study of Cervical and Lumbar Patients," *Archives of Physical Medicine and Rehabilitation* 80 (1999): 20-25.

12. See note 9.

13. K. Williams, et al., "Evaluation of the Effectiveness and Efficacy of Iyegar Yoga Therapy on Chronic Low Back Pain," *Spine* 34 (2009): 2066-2076.

14. J. A. Hides, G. A. Jull, and C. A. Richardson, "Long-Term Effects of Specific Stabilizing Exercises for First-Episode Low Back Pain," *Spine* 26 (2001): E243-E248.

15. "Position Yourself to Stay Well," *Consumer Reports on Health* 18 (February 2006): 8-9.

16. A. Brownstein, "Chronic Back Pain Can Be Beaten," *Bottom Line/Health* 13 (October 1999): 3-4.

Suggested Readings

Alter, M. J. *Science of Flexibility.* Champaign, IL: Human Kinetic Press,2004.

Bracko, M. R. "Can We Prevent Back Injuries?" *ACSM's Health & Fitness Journal* 8, no. 4 (2004): 5-11.

Hoeger, W. W. K. *The Assessment of Muscular Flexibility: Test Protocols and National Flexibility Norms for the Modified Sit-and-Reach Test, Total Body Rotation Test, and Shoulder Rotation Test.* Rockton, IL: Figure Finder Collection Novel Products, Inc., 2006.

Liemohn, W., and G. Pariser. "Core Strength: Implications for Fitness and Low Back Pain." *ACSM's Health and Fitness Journal* 6, no. 5 (2002): 10-16.

McAtee, R. E., and J. Charland. *Facilitated Stretching.* Champaign, IL: Human Kinetics, 2007.

Nelson, A. G., J. Kokkonen, and J. M. McAlexander. *Stretching Anatomy.* Champaign, IL: Human Kinetics, 2007.

Chapter 9:

Notes

1. W. Hoeger, T. A. Spitzer-Gibson, N. Kaluhiokalani, J. Kokonnen, "Comparison of Physiologic Responses to Self-Paced Water Aerobics and Self-Paced Treadmill Running," *Journal of the International Council for Health, Physical Education, Recreation, Sport, and Dance,* 30, no. 4 (2004): 27-30.

2. W. W. K. Hoeger, T. S. Gibson, J. Moore, and D. R. Hopkins, "A Comparison of Selected Training Responses to Low Impact Aerobics and Water Aerobics," *National Aquatics Journal,* 9 (1993), 13-16.

3. E. J. Marcinick, J. Potts, G. Schlabach, S. Will, P. Dawson, and B. F. Hurley, "Effects of Strength Training on Lactate Threshold and Endurance Performance," *Medicine and Science in Sports and Exercise* 23 (1991): 739-743.

4. American College of Sports Medicine, and American Diabetes Association, "Joint Position Statement: Exercise and Type 2 Diabetes," *Medicine and Science in Sports and Exercise* 42 (2010): 2282-2303.

5. American College of Obstetricians and Gynecologists, "Exercise During Pregnancy and the Postpartum Period. ACOG Committee Opinion No. 267, *International Journal of Gynecology and Obstetrics* 77 (2002): 79-81.

6. University of California at Berkeley, *The Wellness Guide to Lifelong Fitness* (New York: Random House, 1993): 198.

7. W. J. Chodzko-Zajko, et al., Exercise and Physical Activity for Older Adults," *Medicine and Science in Sports and Exercise* 41 (2009): 1510-1530.

8. F. W. Kash, J. L. Boyer, S. P. Van Camp, L. S. Verity, and J. P. Wallace, "The Effect of Physical Activity on Aerobic Power in Older Men (A Longitudinal Study)," *Physician and Sports Medicine* 18, no. 4 (1990): 73-83.

9. W. S. Evans, "Exercise, Nutrition and Aging," *Journal of Nutrition* 122 (1992): 796-801.

10. See note 7.

11. J. M. Walker, D. Sue, N. Miles-Elkousy, G. Ford, and H. Trevelyan, "Active Mobility of the Extremities in Older Subjects," *Physical Therapy* 64 (1994): 919-923.

12. J. M. Moore and W. W. Hoeger, "Game On! Preparing Your Clients for Recreational Sports," *ACSM's Health & Fitness Journal* 9 no. 3 (2005): 14-19.

13. J. R. Karp, "Interval training: The New and Better way to train Your Clients?" *IDEA Fitness Journal,* 8, no. 2 (2011): 31-34.

Suggested Readings

American College of Obstetricians and Gynecologists. "Exercise During Pregnancy and the Postpartum Period. ACOG Committee Opinion No. 267." *International Journal of Gynecology and Obstetrics* 77 (2002): 79-81.

Clark, N. *Nancy Clark's Sports Nutrition Guidebook.* Champaign, IL: Human Kinetics, 2008.

Pfeiffer, R. P., and B. C. Mangus. *Concepts of Athletic Training.* Boston: Jones and Bartlett, 2012.

Chapter 10:

Notes

1. U.S. Department of Health and Human Services, Centers for Disease Control and Prevention, National Center for Health Statistics, *National Vital Statistics Reports, Deaths: Preliminary Data for 2008,* 59, no. 2 (December 9, 2010).

2. "Reducing Your Risk of a Stroke: The Latest Tips," *Environmental Nutrition* 29, no. 7 (July 2006): 3.

3. S. N. Blair, H. W. Kohl III, R. S. Paffenbarger, Jr., D. G. Clark, K. H. Cooper, and L. W. Gibbons, "Physical Fitness and All-Cause Mortality: A Prospective Study of Healthy Men and Women," *Journal of the American Medical Association* 262 (1989): 2395-2401.

4. R. S. Paffenbarger, Jr., R. T. Hyde, A. L. Wing, I. Lee, D. L. Jung, and J. B. Kampert, "The Association of Changes in Physical-Activity Level and Other Lifestyle Characteristics with Mortality Among Men," *New England Journal of Medicine* 328 (1993): 538-545.

5. D. P. Swain and B. A. Franklin, "Comparative Cardioprotective Benefits of Vigorous vs. Moderate Intensity Aerobic Exercise," *American Journal of Cardiology* 97, no. 1 (2006): 141-147.

6. "Lipid Research Clinics Program: The Lipid Research Clinic Coronary Primary Prevention Trial Results," *Journal of the American Medical Association* 251 (1984): 351-364.

7. "HDL on the Rise," *HealthNews* (September 10, 1999).

8. M. D. Ozner, "The Ultimate Cholesterol Profile," *Bottom Line/Health* 21 (July 2007): 1-2.

9. R. Singa, et al., "Meat Intake and Mortality: A Prospective Study of Over Half a Million People," *Archives of Internal Medicine* 169 (2009): 562-571

10. A. E. Buyken, et al., "Modifications in Dietary Fat Are Associated with Changes in Serum Lipids of Older Adults Independently of Lipid Medication," *Journal of Nutrition* 140 (2010): 88-94.

11. C. M. Albert, et al., "Blood Levels of Long-Chain n-3 Fatty Acids and the Risk of Sudden Death," *New England Journal of Medicine* 346 (2002): 1113-1118.

12. A. H. Lichtenstein, et al., "Diet and Lifestyle Recommendations Revision 2006: A Scientific Statement from the American Heart Association Nutrition Committee," *Circulation* 114 (2006): 82-96.

13. See note 3.

14. E. B. Rimm, A. Ascherio, E. Giovannucci, M. Spiegelman, M. J. Stampfer, and W. C. Willett, "Vegetable, Fruit, and Cereal Fiber Intake and Risk of Coronary Heart Disease Among Men," *Journal of the American Medical Association* 275 (1996): 447-451.

15. National Cholesterol Education Program Expert Panel, "Summary of the Third Report of the National Cholesterol Education

Program (NCEP) Expert Panel on Detection, Evaluation, and Treatment of High Blood Cholesterol in Adults (Adult Treatment Panel III)," *Journal of the American Medical Association* 285 (2001): 2486-2497.

16. P. W. Siri-Tarino, Q. Sun, F. B. Hu, and R. M. Krauss, "Meta-Analysis of Prospective Cohort Studies Evaluating the Association of Saturated Fat with Cardiovascular Disease," *American Journal of Clinical Nutrition* 91 (2010): 535-546.

17. P. W. Siri-Tarino, Q. Sun, F. B. Hu, and R. M. Krauss, "Saturated Fat, Carbohydrate, and Cardiovascular Disease," *The American Journal of Clinical Nutrition* 91 (2010): 502-509.

18. D. Mozaffarian, R. Micha, and S. Wallace, "Effects on Coronary Heart Disease of Increasing Polyunsaturated Fat in Place of Saturated Fat: A Systematic Review of Meta-Analysis of Randomized Controlled Trials," *PLoS Medicine* 7 (2010): 7:e1000252.

19. A. Jula, et al., "Effects of Diet and Simvastatin on Serum Lipids, Insulin, and Antioxidants in Hypercholesterolemic Men," *Journal of the American Medical Association* 287 (2002): 598-605.

20. "The Homocysteine-CVD Connection," *HealthNews* (October 25, 1999).

21. "Inflammation May Be Key Cause of Heart Disease and More: Diet's Role," *Environmental Nutrition* 27, no. 7 (July 2004): 1, 4.

22. H. R. Superko, "State-of-the-Art Heart Tests," *Bottom Line/ Health* 19 (February 2005): 3-5.

23. P. M. Ridger, et al., "Rosuvastatin to Prevent Vascular Events in Men and Women with Elevated C-Reactive Protein," *New England Journal of Medicine* 359 (2008): 2195-2207.

24. "Predict Heart Disease Better with CRP," *Environmental Nutrition* 28, no. 2 (February 2005): 3.

25. D. M. Nathan, "Navigating the Choices for Diabetes Prevention," *New England Journal of Medicine* 362 (2010): 1533-1535; The Accord Study Group, "Effects of Combination Lipid Therapy in Type 2 Diabetes Mellitus," *New England Journal of Medicine* 362 (2010): 1563-1574; The Accord Study Group, "Effects of Intensive Blood Pressure Control in Type 2 Diabetes Mellitus," *New England Journal of Medicine* 362 (2010): 1575-1585.

26. H. K. Choi, et al., "Dairy Consumption and Risk of Type 2 Diabetes Mellitus in Men," *Archives of Internal Medicine* 165 (2005): 997-1003.

27. S. Liu, et al., "A Prospective Study of Dietary Glycemic Load, Carbohydrate Intake, and Risk of Coronary Heart Disease in the U.S.," *American Journal of Clinical Nutrition* 71 (2000): 1455-1461.

28. G. M. Reaven, T. K. Strom, and B. Fox, *Syndrome X: Overcoming the Silent Killer That Can Give You a Heart Attack* (Englewood Cliffs, NJ: Simon & Schuster, 2000).

29. A. V. Chobanian, et al., "The Seventh Report of the Joint National Committee on Prevention, Detection, Evaluation, and Treatment of High Blood Pressure," *Journal of the American Medical Association* 289 (2003): 2560-2571.

30. L. E. Fields, et al., "The Burden of Adult Hypertension in the United States 1999 to 2000: A Rising Tide," *Hypertension On Line First* (August 23, 2004).

31. "Shake the Salt Habit to Reduce Your Risk of Stroke and Heart Disease," *Health & Nutrition Letter* (March 2010).

32. P. Strazzullo, L. D'Elia, N-B Kandala, and F. P. Cappuccio, "Salt Intake, Stroke, and Cardiovascular Disease: Meta-Analysis of Prospective Studies," *British Medical Journal* 339 (2009): b4567.

33. K. Bibbins-Domingo, et al., "Projected Effect of Dietary Salt Reductions on Future Cardiovascular Disease," *New England Journal of Medicine* 362 (2010): 590-599.

34. "Salt Takes a Licking," *University of California at Berkeley Wellness Letter* (April 2010).

35. See note 3.

36. L. S. Pescatello, et al., "Exercise and Hypertension Position Stand," *Medicine and Science in Sports and Exercise* 36 (2004): 533-553.

37. G. Kelley, "Dynamic Resistance Exercise and Resting Blood Pressure in Adults: A Meta-analysis," *Journal of Applied Physiology* 82 (1997): 1559-1565; G. A. Kelley and Z. Tran, "Aerobic Exercise and Normotensive Adults: A Meta-Analysis," *Medicine and Science in Sports and Exercise* 27 (1995): 1371-1377; G. Kelley and P. McClellan, "Antihypertensive Effects of Aerobic Exercise: A Brief Meta-Analytic Review of Randomized Controlled Trials," *American Journal of Hypertension* 7 (1994): 115-119.

38. R. Collins, et al., "Blood Pressure, Stroke, and Coronary Heart Disease; Part 2, Short-term Reductions in Blood Pressure: Overview of Randomized Drug Trials in Their Epidemiological Context," *Lancet* 335 (1990): 827-838.

39. G. A. Kelley and K. S. Kelley, "Progressive Resistance Exercise and Resting Blood Pressure: A Meta-Analysis of Randomized Controlled Trials," *Hypertension* 35 (2000): 838-843.

40. F. W. Kash, J. L. Boyer, S. P. Van Camp, L. S. Verity, and J. P. Wallace, "The Effect of Physical Activity on Aerobic Power in Older Men (A Longitudinal Study)," *Physician and Sports Medicine* 18, no. 4 (1990): 73-83.

41. S. G. Sheps, "High Blood Pressure Can Often Be Controlled Without Medication," *Bottom Line/Health* (November 1999).

42. J. E. Donnelly, et al., "Appropriate Physical Activity Intervention Strategies for Weight Loss and Prevention of Weight Regain for Adults," *Medicine and Science in Sports and Exercise* 41 (2009): 459-471.

43. C. A. Slentz, et al., "Inactivity, Exercise, and Visceral Fat. STRRIDE: A Randomized, Controlled Study of Exercise Intensity and Amount," *Journal of Applied Physiology* 99 (2005): 1613-1618.

44. S. Kenchaiah, et al., "Body Mass Index and Vigorous Physical Activity and the Risk of Heart Failure among Men," *Circulation* 119 (2009): 44-52.

45. M. Guarneri, "What Most People Don't Know about Heart Disease," *Bottom Line/Health* 21 (July 2007): 11-12.

46. See note 45.

Suggested Readings

American Heart Association. *2011 Heart and Stroke Facts Statistical Update.* Dallas, TX: AHA, 2011.

American Heart Association. *Heart and Stroke Facts.* Dallas, TX: AHA, 2011.

National Cholesterol Education Program Expert Panel. "Summary of the Third Report of the National Cholesterol Education Program (NCEP) Expert Panel on Detection, Evaluation, and Treatment of High Blood Cholesterol in Adults (Adult Treatment Panel III)." *Journal of the American Medical Association* 285 (2001): 2486-2497.

Chapter 11:

Notes

1. American Cancer Society, *Cancer Facts & Figures 2010* (New York: ACS, 2010).

2. Kushi, L. H., et al., American Cancer Society Guidelines on Nutrition and Physical Activity for Cancer Prevention: Reducing the Risk for Cancer with Healthy Food Choices and Physical Activity, *CA: A Cancer Journal for Clinicians* 56, no. 5 (2006): 254-281.

3. J. E. Enstrom, "Health Practices and Cancer Mortality Among Active California Mormons," *Journal of the National Cancer Institute* 81 (1989): 1807-1814.

4. A. S. Ford, et al., "Healthy Living is the Best Revenge: Findings from the European Prospective Investigation into Cancer and Nutrition—Potsdam Study," *Archives of Internal Medicine* 169 (2009): 1355-1362.

5. See note 1.

6. Y. Park, et al., "Dietary Fiber Intake and Risk of Colorectal Cancer," *Journal of the American Medical Association* 294 (2005): 2849-2857.

7. V. W. Setiawan, et al., "Protective Effect of Green Tea on the Risks of Chronic Gastritis and Stomach Cancer," *International Journal of Cancer* 92 (2001): 600-604.

8. L. Mitscher, and V. Dolby, *The Green Tea Book—China's Fountain of Youth* (New York: Avery Press, 1997).

9. "Curbing Cancer's Reach: Little Things That Might Make a Big Difference," *Environmental Nutrition* 29, no. 6 (2006): 1, 6.

10. S. C. Larsson, L. Bergkvist, and A. Wolk, "Consumption of Sugar-Sweetened Foods and the Risk of Pancreatic Cancer in a Prospective Study," *American Journal of Clinical Nutrition* 84 (2006): 1171-1176.

11. N. E. Allen, et al., "Moderate Alcohol Intake and Cancer Incidence in Women," *Journal of the National Cancer Institute* 101 (2009): 296-305.

12. See note 1.

13. E. E. Calle, C. Rodriguez, K. Walker-Thurmond, and M. J. Thun, "Overweight, Obesity, and Mortality from Cancer in a Prospectively Studied Cohort of U.S. Adults," *New England Journal of Medicine* 348 (2003): 1625-1638.

14. American Cancer Society, *1995 Cancer Facts & Figures* (New York: ACS, 1995).

15. S. E. Whitmore, W. L. Morison, C. S. Potten, and C. Chadwick, "Tanning Salon Exposure and Molecular Alterations," *Journal of the American Academy of Dermatology* 44 (2001): 775-780.

16. C. A. Thomson, and P. A. Thomson, "Healthy Lifestyle and Cancer Prevention," *ACSM's Health & Fitness Journal* 12, no. 3 (2008): 18-26.

17. S. W. Farrell, et al., "Cardiorespiratory Fitness, Different Measures of Adiposity, and Cancer Mortality in Men," *Obesity* 15 (2007): 3140-3149.

18. L. Byberg, et al., "Total Mortality After Changes in Leisure Time Physical Activity in 50 Year Old Men: 35 Year Follow-up of Population Based Cohort," *British Medical Journal* (2009): 338:doi:10.1136.

19. E. L. Giovannucci, "A Prospective Study of Physical Activity and Incident and Fatal Prostate Cancer," *Archives of Internal Medicine* 165 (2005): 1005-1010.

20. L. Ratnasinghe, et al., *Exercise and Breast Cancer Risk: A Multinational Study* (Beltsville, MD: Genomic Nanosystems, BioServe Biotechnologies, Ltd.).

21. C. W. Matthews, et al., "Physical Activity and Risk of Endometrial Cancer: A Report from the Shanghai Endometrial Cancer Study," *Cancer Epidemiology Biomarkers & Prevention* 14 (2005): 779-785.

22. M. D. Holmes, et al., "Physical Activity and Survival After Breast Cancer Diagnosis," *Journal of the American Medical Association* 293 (2005): 2479-2486.

23. J. R. Ruiz, "Muscular Strength and Adiposity as Predictors of Adulthood Cancer Mortality in Men," *Cancer Epidemiology, Biomarkers & Prevention* 18 (2009): 1468-1476.

24. D. Servan-Schreiber, "The Anticancer Life Plan," *Bottom Line Health* 23, no. 5 (May 2009).

Suggested Readings

American Cancer Society. *Cancer Facts & Figures 2010*. New York: ACS, 2010.

World Cancer Research Fund and American Institute for Cancer Research. *Food, Nutrition, Physical Activity and the Prevention of Cancer: A Global Perspective*. Washington, DC: WCRF/AICR, 2007.

"Dietary Do's and Don'ts from the Latest Research on Cancer Prevention." *Tufts University Health & Nutrition Letter* 27, no. 5 (July 2009).

"Eating to Beat Cancer." Special Supplement to the *Tufts University Health & Nutrition Letter* 25, no. 3 (May 2007).

U.S. Department of Health and Human Services, National Institutes of Health, National Cancer Institute. *Reducing Environmental Cancer Risk: What We Can Do Now*. Washington, DC: President's Cancer Panel, April 2010.

Chapter 12:

Notes

1. H. Selye, *Stress without Distress* (New York: Signet, 1974).

2. E. Gullete, et al., "Effects of Mental Stress on Myocardial Ischemia during Daily Life," *Journal of the American Medical Association* 277 (1997): 1521-1525; C. A. Lengacher et al., "Psychoneuroimmunology and Immune System Link for Stress, Depression, Health Behaviors, and Breast Cancer," *Alternative Health Practitioner* 4 (1998): 95-108.

3. R. J. Kriegel, and M. H. Kriegel, *The C Zone: Peak Performance Under Stress* (Garden City, NY: Anchor Press/Doubleday, 1985).

4. See note 2. J. Moses, et al., "The Effects of Exercise Training on Mental Well-Being in the Normal Population: A Controlled Trial," *Journal of Psychosomatic Research* 33 (1989): 47-61; C. Shang, "Emerging Paradigms in Mind–Body Medicine," *Journal of Complementary and Alternative Medicine* 7 (2001): 83-91.

5. See note 1.

6. M. Samuels, "Use Your Mind to Heal Your Body," *Bottom Line/Health* 19 (February 2005): 13-14.

7. S. Bodian, "Meditate Your Way to Much Better Health," *Bottom Line/Health* 18 (June 2004): 11-13.

8. D. Mueller, "Yoga Therapy," *ACSM's Health & Fitness Journal* 6 (2002): 18-24.

9. S. C. Manchanda, et al., "Retardation of Coronary Atherosclerosis with Yoga Lifestyle Intervention," *Journal of the Association of Physicians of India* 48 (2000): 687-694.

Suggested Readings

Girdano, D. A., D. E. Dusek, and G. S. Everly. *Controlling Stress and Tension*. San Francisco: Benjamin Cummings, 2009.

Greenberg, J. S. *Comprehensive Stress Management*. New York: McGraw-Hill, 2008.

Olpin, M., and M. Hesson. *Stress Management for Life*. Belmont, CA: Wadsworth/Cengage Learning, 2010.

Schwartz, M. S., and F. Andrasik. *Biofeedback: A Practitioner's Guide*. New York: Guilford Press, 2004.

Selye, H. *The Stress of Life*. New York: McGraw-Hill, 1978.

Chapter 13

Notes

1. U.S. Department of Health and Human Services: Office of Applied Studies, *Results from the 2009 National Survey on Drug Use and Health: National Findings*, available at http://nsduhweb .rti.org (downloaded May 16, 2011).

2. W. W. K. Hoeger, L. W. Turner, and B. Q. Hafen, *Wellness: Guidelines for a Healthy Lifestyle* (Belmont, CA: Wadsworth/Thomson Learning, 2007).

3. R. Goldberg, *Drugs Across the Spectrum* (Belmont, CA: Wadsworth/Cengage Learning, 2010).

4. See note 3.

5. "A Snapshot of Annual High-Risk College Drinking Consequences," available at http://www.collegedrinkingprevention .gov/statssummaries/snapshot.aspx (downloaded May 14, 2011).

6. C. A. Presley, J. S. Leichliter, and P. W. Meilman, *Alcohol and Drugs on American College Campuses: Findings from 1995, 1996, and 1997 (A Report to College Presidents)* (Carbondale: Southern Illinois University, 1999).

7. See note 1.

8. U.S. Department of Agriculture, *Tobacco Outlook Report* (Washington, DC: U.S. Department of Agriculture, Market and Trade Economics Division, Economic Research Service, 2007).

9. American Cancer Society, *Cancer Facts & Figures—2011* (New York: ACS, 2011).

10. U.S. Public Health Service. *The Health Consequences of Involuntary Exposure to Tobacco Smoke: A Report of the Surgeon General—Executive Summary* (Rockville, MD: U.S. Department of Health and Human Services, 2006).

11. American Cancer Society, *World Smoking & Health* (Atlanta, GA: ACS, 1993).

12. American Heart Association, *AHA Public Affairs/Coalition on Smoking: Health Position* (Dallas, TX: AHA, 1996).

13. U.S. Department of Health and Human Services, *Nicotine Addiction, A Report of the Surgeon General* (Atlanta, GA: U.S. Department of Health and Human Services, Centers for Disease Control and Prevention, National Center for Chronic Disease Prevention and Health Promotion, 1988).

14. R. H. Zwick, et al., "Exercise in Addition to Nicotine Replacement Therapy Improves Success Rates in Smoking Cessation," *Chest* 130, no. 4 (2006): 145S.

Suggested Readings

American Cancer Society. *2011 Cancer Facts & Figures—..* New York: ACS, 2011.

Doweiko, H. E. *Concepts of Chemical Dependency.* Belmont, CA: Wadsworth/Thomson Learning, 2009.

Goldberg, R. *Drugs Across the Spectrum.* Belmont, CA: Wadsworth/Thomson Learning, 2010.

U.S. Department of Health and Human Services. *A Report of the Surgeon General: How Tobacco Smoke Causes Disease: The Biology and Behavioral Basis for Smoking-Attributable Disease.* Rockville, MD, USDHHS, 2010.

U.S. Public Health Service. *The Health Consequences of Involuntary Exposure to Tobacco Smoke: A Report of the Surgeon General—Executive Summary.* Rockville, MD: U.S. Department of Health and Human Services, 2006.

Chapter 14:

Notes

1. Centers for Disease Control and Prevention, "Sexually Transmitted Diseases," available at http://www.cdc.gov/STD/ (downloaded May 10, 2011).

2. See note 1.

3. See note 1.

4. See note 1.

5. See note 1.

6. See note 1.

7. See note 1.

8. M. McFarlane, S. S. Bull, and C. A. Rietmeijer, "The Internet as a Newly Emerging Risk Environment for Sexually Transmitted Diseases," *Journal of the American Medical Association* 284 (2000): 443-446.

9. Avert International AIDS Charity, "Worldwide HIV & AIDS Statistics," available at http://www.avert.org/worldstats.htm (downloaded May 10, 2011).

Suggested Readings

Blona, R., and J. Levitan. *Healthy Sexuality.* Belmont, CA: Wadsworth/Thomson Learning, 2006.

Centers for Disease Control and Prevention. "Sexually Transmitted Diseases Treatment Guidelines 2010." *Morbidity and Mortality Weekly Report, Recommendations and Reports* 59, no. RR-12 (December 17, 2010): 1-110.

Hoeger, W. W. K., L. W. Turner, and B. Q. Hafen. *Wellness: Guidelines for a Healthy Lifestyle.* Belmont, CA: Wadsworth/Thomson Learning, 2007.

Chapter 15:

Notes

1. R. J. Donatelle, *Access to Health* (San Francisco: Benjamin Cummings, 2008).

2. National Institutes of Health, National Center for Complementary and Alternative Medicine, *2007 Statistics on CAM Use in the United States*, available at http://nccam.nih.gov/news/camstats/2007/index.htm (downloaded May 20, 2010).

3. National Center for Complementary and Alternative Medicine, National Institutes of Health, *CAM Basics: What Is Complementary and Alternative Medicine?*, available at http://nccam.nih.gov/health/whatiscam/ (downloaded May 16, 2011).

4. National Institutes of Health, National Center for Complementary and Alternative Medicine, *Statistics on CAM Costs*, available at http://nccam.nih.gov/news/camstats/2007/index.htm (downloaded May 20, 2010).

5. D. M. Eisenberg et al., "Trends in Alternative Medicine Use in the United States, 1990–1997," *Journal of the American Medical Association* 280, no. 18 (1998): 1569-1575.

6. *Dynamics of Fitness: The Body in Action*, Film (Pleasantville, NY: Human Relations Media, 1980).

Suggested Readings

American College of Sports Medicine. *ACSM's Health/Fitness Facility Standards and Guidelines.* Champaign, IL: Human Kinetics, 2011.

American College of Sports Medicine. *ACSM's Resources for Guidelines for Exercise Testing and Prescription.* Philadelphia: Wolters Kluwer/Lippincott Williams & Wilkins, 2010.

American College of Sports Medicine. *ACSM's Resources for the Personal Trainer.* Philadelphia: Lippincott Williams & Wilkins, 2009.

Roizen, M. F. *Real Age: Are You as Young as You Can Be?* New York: Cliff Street Books, 1999.

Answer Key

Chapter 1
1. c   2. e   3. d   4. a   5. e   6. d   7. c   8. b   9. a   10. b

Chapter 2
1. a   2. a   3. e   4. d   5. c   6. d   7. a   8. b   9. e   10. e

Chapter 3
1. b   2. e   3. c   4. d   5. d   6. a   7. a   8. c   9. a   10. e

Chapter 4
1. e   2. b   3. d   4. a   5. b   6. e   7. b   8. b   9. e   10. e

Chapter 5
1. b   2. c   3. e   4. a   5. b   6. e   7. a   8. c   9. d   10. e

Chapter 6
1. a   2. d   3. c   4. c   5. c   6. e   7. b   8. d   9. c   10. c

Chapter 7
1. c   2. d   3. a   4. b   5. d   6. a   7. c   8. c   9. e   10. e

Chapter 8
1. b   2. e   3. a   4. a   5. b   6. e   7. c   8. b   9. e   10. d

Chapter 9
1. d   2. a   3. b   4. e   5. d   6. b   7. a   8. e   9. a   10. e

Chapter 10
1. e   2. b   3. a   4. e   5. e   6. e   7. e   8. e   9. e   10. a

Chapter 11
1. b   2. a   3. a   4. e   5. e   6. e   7. b   8. e   9. b   10. e

Chapter 12
1. a   2. c   3. c   4. e   5. e   6. e   7. a   8. a   9. b   10. c

Chapter 13
1. e   2. a   3. c   4. d   5. d   6. d   7. d   8. e   9. e   10. e

Chapter 14
1. c   2. b   3. e   4. e   5. d   6. a   7. a   8. d   9. e   10. c

Chapter 15
1. e   2. c   3. b   4. d   5. e   6. a   7. e   8. c   9. e   10. a

Glossary

Acquired immunodeficiency syndrome (AIDS) Any of a number of diseases that arise when the body's immune system is compromised by HIV; the final stage of HIV infection.

Action stage Stage of change in the transtheoretical model in which the individual is actively changing a negative behavior or adopting a new, healthy behavior.

Activities of daily living Everyday behaviors that people normally do to function in life (cross the street, carry groceries, lift objects, do laundry, sweep floors).

Acupuncture Chinese medical system that requires body piercing with fine needles during therapy to relieve pain and treat ailments and diseases.

Addiction Compulsive and uncontrollable behavior(s) or use of substance(s).

Adenosine triphosphate (ATP) A high-energy chemical compound that the body uses for immediate energy.

Adequate Intake (AI) The recommended amount of a nutrient intake when sufficient evidence is not available to calculate the EAR and subsequent RDA.

Adipose tissue Fat cells in the body.

Aerobic Describes exercise that requires oxygen to produce the necessary energy (ATP) to carry out the activity.

Aerobic dance A series of exercise routines performed to music.

Air displacement Technique to assess body composition by calculating the body volume from the air replaced by an individual sitting inside a small chamber.

Alcohol (ethyl alcohol) A depressant drug that affects the brain and slows down central nervous system activity; has strong addictive properties.

Alcoholism Disease in which an individual loses control over drinking alcoholic beverages.

Altruism Unselfish concern for the welfare of others.

Alveoli Air sacs in the lungs where oxygen is taken up and carbon dioxide (produced by the body) is released from the blood.

Amenorrhea Cessation of regular menstrual flow.

Amino acids Chemical compounds that contain nitrogen, carbon, hydrogen, and oxygen; the basic building blocks the body uses to build different types of protein.

Amotivational syndrome A condition characterized by loss of motivation, dullness, apathy, and no interest in the future.

Amphetamines A class of powerful central nervous system stimulants.

Anabolic steroids Synthetic versions of the male sex hormone testosterone, which promotes muscle development and hypertrophy.

Anaerobic Describes exercise that does not require oxygen to produce the necessary energy (ATP) to carry out the activity.

Anaerobic threshold The highest percentage of the VO_{2max} at which an individual can exercise (maximal steady state) for an extended time without accumulating significant amounts of lactic acid (accumulation of lactic acid forces an individual to slow down the exercise intensity or stop altogether).

Android obesity Obesity pattern seen in individuals who tend to store fat in the trunk or abdominal area.

Angina pectoris Chest pain associated with coronary heart disease.

Angiogenesis Formation of blood vessels (capillaries).

Angioplasty A procedure in which a balloon-tipped catheter is inserted, then inflated, to widen the inner lumen of the artery.

Anorexia nervosa An eating disorder characterized by self-imposed starvation to lose weight and maintain very low body weight.

Anthropometric measurement Techniques to measure body girths at different sites.

Antibodies Substances produced by the white blood cells in response to an invading agent.

Anticoagulant Any substance that inhibits blood clotting.

Antioxidants Compounds such as vitamins C and E, beta-carotene, and selenium that prevent oxygen from combining with other substances in the body to form harmful compounds.

Aquaphobic Having a fear of water.

Arrhythmias Irregular heart rhythms.

Arterial-venous oxygen difference (a-vO₂diff) The amount of oxygen removed from the blood as determined by the difference in oxygen content between arterial and venous blood.

Atherosclerosis Fatty/cholesterol deposits in the walls of the arteries leading to formation of plaque.

Atrophy Decrease in the size of a cell.

Autogenic training A stress management technique using a form of self-suggestion, wherein individuals are able to place themselves in an autohypnotic state by repeating and concentrating on feelings of heaviness and warmth in the extremities.

Ayurveda Hindu system of medicine based on herbs, diet, massage, meditation, and yoga to help the body boost its own natural healing.

Ballistic (dynamic) stretching Exercises done with jerky, rapid, bouncy movements, or slow, short, and sustained movements.

Basal metabolic rate (BMR) The lowest level of oxygen consumption necessary to sustain life.

Behavior modification The process of permanently changing negative behaviors to positive behaviors that will lead to better health and well-being.

Benign Noncancerous.

Binge-eating disorder An eating disorder characterized by uncontrollable episodes of eating excessive amounts of food within a relatively short time.

Bioelectrical impedance Technique to assess body composition by running a weak electrical current through the body.

Biofeedback A stress management technique in which a person learns to influence physiological responses that are not typically under voluntary control or responses that typically are regulated but for which regulation has broken down as a result of injury, trauma, or illness.

Blood lipids (fat) Cholesterol and triglycerides.

Blood pressure A measure of the force exerted against the walls of the vessels by the blood flowing through them.

Bod Pod Commercial name of the equipment used to assess body composition through the air displacement technique.

Body composition The fat and nonfat components of the human body; important in assessing recommended body weight.

Body mass index (BMI) Parameter to determine thinness or excessive fatness that incorporates height and weight to estimate critical fat values at which the risk for disease increases.

Bone integrity A component of physiological fitness used to determine risk for osteoporosis based on bone mineral density.

Bradycardia Slower heart rate than normal.

Breathing exercises A stress management technique wherein the individual concentrates on "breathing away" the tension and inhaling fresh air to the entire body.

Bulimia nervosa An eating disorder characterized by a pattern of binge eating and purging in an attempt to lose weight and maintain low body weight.

Calorie The amount of heat necessary to raise the temperature of 1 gram of water 1 degree centigrade; used to measure the energy value of food and cost (energy expenditure) of physical activity.

Cancer Group of diseases characterized by uncontrolled growth and spread of abnormal cells.

Capillaries Smallest blood vessels carrying oxygenated blood to the tissues in the body.

Carbohydrate loading Increasing intake of carbohydrates during heavy aerobic training or prior to aerobic endurance events that last longer than 90 minutes.

Carbohydrates A classification of a dietary nutrient containing carbon, hydrogen, and oxygen; the major source of energy for the human body.

Carcinogens Substances that contribute to the formation of cancers.

Carcinoma in situ Encapsulated malignant tumor that has not spread.

Cardiac output Amount of blood pumped by the heart in one minute.

Cardiomyopathy A disease affecting the heart muscle.

Cardiorespiratory endurance The ability of the lungs, heart, and blood vessels to deliver adequate amounts of oxygen to the cells to meet the demands of prolonged physical activity.

Cardiorespiratory training zone Recommended training intensity range, in terms of exercise heart rate, to obtain adequate cardiorespiratory endurance development.

Cardiovascular diseases The array of conditions that affect the heart and the blood vessels.

Carotenoids Pigment substances in plants, some of which are precursors to vitamin A. More than 600 carotenoids are found in nature, about 50 of which are precursors to vitamin A, the most potent being beta-carotene.

Catecholamines "Fight-or-flight" hormones, including epinephrine and norepinephrine.

Cellulite Term frequently used in reference to fat deposits that bulge in layers or streaks; these deposits are enlarged fat cells from excessive accumulation of body fat.

Chiropractics Health care system that proposes that many diseases and ailments are related to misalignments of the vertebrae and emphasizes the manipulation of the spinal column.

Chlamydia A sexually transmitted disease, caused by a bacterial infection, that can cause significant damage to the reproductive system.

Cholesterol A waxy substance, technically a steroid alcohol, found only in animal fats and oil; used in making cell membranes, as a building block for some hormones, in the fatty sheath around nerve fibers, and other necessary substances.

Chronic diseases Illnesses that develop as a result of an unhealthy lifestyle and last a long time.

Chronological age Calendar age.

Chylomicrons Triglyceride-transporting molecules.

Circuit training Alternating exercises by performing them in a sequence of three to six or more.

Cirrhosis A disease characterized by scarring of the liver.

Cocaine 2-beta-carbomethoxy-3-betabenozoxytropane, the primary psychoactive ingredient derived from coca plant leaves.

Cold turkey Eliminating a negative behavior all at once.

Complementary and alternative medicine (CAM) A group of diverse medical and health care systems, practices, and products that are not presently considered to be part of conventional medicine; also called unconventional or nonallopathic medicine.

Complex carbohydrates Carbohydrates formed by three or more simple sugar molecules linked together; also referred to as polysaccharides.

Concentric Describes shortening of a muscle during muscle contraction.

Contemplation stage Stage of change in the transtheoretical model in which the individual is considering changing behavior within the next six months.

Contraindicated exercises Exercises that are not recommended because they may cause injury to a person.

Controlled ballistic stretching Exercises done with slow, short, gentle, and sustained movements.

Conventional Western medicine Traditional medical practice based on methods that are tested through rigorous scientific trials; also called allopathic medicine.

Cool-down Tapering off an exercise session slowly.

Core strength training A program designed to strengthen the abdominal, hip, and spinal muscles (the core of the body).

Coronary heart disease (CHD) Condition in which the arteries that supply the heart muscle with oxygen and nutrients are narrowed by fatty deposits, such as cholesterol and triglycerides.

C-reactive protein (CRP) A protein whose blood levels increase with inflammation, at times hidden deep in the body; elevation of this protein is an indicator of potential cardiovascular events.

Creatine An organic compound derived from meat, fish, and amino acids that combines with inorganic phosphate to form creatine phosphate.

Creatine phosphate (CP) A high-energy compound that the cells use to resynthesize ATP during all-out activities of very short duration.

Cross-training Training modality that uses a combination of aerobic activities to promote to overall fitness.

Cruciferous vegetables Plants that produce cross-shaped leaves (cauliflower, broccoli, cabbage, Brussels sprouts, kohlrabi), which seem to have a protective effect against cancer.

Daily Values (DVs) Reference values for nutrients and food components used in food labels.

Dentist Practitioner who specializes in diseases of the teeth, gums, and oral cavity.

Deoxyribonucleic acid (DNA) Genetic substance of which genes are made; molecule that contains cell's genetic code.

Diabetes mellitus A disease in which the body doesn't produce or utilize insulin properly.

Diastolic blood pressure Pressure exerted by blood against walls of arteries during relaxation phase (diastole) of the heart; lower of the two numbers in blood pressure readings.

Dietary fiber A complex carbohydrate in plant foods that is not digested but is essential to digestion.

Dietary Reference Intake (DRI) A general term that describes four types of nutrient standards that establish adequate amounts and maximum safe nutrient intakes in the diet: Estimated Average Requirement (EAR), Recommended Dietary Allowance (RDA), Adequate Intake (AI), and Tolerable Upper Intake Level (UL).

Disaccharides Simple carbohydrates formed by two monosaccharide units linked together, one of which is glucose. The major disaccharides are sucrose, lactose, and maltose.

Distress Negative stress; unpleasant or harmful stress under which health and performance begin to deteriorate.

Dopamine A neurotransmitter that affects emotional, mental, and motor functions.

Dual energy X-ray absorptiometry (DXA) Method to assess body composition that uses very low dose beams of X-ray energy to measure total body fat mass, fat distribution pattern, and bone density.

Dynamic constant external resistance (DCER) See fixed resistance.

Dynamic training Strength-training method referring to a muscle contraction with movement.

Dysmenorrhea Painful menstruation.

Eccentric Describes lengthening of a muscle during muscle contraction.

Ecosystem A community of organisms interacting with each other in an environment.

Elastic elongation Temporary lengthening of soft tissue.

Electrocardiogram (ECG or EKG) A recording of the electrical activity of the heart.

Electrolytes Substances that become ions in solution and are critical for proper muscle and neuron activation (include sodium, potassium, chloride, calcium, magnesium, phosphate, and bicarbonate, among others).

Emotional eating The consumption of large quantities of food to suppress negative emotions.

Emotional wellness The ability to understand your own feelings, accept your limitations, and achieve emotional stability.

Endorphins Morphine-like substances released from the pituitary gland in the brain during prolonged aerobic exercise, thought to induce feelings of euphoria and natural well-being.

Energy-balancing equation A principle holding that as long as caloric input equals caloric output, the person will not gain or lose weight. If caloric input exceeds output, the person gains weight; if output exceeds input, the person loses weight.

Environmental wellness The capability to live in a clean and safe environment that is not detrimental to health.

Enzymes Catalysts that facilitate chemical reactions in the body.

Essential fat Minimal amount of body fat needed for normal physiological functions; constitutes about 3 percent of total weight in men and 12 percent in women.

Estimated Average Requirement (EAR) The amount of a nutrient that meets the dietary needs of half the people.

Estimated Energy Requirement (EER) The average dietary energy (caloric) intake that is predicted to maintain energy balance in a healthy adult of defined age, gender, weight, height, and level of physical activity, consistent with good health.

Estrogen Female sex hormone essential for bone formation and conservation of bone density.

Eustress Positive stress; health and performance continue to improve, even as stress increases.

Exercise A type of physical activity that requires planned, structured, and repetitive bodily movement with the intent of improving or maintaining one or more components of physical fitness.

Exercise intolerance Inability to function during exercise because of excessive fatigue or extreme feelings of discomfort.

Explanatory style The way people perceive the events in their lives, from an optimistic or a pessimistic perspective.

Fast-twitch fibers Muscle fibers with greater anaerobic potential and fast speed of contraction.

Fats A classification of nutrients containing carbon, hydrogen, some oxygen, and sometimes other chemical elements.

Ferritin Iron stored in the body.

Fighting spirit Determination; the open expression of emotions, whether negative or positive.

Fight or flight Physiological response of the body to stress that prepares the individual to take action by stimulating the body's vital defense systems.

FITT An acronym used to describe the four cardiorespiratory exercise prescription variables: frequency, intensity, type (mode), and time (duration).

Fixed resistance Type of exercise in which a constant resistance is moved through a joint's full range of motion (dumbbells, barbells, machines using a constant resistance).

Folate One of the B vitamins.

Fortified foods Foods that have been modified by the addition or increase of nutrients that either were not present or were present in insignificant amounts with the intent of preventing nutrient deficiencies.

Free weights Barbells and dumbbells.

Frequency Number of times per week a person engages in exercise.

Functional capacity The ability to perform the ordinary and unusual demands of daily living without limitations, excessive fatigue, or injury.

Functional foods Foods or food ingredients containing physiologically active substances that provide specific health benefits beyond those supplied by basic nutrition.

Functional independence Ability to carry out activities of daily living without assistance from other individuals.

General adaptation syndrome (GAS) A theoretical model that explains the body's adaptation to sustained stress; includes three stages: Alarm reaction, resistance, and exhaustion/recovery.

Genetically modified (GM) foods Foods whose basic genetic material (DNA) is manipulated by inserting genes with desirable traits from one plant, animal, or microorganism into another one either to introduce new traits or to enhance existing ones.

Genital herpes A sexually transmitted disease caused by a viral infection of the herpes simplex virus types 1 and 2. The virus can attack different areas of the body but typically causes blisters on the genitals.

Genital warts A sexually transmitted disease caused by a viral infection.

Gonorrhea A sexually transmitted disease caused by a bacterial infection.

Girth measurements Technique to assess body composition by measuring circumferences at specific body sites.

Glucose intolerance A condition characterized by slightly elevated blood glucose levels.

Glycemic index A measure that is used to rate the plasma glucose response of carbohydrate-containing foods with the response produced by the same amount of carbohydrate from a standard source, usually glucose or white bread.

Glycogen Form in which glucose is stored in the body.

Goals The ultimate aims toward which effort is directed.

Gynoid obesity Obesity pattern seen in people who store fat primarily around the hips and thighs.

Hatha yoga A form of yoga that incorporates specific sequences of static-stretching postures to help induce the relaxation response.

Health A state of complete well-being—not just the absence of disease or infirmity.

Health fitness standards The lowest fitness requirements for maintaining good health, decreasing the risk for chronic diseases, and lowering the incidence of muscular-skeletal injuries.

Health promotion The science and art of enabling people to increase control over their lifestyles to move toward a state of wellness.

Health-related fitness Fitness programs that are prescribed to improve the individual's overall health.

Healthy life expectancy (HLE) Number of years a person is expected to live in good health; this number is obtained by subtracting ill-health years from the overall life expectancy.

Heart rate reserve (HRR) The difference between maximal heart rate and resting heart rate.

Heat cramps Muscle spasms caused by heat-induced changes in electrolyte balance in muscle cells.

Heat exhaustion Heat-related fatigue.

Heat stroke Emergency situation resulting from the body being subjected to high atmospheric temperatures.

Hemoglobin Protein–iron compound in red blood cells that transports oxygen in the blood.

Herbal medicine Unconventional system that uses herbs to treat ailments and disease.

Heroin A potent drug that is a derivative of opium.

High-density lipoprotein (HDL) Cholesterol-transporting molecule in the blood ("good" cholesterol) that helps clear cholesterol from the blood.

High-impact aerobics Exercises incorporating movements in which both feet are off the ground at the same time momentarily.

Homeopathy System of treatment based on the use of minute quantities of remedies that in large amounts produce effects similar to the disease being treated.

Homeostasis A natural state of equilibrium; the body attempts to maintain this equilibrium by constantly reacting to external forces that attempt to disrupt this fine balance.

Homocysteine An amino acid that, when allowed to accumulate in the blood, may lead to plaque formation and blockage of arteries.

Human immunodeficiency virus (HIV) Virus that leads to AIDS.

Human papillomavirus (HPV) A group of viruses that can cause sexually transmitted diseases.

Hydrostatic weighing Underwater technique to assess body composition; considered the most accurate of the body composition assessment techniques.

Hypertension Chronically elevated blood pressure.

Hypertrophy An increase in the size of the cell, as in muscle hypertrophy.

Hypokinetic diseases "Hypo" denotes "lack of"; therefore, lack of physical activity.

Hyponatremia A low sodium concentration in the blood caused by overhydration with water.

Hypotension Low blood pressure.

Hypothermia A breakdown in the body's ability to generate heat; a drop in body temperature below 95°F.

Imagery Mental visualization of relaxing images and scenes to induce body relaxation in times of stress or as an aid in the treatment of certain medical conditions such as cancer, hypertension, asthma, chronic pain, and obesity.

Immunity The function that guards the body from invaders, both internal and external.

Insulin A hormone secreted by the pancreas; essential for proper metabolism of blood glucose (sugar) and maintenance of blood glucose level.

Insulin resistance Inability of the cells to respond appropriately to insulin.

Intensity In cardiorespiratory exercise, how hard a person has to exercise to improve or maintain fitness.

Intensity (for flexibility exercises) Degree of stretch when doing flexibility exercises.

International units (IU) Measure of nutrients in foods.

Interval training A system of exercise wherein a short period of intense effort is followed by a specified recovery period according to a prescribed ratio; for instance, a 1:3 work-to-recovery ratio.

Isokinetic training Strength-training method in which the speed of the muscle contraction is kept constant because the equipment (machine) provides an accommodating resistance to match the user's force (maximal) through the range of motion.

Isometric training Strength-training method referring to a muscle contraction that produces little or no movement, such as pushing or pulling against an immovable object.

Lactic acid End product of anaerobic glycolysis (metabolism).

Lactovegetarians Vegetarians who eat foods from the milk group.

Lapse (v.) To slip or fall back temporarily into unhealthy behavior(s); (n.) short-term failure to maintain healthy behaviors.

Lean body mass Body weight without body fat.

Learning theories Behavioral modification perspective stating that most behaviors are learned and maintained under complex schedules of reinforcement and anticipated outcomes.

Life expectancy Number of years a person is expected to live based on the person's birth year.

Life Experiences Survey A questionnaire used to assess sources of stress in life.

Lipoproteins Lipids covered by proteins; these transport fats in the blood. Types are LDL, HDL, and VLDL.

Locus of control A concept examining the extent to which a person believes that he or she can influence the external environment.

Low-density lipoprotein (LDL) Cholesterol-transporting molecule in the blood ("bad" cholesterol) that tends to increase blood cholesterol.

Low-impact aerobics Exercises in which at least one foot is in contact with the ground or floor at all times.

Lymphocytes Immune system cells responsible for waging war against disease or infection.

Magnetic therapy Unconventional treatment that relies on magnetic energy to promote healing.

Maintenance stage Stage of change in the transtheoretical model in which the individual maintains behavioral change for up to five years.

Malignant Cancerous.

Mammogram Low-dose X-rays of the breasts used as a screening technique for the early detection of breast cancer.

Marijuana A psychoactive drug prepared from a mixture of crushed leaves, flowers, small branches, stems, and seeds from the hemp plant *Cannabis sativa*.

Massage therapy The rubbing or kneading of body parts to treat ailments.

Mastery experiences Moments when an individual has repeated successes in the performance of a task.

Maximal heart rate (MHR) Highest heart rate for a person, related primarily to age.

Maximal oxygen uptake (VO_{2max}) Maximum amount of oxygen the body is able to utilize per minute of physical activity, commonly expressed in mL/kg/min; the best indicator of cardiorespiratory or aerobic fitness.

MDA A hallucinogenic drug that is structurally similar to amphetamine.

MDMA A synthetic hallucinogenic drug with a chemical structure that closely resembles MDA and methamphetamine; also known as Ecstasy.

Meditation A stress management technique used to gain control over one's attention by clearing the mind and blocking out the stressor(s) responsible for the increased tension.

Mediterranean diet Typical diet of people around the Mediterranean region, focusing on olive oil, red wine, grains, legumes, vegetables, and fruits, with limited amounts of meat, fish, milk, and cheese.

Megadoses For most vitamins, 10 times the RDA or more; for vitamins A and D, 5 and 2 times the RDA, respectively.

Melanoma The most virulent, rapidly spreading form of skin cancer.

Mental wellness A state in which your mind is engaged in lively interaction with the world around you.

MET Short for *metabolic equivalent*, the rate of energy expenditure at rest; 1 MET is the equivalent of a VO_2 of 3.5 mL/kg/min.

Metabolic fitness A component of physiological fitness that denotes reduction in the risk for diabetes and cardiovascular disease through a moderate-intensity exercise program in spite of little or no improvement in cardiorespiratory fitness.

Metabolic profile A measurement of plasma insulin, glucose, lipid, and lipoprotein levels to assess risk for diabetes and cardiovascular disease.

Metabolic syndrome An array of metabolic abnormalities that contribute to the development of atherosclerosis triggered by insulin resistance. These conditions include low HDL cholesterol, high triglycerides, high blood pressure, and an increased blood-clotting mechanism.

Metabolism All energy and material transformations that occur within living cells; necessary to sustain life.

Metastasis The movement of cells from one part of the body to another.

Methamphetamine A potent form of amphetamine.

Minerals Inorganic nutrients essential for normal body functions; found in the body and in food.

Mitochondria Structures within the cells where energy transformations take place.

Mode Form or type of exercise.

Moderate physical activity Activity that uses 150 calories of energy per day, or 1,000 calories per week.

Monogamous A relationship in which two people have sexual relations only with each other.

Monosaccharides The simplest carbohydrates (sugars), formed by five- or six-carbon skeletons. The three most common monosaccharides are glucose, fructose, and galactose.

Morbidity A condition related to or caused by illness or disease.

Morphological fitness A component of physiological fitness used in reference to body composition factors such as percent body fat, body fat distribution, and body circumference.

Motivation The desire and will to do something.

Motor neurons Nerves connecting the central nervous system to the muscle.

Motor unit The combination of a motor neuron and the muscle fibers that neuron innervates.

Muscular endurance The ability of a muscle to exert submaximal force repeatedly over time.

Muscular fitness A term that is used to define good levels of both muscular strength and muscular endurance.

Muscular strength The ability of a muscle to exert maximum force against resistance (for example, 1 repetition maximum [or 1 RM] on the bench press exercise).

Myocardial infarction Heart attack; damage to or death of an area of the heart muscle as a result of an obstructed artery to that area.

Myocardium Heart muscle.

Naturopathic medicine Unconventional system of medicine that relies exclusively on natural remedies to treat disease and ailments.

Negative resistance The lowering or eccentric phase of a repetition during a strength-training exercise.

Neustress Neutral stress; stress that is neither harmful nor helpful.

Nicotine Addictive compound found in tobacco leaves.

Nitrosamines Potentially cancer-causing compounds formed when nitrites and nitrates, which prevent the growth of harmful bacteria in processed meats, combine with other chemicals in the stomach.

Nonmelanoma skin cancer Cancer that spreads or grows at the original site but does not metastasize to other regions of the body.

Nonresponders Individuals who exhibit small or no improvements in fitness as compared with others who undergo the same training program.

Nurse Health care practitioner who assists in the diagnosis and treatment of health problems and provides many services to patients in a variety of settings.

Nutrient density A measure of the amount of nutrients and calories in various foods.

Nutrients Substances found in food that provide energy, regulate metabolism, and help with growth and repair of body tissues.

Nutrition Science that studies the relationship of foods to optimal health and performance.

Obesity An excessive accumulation of body fat, usually at least 30 percent above recommended body weight.

Occupational wellness The ability to perform your job skillfully and effectively under conditions that provide personal and team satisfaction and adequately reward each individual.

Oligomenorrhea Irregular menstrual cycles.

Omega-6 fatty acids Polyunsaturated fatty acids found primarily in corn and sunflower oils and most oils in processed foods.

Omega-3 fatty acids Polyunsaturated fatty acids found primarily in cold-water seafood and flaxseeds; thought to lower blood cholesterol and triglycerides.

Oncogenes Genes that initiate cell division.

One repetition maximum (1 RM) The maximum amount of resistance an individual is able to lift in a single effort.

Ophthalmologist Medical specialist concerned with diseases of the eye and prescription of corrective lenses.

Opportunistic infections Infections that arise in the absence of a healthy immune system, which would fight them off in healthy people.

Optometrist Health care practitioner who specializes in the prescription and adaptation of lenses.

Oral surgeon A dentist who specializes in surgical procedures of the oral-facial complex.

Orthodontist A dentist who specializes in the correction and prevention of teeth irregularities.

Osteopath A medical practitioner with specialized training in musculoskeletal problems who uses diagnostic and therapeutic methods of conventional medicine in addition to manipulative measures.

Osteoporosis A condition of softening, deterioration, or loss of bone mineral density that leads to disability, bone fractures, and even death from medical complications.

Overload principle Training concept in which the demands placed on a system (cardiorespiratory or muscular) must be increased systematically and progressively over time to cause physiological adaptation (development or improvement).

Overtraining An emotional, behavioral, and physical condition marked by increased fatigue, decreased performance, persistent muscle soreness, mood disturbances, and feelings of "staleness" or "burnout" as a result of excessive physical training.

Overweight An excess amount of weight against a given standard, such as height or recommended percent body fat.

Ovolactovegetarians Vegetarians who include eggs and milk products in their diet.

Ovovegetarians Vegetarians who allow eggs in their diet.

Oxygen free radicals Substances formed during metabolism that attack and damage proteins and lipids, in particular the cell membrane and DNA, leading to diseases such as heart disease, cancer, and emphysema.

Oxygen uptake (VO$_2$) The amount of oxygen the human body uses.

Pedometer An electronic device that senses body motion and counts footsteps. Some pedometers also record distance, calories burned, speeds, "aerobic steps," and time spent being physically active.

Pelvic inflammatory disease (PID) An overall designation referring to the effects of other STIs, primarily chlamydia and gonorrhea.

Percent body fat Proportional amount of fat in the body based on the person's total weight; includes both essential fat and storage fat; also termed *fat mass*.

Periodization A training approach that divides the season into three cycles (macrocycles, mesocycles, and microcycles) using a systematic variation in intensity and volume of training to enhance fitness and performance.

Peripheral vascular disease Narrowing of the peripheral blood vessels.

Peristalsis Involuntary muscle contractions of intestinal walls that facilitate excretion of wastes.

Personal trainer A health/fitness professional who evaluates, motivates, educates, and trains clients to help them meet individualized, healthy lifestyle goals.

Physical activity Bodily movement produced by skeletal muscles; requires expenditure of energy and produces progressive health benefits. Examples include walking, taking the stairs, dancing, gardening, doing yard work, house cleaning, snow shoveling, washing the car, and all forms of structured exercise.

Physical activity perceived exertion (H-PAPE) scale A perception scale to monitor or interpret the intensity of physical activity and exercise.

Physical fitness The ability to meet the ordinary as well as the unusual demands of daily life safely and effectively without being overly fatigued and still have energy left for leisure and recreational activities.

Physical fitness standards A fitness level that allows a person to sustain moderate-to-vigorous physical activity without undue fatigue and the ability to closely maintain this level throughout life.

Physical wellness Good physical fitness and confidence in your personal ability to take care of health problems.

Physician assistant Health care practitioner trained to treat most standard cases of care.

Physiological age The biological and functional capacity of the body in relation to the person's maximal potential at any given age in the lifespan.

Physiological fitness A term used primarily in the field of medicine to mean biologic systems affected by physical activity and the role of activity in preventing disease.

Phytonutrients Compounds thought to prevent and fight cancer; found in large quantities in fruits and vegetables.

Pilates A training program that uses exercises designed to help strengthen the body's core by developing pelvic stability and abdominal control; exercises are coupled with focused breathing patterns.

Plastic elongation Permanent lengthening of soft tissue.

Plyometric exercise Explosive jump training, incorporating speed and strength training to enhance explosiveness.

Plyometric training A form of aerobic exercise that requires forceful jumps or springing off the ground immediately after landing from a previous jump.

Positive resistance The lifting, pushing, or concentric phase of a repetition during a strength-training exercise.

Prayer Sincere and humble communication with a higher power.

Precontemplation stage Stage of change in the transtheoretical model in which an individual is unwilling to change behavior.

Preparation stage Stage of change in the transtheoretical model in which the individual is getting ready to make a change within the next month.

Primary care physician A medical practitioner who provides routine treatment of ailments; typically, the patient's first contact for health care.

Principle of individuality Training concept holding that genetics plays a major role in individual responses to exercise training and that these differences must be considered when designing exercise programs for different people.

Probiotics Healthy bacteria (abundant in yogurt) that help break down foods and prevent disease-causing organisms from settling in the intestines.

Problem-solving model Behavioral modification model proposing that many behaviors are the result of making decisions as the individual seeks to solve the problem behavior.

Processes of change Actions that help you achieve change in behavior.

Progressive muscle relaxation A stress management technique that involves sequential contraction and relaxation of muscle groups throughout the body.

Progressive resistance training A gradual increase of resistance over a period of time.

Proprioceptive neuromuscular facilitation (PNF) Mode of stretching that uses reflexes and neuromuscular principles to relax the muscles being stretched.

Proteins A classification of nutrients consisting of complex organic compounds containing nitrogen and formed by combinations of amino acids; the main substances used in the body to build and repair tissues.

Quackery/fraud The conscious promotion of unproven claims for profit.

Range of motion Entire arc of movement of a given joint.

Recommended body weight Body weight at which there seems to be no harm to human health; healthy weight.

Recommended Dietary Allowance (RDA) The daily amount of a nutrient (statistically determined from the EARs) that is considered adequate to meet the known nutrient needs of almost 98 percent of all healthy people in the United States.

Recovery time Amount of time the body takes to return to resting levels after exercise.

Registered dietitian (RD) A person with a college degree in dietetics who meets all certification and continuing education requirements of the American Dietetic Association or Dietitians of Canada.

Relapse (v.) To slip or fall back into unhealthy behavior(s) over a longer time; (n.) longer-term failure to maintain healthy behaviors.

Relapse prevention Behavioral modification model based on the principle that high-risk situations can be anticipated through the development of strategies to prevent lapses and relapses.

Repetitions Number of times a given stretching exercise is performed.

Resistance Amount of weight lifted.

Responders Individuals who exhibit improvements in fitness as a result of exercise training.

Resting heart rate (RHR) Heart rate after a person has been sitting quietly for 15–20 minutes.

Resting metabolic rate (RMR) The energy requirement to maintain the body's vital processes in the resting state.

Resting metabolism Amount of energy (expressed in milliliters of oxygen per minute or total calories per day) an individual requires during resting conditions to sustain proper body function.

Reverse cholesterol transport A process in which HDL molecules attract cholesterol and carry it to the liver, where it is changed to bile and eventually excreted in the stool.

Ribonucleic acid (RNA) Genetic material that guides the formation of cell proteins.

RICE An acronym used to describe the standard treatment procedure for acute sports injuries: *r*est, *i*ce (cold application), *c*ompression, and *e*levation.

Risk factors Lifestyle and genetic variables that may lead to disease.

RM zone A range of repetitions that are to be performed maximally during one set. For example, an 8 to 12 RM zone implies that the individual will perform anywhere from 8 to 12 repetitions, but could not perform any more following the completion of the final repetition (e.g., 9 RM and could not perform a 10th repetition).

Sarcopenia Age-related loss of lean body mass, strength, and function.

Sedentary Description of a person who is relatively inactive and whose lifestyle is characterized by a lot of sitting.

Sedentary Death Syndrome (SeDS) Cause of death attributed to a lack of regular physical activity.

Self-efficacy The belief in one's own ability to perform a given task.

Self-esteem A sense of positive self-regard and self-respect.

Semivegetarians Vegetarians who include milk products, eggs, and fish and poultry in the diet.

Set A fixed number of repetitions; one set of bench presses might be 10 repetitions.

Setpoint Weight control theory that the body has an established weight that it strongly attempts to maintain.

Sexually transmitted infections (STIs) Communicable diseases spread through sexual contact.

Shin splints Injury to the lower leg characterized by pain and irritation in the shin region of the leg.

Side stitch A sharp pain in the side of the abdomen.

Simple carbohydrates Formed by simple or double sugar units with little nutritive value; divided into monosaccharides and disaccharides.

Skill-related fitness Fitness components important for success in skillful activities and athletic events; encompasses agility, balance, coordination, power, reaction time, and speed.

Skinfold thickness Technique to assess body composition by measuring a double thickness of skin at specific body sites.

Slow-sustained stretching Exercises in which the muscles are lengthened gradually through a joint's complete range of motion.

Slow-twitch fibers Muscle fibers with greater aerobic potential and slow speed of contraction.

SMART goals *S*pecific, *m*easurable, *a*ttainable, *r*ealistic, and *t*ime-specific goals.

Social cognitive theory Behavioral modification model holding that behavior change is influenced by the environment, self-efficacy, and characteristics of the behavior itself.

Social wellness The ability to relate well to others, both within and outside the family unit.

Specific adaptation to imposed demand (SAID) training Training principle stating that, for improvements to occur in a specific activity, the exercises performed during a strength-training program should resemble as closely as possible the movement patterns encountered in that particular activity.

Specificity of training Principle that training must be done with the specific muscle the person is attempting to improve.

Sphygmomanometer Inflatable bladder contained within a cuff and a mercury gravity manometer (or aneroid manometer) from which blood pressure is read.

Spiritual wellness The sense that life is meaningful and has purpose and that some power brings all humanity together; the ethics, values, and morals that guide you and give meaning and direction to life.

Spontaneous remission Inexplicable recovery from incurable disease.

Spot reducing Fallacious theory proposing that exercising a specific body part will result in significant fat reduction in that area.

Step aerobics A form of exercise that combines stepping up and down from a bench with arm movements.

Sterols Derived fats, of which cholesterol is the best-known example.

Storage fat Body fat in excess of essential fat; stored in adipose tissue.

Strength training A program designed to improve muscular strength and/or endurance through a series of progressive resistance (weight) training exercises that overload the muscle system and cause physiological development.

Stress The mental, emotional, and physiological response of the body to any situation that is new, threatening, frightening, or exciting.

Stress electrocardiogram An exercise test during which the workload is increased gradually until the individual reaches maximal fatigue, with blood pressure and 12-lead electrocardiographic monitoring throughout the test.

Stressor Stress-causing event.

Stretching Moving the joints beyond the accustomed range of motion.

Stroke Condition in which a blood vessel that feeds the brain ruptures or is clogged, leading to blood flow disruption to the brain.

Stroke volume Amount of blood pumped by the heart in one beat.

Structured interview Assessment tool used to determine behavioral patterns that define Type A and B personalities.

Subcutaneous fat Deposits of fat directly under the skin.

Subluxation Partial dislocation of a joint.

Substrates Substances acted upon by an enzyme (examples: carbohydrates, fats).

Sun protection factor (SPF) Degree of protection offered by ingredients in sunscreen lotion; at least SPF 15 is recommended.

Supplements Tablets, pills, capsules, liquids, or powders that contain vitamins, minerals, antioxidants, amino acids, herbs, or fiber that individuals take to increase their intake of these nutrients.

Suppressor genes Genes that deactivate cell division.

Synergistic action The effect of mixing two or more drugs, which can be much greater than the sum of two or more drugs acting by themselves.

Synergy A reaction in which the result is greater than the sum of its two parts.

Syphilis A sexually transmitted disease caused by a bacterial infection.

Systolic blood pressure Pressure exerted by blood against walls of arteries during forceful contraction (systole) of the heart; higher of the two numbers in blood pressure readings.

Tachycardia Faster than normal heart rate.

Tar Chemical compound that forms during the burning of tobacco leaves.

Techniques of change Methods or procedures used during each process of change.

Telomerase An enzyme that allows cells to reproduce indefinitely.

Telomeres A strand of molecules at both ends of a chromosome.

Termination/adoption stage Stage of change in the transtheoretical model in which the individual has eliminated an undesirable behavior or maintained a positive behavior for more than five years.

Thermogenic response Amount of energy required to digest food.

Trans fatty acid Solidified fat formed by adding hydrogen to monounsaturated and polyunsaturated fats to increase shelf life.

Transtheoretical model Behavioral modification model proposing that change is accomplished through a series of progressive stages in keeping with a person's readiness to change.

Triglycerides Fats formed by glycerol and three fatty acids; also called free fatty acids.

Type A Behavior pattern characteristic of a hard-driving, overambitious, aggressive, at times hostile, and overly competitive person.

Type B Behavior pattern characteristic of a calm, casual, relaxed, and easygoing individual.

Type C Behavior pattern of individuals who are just as highly stressed as Type A people but do not seem to be at higher risk for disease than Type B.

Type 1 diabetes Insulin-dependent diabetes mellitus (IDDM), a condition in which the pancreas produces little or no insulin; also known as juvenile diabetes.

Type 2 diabetes Non-insulin-dependent diabetes mellitus (NIDDM), a condition in which insulin is not processed properly; also known as adult-onset diabetes.

Ultraviolet A (UVA) rays Ultraviolet rays that pass deeper into the skin and are believed to cause skin damage and skin cancers.

Ultraviolet B (UVB) rays Ultraviolet rays that cause sunburn and encourage skin cancers.

Underweight Extremely low body weight.

Upper Intake Level (UL) The highest level of nutrient intake that seems safe for most healthy people, beyond which exists an increased risk of adverse effects.

Variable resistance Training using special machines equipped with mechanical devices that provide differing amounts of resistance through the range of motion.

Vegans Vegetarians who eat no animal products at all.

Vegetarians Individuals whose diet is of vegetable or plant origin.

Very low calorie diet A diet that allows an energy intake (consumption) of only 800 calories or less per day.

Very low density lipoproteins (VLDLs) Triglyceride, cholesterol, and phospholipid-transporting molecules in the blood that tend to increase blood cholesterol.

Vicarious experiences Developing a belief that one can perform a task by observing peers of similar ability perform that task.

Vigorous activity Any exercise that requires a metabolic equivalent (MET) level equal to or greater than 6 METs (21 mL/kg/min). One MET is the energy expenditure at rest, 3.5 mL/kg/min, and METs are defined as multiples of this resting metabolic rate (examples of activities that require a 6 MET level include aerobics, walking uphill at 3.5 mph, cycling at 10 to 12 mph, playing doubles in tennis, and vigorous strength training).

Vigorous exercise Cardiorespiratory exercise that requires an intensity level above 60 percent of maximal capacity.

Vitamins Organic nutrients essential for normal metabolism, growth, and development of the body.

Volume The total amount of training performed in a given work period (day, week, month, or season).

Volume (in strength training) The sum of all the repetitions performed multiplied by the resistances used during a strength-training session.

Waist circumference (WC) A waist girth measurement to assess potential risk for disease based on intra-abdominal fat content.

Warm-up Starting a workout slowly.

Water The most important classification of essential body nutrients, involved in almost every vital body process.

Weight-regulating mechanism (WRM) A feature of the hypothalamus of the brain that controls how much the body should weigh.

Wellness The constant and deliberate effort to stay healthy and achieve the highest potential for well-being. It encompasses seven dimensions—physical, emotional, mental, social, environmental, occupational, and spiritual—and integrates them all into a quality life.

Workload Load (or intensity) placed on the body during physical activity.

Yoga A school of thought in the Hindu religion that seeks to help the individual attain a higher level of spirituality and peace of mind.

Index

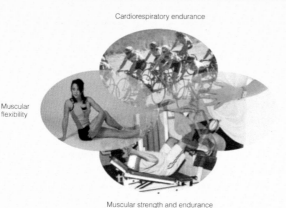

Cardiorespiratory endurance

Muscular flexibility

Body composition

Muscular strength and endurance

Research indicates that adhering to the following 12 lifestyle habits will significantly improve health and extend life.

❑ 1. Participate in a lifetime physical activity program.

❑ 2. Do not smoke cigarettes.

❑ 3. Eat right.

❑ 4. Avoid snacking.

❑ 5. Maintain recommended body weight through adequate nutrition and exercise.

❑ 6. Get enough rest.

❑ 7. Lower your stress levels.

❑ 8. Be wary of alcohol.

❑ 9. Surround yourself with healthy friendships.

❑ 10. Be informed about the environment.

❑ 11. Increase education.

❑ 12. Take personal safety measures.

- **Cardiorespiratory endurance** The ability of the lungs, heart, and blood vessels to deliver adequate amounts of oxygen to the cells to meet the demands of prolonged physical activity.

- **Body composition** The fat and non-fat components of the human body; important in assessing recommended body weight.

- **Muscular strength** The ability of a muscle to exert maximum force against resistance (for example, 1 repetition maximum [or 1 RM] on the bench press exercise).

- **Muscular endurance** The ability of a muscle to exert submaximal force repeatedly over time.

- **Flexibility** The achievable range of motion at a joint or group of joints without causing injury.

	Pace (min/Mile)				
	Walking		**Jogging**		
Height	20	15	12	10	8
Women					
5'0"	2,371	2,054	1,997	1,710	1,423
5'4"	2,315	1,998	1,943	1,656	1,369
5'8"	2,258	1,941	1,889	1,602	1,315
6'0"	2,202	1,885	1,835	1,548	1,261
Men					
5'2"	2,310	1,993	1,970	1,683	1,396
5'6"	2,253	1,937	1,916	1,629	1,342
5'10"	2,197	1,880	1,862	1,575	1,288
6'2"	2,141	1,824	1,808	1,521	1,234

Prediction Equations (pace in min/mile and height in inches):
Walking
Women: Steps/mile = $1{,}949 + [(63.4 \times \text{pace}) - (14.1 \times \text{height})]$
Men: Steps/mile = $1{,}916 + [(63.4 \times \text{pace}) - (14.1 \times \text{height})]$
Running
Women and Men: Steps/mile = $1{,}084 + [(143.6 \times \text{pace}) - (13.5 \times \text{height})]$
Source: Werner W. K. Hoeger et al., "One- mile step count at walking and running speeds." *ACSM's Health & Fitness Journal,* Vol 12(1):14–19, 2008.

Stages of Change: Model of Progression and Relapse

Steps for Successful Behavior Modification

- ❑ 1. Acknowledge that you have a problem.
- ❑ 2. Describe the behavior to change (increase physical activity, stop overeating, quit smoking).
- ❑ 3. List advantages and disadvantages of changing the specified behavior.
- ❑ 4. Decide positively that you will change.
- ❑ 5. Identify your stage of change.
- ❑ 6. Set a realistic goal (SMART goal), completion date, and sign a behavioral contract.
- ❑ 7. Define your behavioral change plan: List processes of change, techniques of change, and objectives that will help you reach your goal.
- ❑ 8. Implement the behavior change plan.
- ❑ 9. Monitor your progress toward the desired goal.
- ❑ 10. Periodically evaluate and reassess your goal.
- ❑ 11. Reward yourself when you achieve your goal.
- ❑ 12. Maintain the successful change for good.

Computation for Fat Content in Food

Nutrition Facts

Serving Size 1 cup (240 ml)
Servings Per Container 4

Amount Per Serving

Calories 120	Calories from Fat 45

	% Daily Value*
Total Fat 5g	**8%**
Saturated Fat 3g	**15%**
Trans Fat 0g	**0%**
Cholesterol 20mg	**7%**
Sodium 120mg	**5%**
Total Carbohydrate 12g	**4%**
Dietary Fiber 0g	**0%**
Sugars 12g	
Protein 8g	

Vitamin A	10%	•	Vitamin C	4%
Calcium	30%	•	Iron	0%

* Percent Daily Values are based on a 2,000 calorie diet. Your daily values may be higher or lower depending on your calorie needs:

	Calories	2,000	2,500
Total Fat	Less than	65g	80g
Sat Fat	Less than	20g	25g
Cholesterol	Less than	300mg	300mg
Sodium	Less than	2,300mg	2,300mg
Total Carbohydrate		300g	375g
Fiber		25g	30g

Calories per gram:
Fat 9 • Carbohydrate 4 • Protein 4

Percent fat calories = (grams of fat × 9) ÷ calories per serving × 100

5 grams of fat × 9 calories per grams of fat = 45 calories from fat

45 calories from fat ÷ 120 calories per serving × 100 = 38% fat

Good Sources of Vitamin D

Food	Amount	IU*
Multivitamins (most brands)	daily dose	400
Salmon	3.5 oz	360
Mackerel	3.5 oz	345
Sardines (oil/drained)	3.5 oz	250
Shrimp	3.5 oz	200
Orange juice (D-fortified)	8 oz	100
Milk (any type/D-fortified)	8 oz	100
Margarine (D-fortified)	1 tbsp	60
Yogurt (D-fortified)	6–8 oz	60
Cereal (D-fortified)	¾–1 c	40
Egg	1	20

*IU = international units

Burgers

	Calories	Total Fat (grams)	Saturated Fat (grams)	Percent Fat Calories
McDonald's Big Mac	590	34	11	52
McDonald's Big N' Tasty with Cheese	590	37	12	56
McDonald's Quarter Pounder with Cheese	530	30	13	51
Burger King Whopper	760	46	15	54
Burger King Bacon Double Cheeseburger	580	34	18	53
Burger King BK Smokehouse Cheddar Griller	720	48	19	60
Burger King Whopper with Cheese	850	53	22	56
Burger King Double Whopper	1,060	69	27	59
Burger King Double Whopper with Cheese	1,150	76	33	59
Wendy's Baconator	830	51	22	55

Continued on back

Mexican

	Calories	Total Fat (grams)	Saturated Fat (grams)	Percent Fat Calories
Taco Bell Crunchy Taco	170	10	4	53
Taco Bell Taco Supreme	220	14	6	57
Taco Bell Soft Chicken Taco	190	7	3	33
Taco Bell Bean Burrito	370	12	4	29
Taco Bell Fiesta Steak Burrito	370	12	4	29
Taco Bell Grilled Steak Soft Taco	290	17	4	53
Taco Bell Double Decker Taco	340	14	5	37

French Fries

	Calories	Total Fat (grams)	Saturated Fat (grams)	Percent Fat Calories
Wendy's, biggie (5½ oz)	440	19	7	39
McDonald's, large (6 oz)	540	26	9	43
Burger King, large (5½ oz)	500	25	13	45

Continued on back

Do you regularly follow the habits below?

To select nutritious foods:

❑ 1. Given the choice between whole foods and refined, processed foods, choose the former (apples rather than apple pie, potatoes rather than potato chips). No nutrients have been refined out of the whole foods, and they contain less fat, salt, and sugar.

❑ 2. Choose the leaner cuts of meat. Select fish or poultry often, beef seldom. Ask for broiled, not fried, to control your fat intake.

❑ 3. Use both raw and cooked vegetables and fruits. Raw foods offer more fiber and vitamins, such as folate and thiamin, that are destroyed by cooking. Cooking foods frees other vitamins and minerals for absorption.

❑ 4. Include milk, milk products, or other calcium sources for the calcium you need. Use low-fat or non-fat items to reduce fat and calories.

❑ 5. Learn to use margarine, butter, and oils sparingly. A little gives flavor, a lot overloads you with fat and calories, and increases disease risk.

Continued on back

The following "super" foods that fight disease and promote health should be included often in your diet. Are you eating these foods regularly?

❑ Acai berries
❑ Avocados
❑ Bananas
❑ Barley
❑ Beans
❑ Beets
❑ Blueberries
❑ Broccoli
❑ Butternut squash
❑ Carrots
❑ Flaxseeds
❑ Goji berries
❑ Grapes
❑ Kale
❑ Kiwifruit
❑ Lentils
❑ Nuts (Brazil, walnuts)
❑ Oats and oatmeal
❑ Olives and olive oil
❑ Onions
❑ Oranges
❑ Peppers
❑ Pomegranites
❑ Salmon (wild)
❑ Soy
❑ Strawberries
❑ Spinach
❑ Sweet potatoes
❑ Tea (green, black, red)
❑ Tomatoes
❑ Yogurt

Sandwiches	Calories	Total Fat (grams)	Saturated Fat (grams)	Percent Fat Calories
Arby's Regular Roast Beef	350	16	6	41
Arby's Super Roast Beef	470	23	7	44
Arby's Roast Chicken Club	520	28	7	48
Arby's Market Fresh Roast Beef & Swiss	810	42	13	47
McDonald's Crispy Chicken	430	21	8	43
McDonald's Filet-O-Fish	470	26	5	50
McDonald's Chicken McGrill	400	17	3	38
Wendy's Chicken Club	470	19	4	36
Wendy's Breast Fillet	430	16	3	34
Wendy's Grilled Chicken	300	7	2	21
Burger King Specialty Chicken	560	28	6	45
Subway Veggie Delight*	226	3	1	12
Subway Turkey Breast	281	5	2	16
Subway Sweet Onion Chicken Teriyaki	374	5	2	12
Subway Steak & Cheese	390	14	5	32
Subway Cold Cut Trio	440	21	7	43
Subway Tuna	450	22	6	44

Shakes	Calories	Total Fat (grams)	Saturated Fat (grams)	Percent Fat Calories
Wendy's Frosty, medium (16 oz)	440	11	7	23
McDonald's McFlurry, small (12 oz)	610	22	14	32
Burger King, Old Fashioned Ice Cream Shake, medium (22 oz)	760	41	29	49
Hash Browns				
McDonald's Hash Browns (2 oz)	130	8	4	55
Burger King, Hash Browns, small (2½ oz)	230	15	9	59

*6-inch sandwich with no mayo

Source: Adapted from Restaurant Confidential by Michael F. Jacobson and Jayne Hurley (Workman, 2002), by permission of Center for Science in the Public Interest.

❑ Base your diet on a large variety of foods.

❑ Consume ample amounts of green, yellow, and orange fruits and vegetables.

❑ Eat foods high in complex carbohydrates, including at least three 1-ounce servings of whole-grain foods per day.

❑ Obtain most of your vitamins and minerals from food sources.

❑ Eat foods rich in vitamin D.

❑ Maintain adequate daily calcium intake and consider a bone supplement with vitamin D_3.

❑ Consume protein in moderation.

❑ Limit meat consumption to 3 to 6 ounces per day.

❑ Limit daily fat, trans fat, and saturated fat intake.

❑ Limit cholesterol consumption to less than 300 mg per day.

❑ Limit sodium intake to 2,300 mg per day.

❑ Limit sugar intake.

❑ If you drink alcohol, do so in moderation (one daily drink for women and two for men).

❑ Consider taking a daily multivitamin (preferably one that includes vitamin D_3).

❑ 6. Vary your choices. Eat broccoli today, carrots tomorrow, and corn the next day. Eat Chinese today, Italian tomorrow, and broiled fish with brown rice and steamed vegetables the third day.

❑ 7. Load your plate with vegetables and unrefined starchy foods. A small portion of meat or cheese is all you need for protein.

❑ 8. When choosing breads and cereals, choose the whole-grain varieties.

To select nutritious fast foods:

❑ 9. Choose the broiled sandwich with lettuce, tomatoes, and other goodies—and hold the mayo—rather than the fish or chicken patties coated with breadcrumbs and cooked in fat.

❑ 10. Select a salad—and use more plain vegetables than those mixed with oily or mayonnaise-based dressings.

❑ 11. Order chili with more beans than meat. Choose a soft bean burrito over tacos with fried shells.

❑ 12. Drink low-fat milk rather than a cola beverage.

When choosing from a vending machine:

❑ 13. Choose cracker sandwiches over chips and pork rinds (virtually pure fat). Choose peanuts, pretzels, and popcorn over cookies and candy.

❑ 14. Choose milk and juices over cola beverages.

BMI	Disease Risk	Classification
<18.5	Increased	Underweight
18.5–21.99	Low	Acceptable
22.0–24.99	Very Low	Acceptable
25.0–29.99	Increased	Overweight
30.0–34.99	High	Obesity I
35.0–39.99	Very High	Obesity II
≥40.00	Extremely High	Obesity III

See page 125 to look up your BMI

Maintenance of recommended body composition is one of the most significant health issues of the 21st century. If you are committed to lifetime weight management, the following strategies will help:

❏ Accumulate 60 to 90 minutes of physical activity daily.

❏ Exercise at a vigorous aerobic pace for a minimum of 20 minutes three times per week.

❏ Strength train two to three times per week.

❏ Use common sense and moderation in your daily diet.

❏ Manage daily caloric intake by keeping in mind long-term benefits (recommended body weight) instead of instant gratification (overeating).

❏ "Junior-size" instead of "super-size."

❏ Regularly monitor body weight, body composition, body mass index, and waist circumference.

❏ Do not allow increases in body weight (percent fat) to accumulate; deal immediately with the problem through moderate reductions in caloric intake and maintenance of physical activity and exercise habits.

The following physical activity guidelines are recommended to effectively manage body weight:

❏ 30 minutes of physical activity on most days of the week if you do not have difficulty maintaining body weight (more minutes and/or higher intensity if you choose to reach a high level of physical fitness).

❏ 60 minutes of daily activity if you want to prevent weight gain.

❏ Between 60 and 90 minutes each day if you are trying to lose weight or attempting to keep weight off following extensive weight loss (30 pounds of weight loss or more). Be sure to include some high-intensity/low-impact activities at least twice a week in your program.

Intensity of Exercise

1. Estimate your own maximal heart rate (MHR)

    $\text{MHR} = 207 - (.70 \times \text{age})$

    $\text{MHR} = 207 - \boxed{} \times \boxed{} = \boxed{}$ bpm

2. Resting Heart Rate (RHR) = $\boxed{}$ bpm

3. Heart Rate Reserve (HRR) = MHR − RHR

    $\text{HRR} = \boxed{} - \boxed{} = \boxed{}$ beats

4. Training Intensities (TI) = HRR × TI + RHR

    30 Percent TI = $\boxed{} \times .30 + \boxed{} = \boxed{}$ bpm

    40 Percent TI = $\boxed{} \times .40 + \boxed{} = \boxed{}$ bpm

    60 percent TI = $\boxed{} \times .60 + \boxed{} = \boxed{}$ bpm

    85 Percent TI = $\boxed{} \times .85 + \boxed{} = \boxed{}$ bpm

5. Light-Intensity Cardiorespiratory Training Zone:

    $\boxed{}$ (30% TI) to $\boxed{}$ (40% TI)

6. Moderate-Intensity Cardiorespiratory Training Zone:

    $\boxed{}$ (40% TI) to $\boxed{}$ (85% TI)

7. Vigorous-Intensity Cardiorespiratory Training Zone:

    $\boxed{}$ (60% TI) to $\boxed{}$ (85% TI)

Mode: Moderate- or vigorous-intensity aerobic activity (examples: walking, jogging, stair climbing, elliptical activity, aerobics, water aerobics, cycling, stair climbing, swimming, cross-country skiing, racquetball, basketball, and soccer)

Intensity: 30% to 85% of heart rate reserve (the training intensity is based on age, health status, initial fitness level, exercise tolerance, and exercise program goals)

Duration: Be active 20 to 90 minutes. At least 20 minutes of continuous vigorous-intensity or 30 minutes of moderate-intensity aerobic activity (the latter may be accumulated in segments of at least 10 minutes in duration each over the course of the day)

Frequency: 3 to 5 days per week for vigorous-intensity aerobic activity to accumulate at least 75 minutes per week, or 5 days per week of moderate-intensity aerobic activity for a minimum total of 150 minutes weekly

Rate of progression:
- Start with three training sessions per week of 15 to 20 minutes
- Increase the duration by 5 to 10 minutes per week and the frequency so that by the fourth or fifth week you are exercising five times per week
- Progressively increase frequency, duration, and intensity of exercise until you reach your fitness goal prior to exercise maintenance

Source: American College of Sports Medicine, *ACSM's Guidelines for Exercise Testing and Prescription* (Philadelphia: Lippincott Williams & Wilkins, 2006).

Mode: Select 8 to 10 dynamic strength-training exercises that involve the body's major muscle groups and include opposing muscle groups (chest and upper back, abdomen and lower back, front and back of the legs).

Resistance: Sufficient resistance to perform 8 to 12 repetitions maximum for muscular strength and 15 to 25 repetitions to near fatigue for muscular edurance. Older adults and injury prone individuals should use 10 to 15 repetitions with moderate resistance (50% to 60% of their 1 RM).

Sets: 2 to 4 sets per exercise with 2 to 3 minutes recovery between sets for optimal strength development. Less than 2 minutes per set if exercises are alternated that require different muscle groups (chest and upper back) or between muscular endurance sets.

Frequency: 2 to 3 days per week on nonconsecutive days. More frequent training can be done if different muscle groups are exercised on different days. (Allow at least 48 hours between strength-training sessions of the same muscle group.)

Adapted from American College of Sports Medicine, *Guidelines for Exercise Testing and Prescription* (Baltimore: Lippincott Williams & Wilkins, 2006).

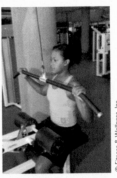

© Fitness & Wellness, Inc.

- ❑ Make a progressive resistance strength-training program a priority in your weekly schedule.
- ❑ Strength train at least once a week; even better, twice a week.
- ❑ Find a facility where you feel comfortable training and where you can get good professional guidance.
- ❑ Learn the proper technique for each exercise.
- ❑ Train with a friend or group of friends.
- ❑ Consume a pre-exercise snack consisting of a combination of carbohydrates and some protein about 30 to 60 minutes before each strength-training session.
- ❑ Use a minimum of 8 to 10 exercises that involve all major muscle groups of your body.
- ❑ Perform at least one set of each exercise to near muscular fatigue.
- ❑ To enhance protein synthesis, consume one post-exercise snack with a 4-to-1 gram ratio of carbohydrates to protein immediately following strength training; and a second snack one hour thereafter.
- ❑ Allow at least 48 hours between strength-training sessions that involve the same muscle groups.

Mode: Static, dynamic, or proprioceptive neuromuscular facilitation (PNF) stretching to include all major muscle/tendon groups of the body

Intensity: To the point of mild tension or limits of discomfort

Repetitions: Repeat each exercise 4 times, holding the final position between 15 and 30 seconds

Frequency: At least 2 or 3 days per week
Ideal, 5 to 7 days per week

Source: Adapted from American College of Sports Medicine, *ACSM's Guidelines for Exercise Testing and Prescription* (Baltimore: Williams & Wilkins, 2006).

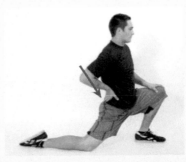

❑ Be physically active.

❑ Maintain recommended body weight (excess weight strains the back).

❑ Stretch often using spinal exercises through a functional range of motion.

❑ Regularly strengthen the core of the body using sets of 10 to 12 repetitions to near fatigue with isometric contractions when applicable.

❑ Lift heavy objects by bending at the knees and carry them close to the body. Place one foot forward, and keep your knees slightly bent while standing.

❑ Avoid sitting (over 50 minutes) or standing in one position for lengthy periods of time.

❑ Maintain correct posture.

❑ Sleep on your back with a pillow under the knees or on your side with the knees drawn up and a small pillow between the knees.

❑ Try out different mattresses of firm consistency before selecting a mattress.

❑ Warm up properly using mild stretches before engaging in physical activity.

❑ Practice adequate stress management techniques.

❑ Don't smoke (it reduces blood flow to the spine, increasing back pain risk).

Stop exercise and seek medical advice if you experience any of the following symptoms:

• Unusual pain or discomfort, especially in the chest or abdominal area

• Cramping, primarily in the pelvic or lower back areas

• Muscle weakness, excessive fatigue, or shortness of breath

• Abnormally high heart rate or a pounding (palpitations) heart rate

• Decreased fetal movement

• Insufficient weight gain

• Amniotic fluid leakage

• Nausea, dizziness, or headaches

• Persistent uterine contractions

• Vaginal bleeding or rupture of the membranes

• Swelling of ankles, calves, hands, or face

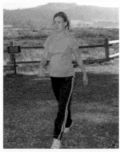

© Fitness & Wellness, Inc.

I. Increase intake of phytonutrients, fiber, cruciferous vegetables and more antioxidants by:

• Eating a predominantly vegetarian diet

• Eating more fruits and vegetables every day (six to eight servings per day maximize anticancer benefits)

• Increasing the consumption of broccoli, cauliflower, kale, turnips, cabbage, kohlrabi, Brussels sprouts, hot chili peppers, red and green peppers, carrots, sweet potatoes, winter squash, spinach, garlic, onions, strawberries, tomatoes, pineapple, and citrus fruits in your regular diet

• Eating vegetables raw or quickly cooked by steaming or stir-frying

• Substituting tea and fruit and vegetable juices for coffee and soda

• Eating whole-grain breads

• Including calcium in the diet (or from a supplement)

• Including soy products in the diet

• Using whole-wheat flour instead of refined white flour in baking

• Using brown (unpolished) rice instead of white (polished) rice

Rating	Systolic	Diastolic
Normal	<120	<80
Prehypertension	121–139	81–89
Stage 1 hypertension	140–159	90–99
Stage 2 hypertension	≥160	≥100

Source: National High Blood Pressure Education Program.

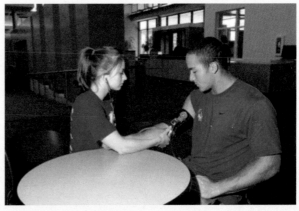

© Fitness & Wellness, Inc.

Continued on back

Any or all of the following signs may occur during a heart attack or a stroke. If you experience any of these and they last longer than a few minutes, call 911 and seek medical attention immediately. Failure to do so may cause irreparable damage and even result in death.

Warning Signs of a Heart Attack

- Chest pain, discomfort, pressure, or squeezing that lasts for several minutes. These feelings may go away and return later.
- Pain or discomfort in the shoulders, neck, or arms or between the shoulder blades
- Chest discomfort with shortness of breath, lightheadedness, cold sweats, nausea and/or vomiting, a feeling of indigestion, sudden fatigue or weakness, fainting, or sense of impending doom

Warning Signs of Stroke

- Sudden weakness or numbness of the face, arm, or leg—particularly on one side of the body
- Sudden severe headache
- Sudden confusion, dizziness, or difficulty with speech and understanding
- Sudden difficulty walking; loss of balance or coordination
- Sudden visual difficulty

- ❏ Balance caloric intake and physical activity to achieve or maintain a healthy body weight.
- ❏ Consume a diet rich in vegetables and fruits.
- ❏ Consume whole-grain, high-fiber foods.
- ❏ Consume fish, especially oily fish, at least twice a week.
- ❏ Limit your intake of saturated fat to less than 7 percent and trans fat to less than 1 percent of total daily caloric intake.
- ❏ Limit cholesterol intake to less than 300 mg per day.
- ❏ Minimize your intake of beverages and foods with added sugars.
- ❏ Choose and prepare foods with little or no salt.
- ❏ If you consume alcohol, do so in moderation.
- ❏ When you eat food that is prepared outside of the home, follow the above recommendations.
- ❏ Avoid use of and exposure to tobacco products.

Components	Men	Women
Waist circumference	>40 inches	>35 inches
Blood pressure	>130/85 mm Hg	>130/85 mm Hg
Fasting blood glucose	>110 mg/dL	>110 mg/dL
Fasting HDL cholesterol	<40 mg/dL	<50 mg/dL
Fasting triglycerides	>150 mg/dL	>150 mg/dL

Note: Metabolic syndrome is identified by the presence of at least three of the above components.

Increase intake of phytonutrients, fiber, cruciferous vegetables, and more antioxidants by

- ❏ Eating a predominantly vegetarian diet
- ❏ Eating more fruits and vegetables every day (six to eight servings per day maximize anticancer benefits)
- ❏ Increasing the consumption of broccoli, cauliflower, kale, turnips, cabbage, kohlrabi, Brussels sprouts, hot chili peppers, red and green peppers, carrots, sweet potatoes, winter squash, spinach, garlic, onions, strawberries, tomatoes, pineapple, and citrus fruits in your regular diet
- ❏ Eating vegetables raw or quickly cooked by steaming or stir-frying
- ❏ Substituting tea and fruit and vegetable juices for coffee and soda
- ❏ Eating whole-grain breads
- ❏ Including calcium in the diet (or from a supplement)
- ❏ Including soy products in the diet

Continued on back

Do you have these healthy lifestyle factors working in your favor?

Factor	Function
❑ Physical activity	Controls body weight, may influence hormone levels, strengthens the immune system.
❑ Fiber	Contains anti-cancer substances, increases stool movement, blunts insulin secretion.
❑ Fruits and vegetables	Contain phytonutrients and vitamins that thwart cancer.
❑ Recommended weight	Helps control hormones that promote cancer.
❑ Healthy grilling	Prevents formation of carcinogenic substances.
❑ Tea	Contains polyphenols that neutralize free radicals.
❑ Spices	Provide phytonutrients and strengthen the immune system.
❑ Vitamin D	Disrupts abnormal cell growth.
❑ Monounsaturated fat	May contribute to cancer cell destruction.

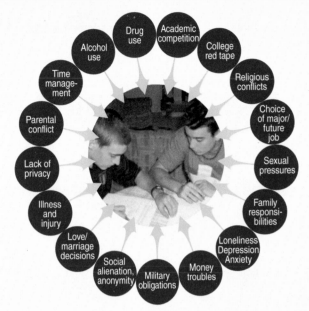

Drug use
Academic competition
Alcohol use
College red tape
Time management
Religious conflicts
Parental conflict
Choice of major/ future job
Lack of privacy
Sexual pressures
Illness and injury
Family responsibilities
Love/ marriage decisions
Loneliness Depression Anxiety
Social alienation, anonymity
Military obligations
Money troubles

Adapted from W. W. K. Hoeger, L. W. Turner, and B. Q. Hafen. *Wellness Guidelines for a Healthy Lifestyle.* Wadsworth/Thomson Learning, 2007.

II. Limit saturated and trans fats by:

- Limiting red meat intake to two 3-ounce servings of lean meat per week

- Consuming low-fat or nonfat dairy products only

- Using primarily omega-3 fats found in cold water fish at least twice per week as well as poultry, nuts, and legumes as the main protein sources in the diet

III. Balancing caloric input with caloric output to maintain recommended body weight

Check those symptoms you experience regularly.

❑ Headaches

❑ Muscular aches (mainly in neck, shoulders, and back)

❑ Grinding teeth

❑ Nervous tic, finger tapping, toe tapping

❑ Increased sweating

❑ Increase in or loss of appetite

❑ Insomnia

❑ Nightmares

❑ Fatigue

❑ Dry mouth

❑ Stuttering

❑ High blood pressure

❑ Tightness or pain in the chest

❑ Impotence

❑ Hives

❑ Dizziness

❑ Depression

❑ Irritation

❑ Anger

❑ Hostility

❑ Fear, panic, anxiety

❑ Stomach pain, flutters

❑ Nausea

❑ Cold, clammy hands

❑ Poor concentration

❑ Pacing

❑ Restlessness

❑ Rapid heart rate

❑ Low-grade infection

❑ Loss of sex drive

❑ Rash or acne

CHAPTER 12 CHECK YOURSELF

Tips to Manage Anger

- ❑ Commit to change and gain control over the behavior.
- ❑ Remind yourself that chronic anger leads to illness and disease and may eventually kill you.
- ❑ Recognize when feelings of anger are developing and ask yourself the following questions:
  - Is the matter really that important?
  - Is the anger justified?
  - Can I change the situation without getting angry?
  - Is it worth risking my health over it?
  - How will I feel about the situation in a few hours?
- ❑ Tell yourself, "Stop, my health is worth it" every time you start to feel anger.
- ❑ Prepare for a positive response: Ask for an explanation or clarification of the situation, walk away and evaluate the situation, exercise, or use appropriate stress management techniques (breathing, meditation, imagery) before you become angry and hostile.
- ❑ Manage anger at once; do not let it build up.
- ❑ Never attack anyone verbally or physically.
- ❑ Keep a journal and ponder the situations that cause you to be angry.
- ❑ Seek professional help if you are unable to overcome anger by yourself: You are worth it.

CHAPTER 13 CHECK YOURSELF

American Medical Association Alcohol Abuse Questionnaire

- ❑ When you are holding an empty glass at a party, do you always actively look for a refill instead of waiting to be offered one?
- ❑ If given the chance, do you frequently pour out a more generous drink for yourself than seems to be the "going" amount for others?
- ❑ Do you often have a drink or two when you are alone, either at home or in a bar?
- ❑ Is your drinking ever the direct cause of an argument, or do arguments often seem to occur, if only by coincidence, when you have had a drink or two?
- ❑ Do you feel that you must have a drink at a specific time every day?
- ❑ When worried or under unusual stress, do you almost automatically take a stiff drink to "settle your nerves"?
- ❑ Are you untruthful about how much you have had to drink when questioned on the subject?
- ❑ Does drinking ever cause you to take time off work or to miss class, scheduled meetings, or appointments?
- ❑ Do you feel physically deprived if you cannot have at least one drink every day?
- ❑ Do you sometimes crave a drink in the morning?
- ❑ Do you sometimes have "mornings after" when you cannot remember what happened the night before?

Even one checked box is a warning sign that you may have a problem with alcohol.

CHAPTER 14 CHECK YOURSELF

Protecting Yourself and Others from STI's

Are you sexually active? If you are not, read the following items to better educate yourself regarding intimacy. If you are sexually active, continue through all the questions below.

- ❑ Do you plan ahead before you get into a sexual situation?
- ❑ Do you know whether your partner now has or has ever had an STI? Are you comfortable asking your partner this question?
- ❑ Are you in a mutually monogamous sexual relationship and you know that your partner does not have an STI?
- ❑ Do you have multiple sexual partners? If so, do you *always* practice safe sex?
- ❑ Do you avoid alcohol and drugs in situations where you may end up having planned or unplanned sex?
- ❑ Do you abstain from sexual activity if you know or suspect that you have an STI? Do you seek medical care and advice as to when you can safely resume sexual activity?

CHAPTER 15 CHECK YOURSELF

Healthy Lifestyle Guidelines

- ❑ 1. Accumulate a minimum of 30 minutes of moderate-intensity physical activity at least five days per week.
- ❑ 2. Exercise aerobically in the proper cardiorespiratory training zone at least three times per week for a minimum of 20 minutes.
- ❑ 3. Strength train at least once a week (preferably twice per week) using a minimum of eight exercises that involve all major muscle groups of the body.
- ❑ 4. Perform flexibility exercises that involve all major joints of the body at least two to three times per week.
- ❑ 5. Eat a healthy diet that is rich in whole-wheat grains, fruits, and vegetables and is low in saturated and trans fats.
- ❑ 6. Eat a healthy breakfast every day.
- ❑ 7. Do not use tobacco in any form, avoid secondhand smoke, and avoid all other forms of substance abuse.
- ❑ 8. Maintain healthy body weight (achieve a range between the high-physical fitness and health-fitness standards for percent body fat).
- ❑ 9. Get 7 to 8 hours of sleep per night.
- ❑ 10. Get 10 to 20 minutes of safe sun exposure on most days of the week.
- ❑ 11. Manage stress effectively.
- ❑ 12. Limit daily alcohol intake to two or less drinks per day if you are a man or one drink or less per day if you are a woman (or do not consume any alcohol at all).
- ❑ 13. Seek proper medical evaluations as necessary.